# ANATOMY & YOGA

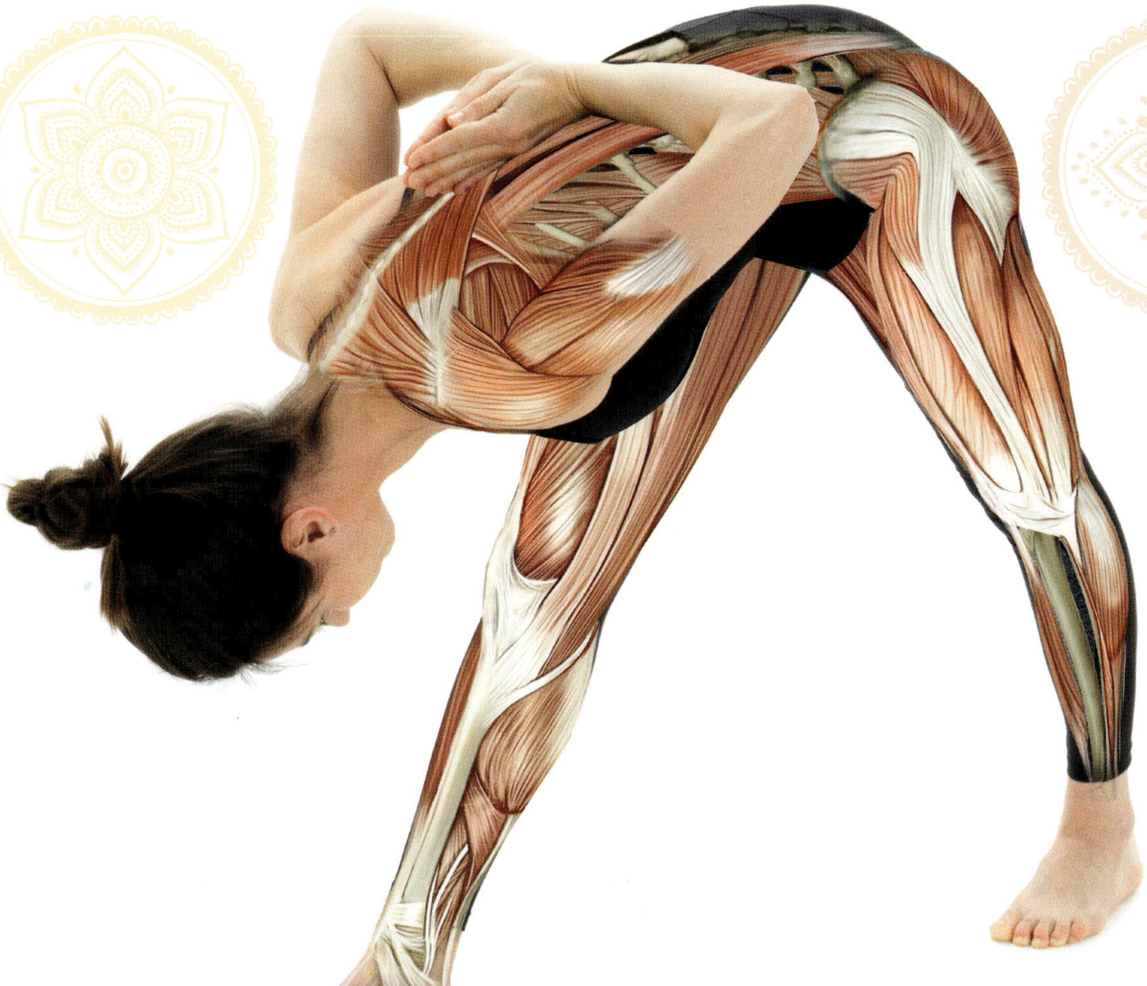

**Paidotribo**

# ANATOMY & YOGA

**Production and development:**
Paidotribo Publishing

**Head of Publishing:** María Fernanda Canal
**Texts:** Mireia Patiño Coll
**Phisiotherapy:** Joana Sánchez
**Advising:** Mª José Portal
**Review:** Roser Pérez
**Scientific Review:** Victor Gotzens
**Graphic design:** Toni Inglès
**Illustrations:** Myriam Ferrón
**Photography:** Nos i Soto
**Layout:** Estudi Toni Inglès
**Typesetting:**
www.satzstudio-hilger.de
**Translation:** AAA Translation,
St. Louis, Missouri
**Models:** Joana Sánchez
Alba Garcia Patiño
Christian Garcia Vilar

Spanish original title:
Anatomía & Yoga
© 2018 Editorial Paidotribo—World Rights
Published by Editorial Paidotribo, Spain

First edition
© 2018 Paidotribo Publishing
Printed in Spain

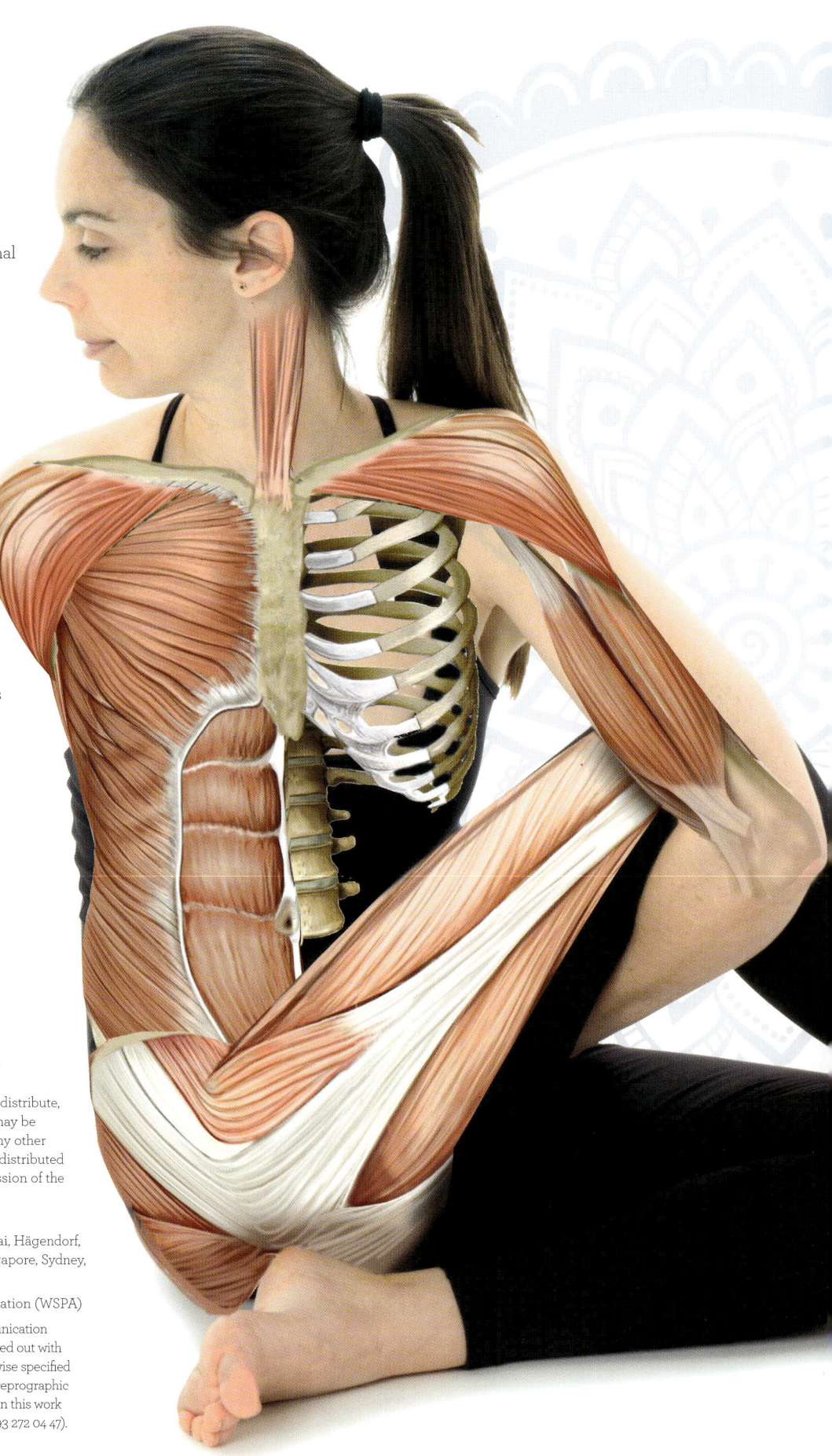

Anatomy & Yoga
British Library Cataloguing in Publication Data
A catalogue record for this book is available from the British Library

Maidenhead: Meyer & Meyer Sport (UK) Ltd., 2018
ISBN: 978-1-78255-152-2
All rigts reserved, especially the right to copy and distribute, including translation rights. No part of this work may be produced–including by photocopy, microfilm or any other means–processed, stored electronically, copied or distributed in any form whatsoever without the written permission of the publisher.

© 2018 by Meyer & Meyer Sport (UK) Ltd.
Aachen, Auckland, Beirut, Cairo, Cape Town, Dubai, Hägendorf, Hong Kong, Indianapolis, Manila, New Delhi, Singapore, Sydney, Tehran, Vienna

Member of the World Sport Publishers' Association (WSPA)

Any form of reproduction, distribution, public communication or similar processing of this work should only be carried out with the express permission of the publisher, unless otherwise specified by law. Please refer to CEDAR (the Spanish center of reprographic rights, www.cedro.org) if you wish to photocopy or scan this work in whole or part (www.conlicencia.com 91 702 19 70 / 93 272 04 47).

# Introduction

Yoga is a thousand-year-old practice that appeared in India more than 4,000 years ago and has endured until today. Currently, millions of people throughout the world practice some form of yoga: Hatha Yoga, Raja Yoga, Ashtanga Yoga, Bhakti Yoga, Kundalini Yoga, Iyengar Yoga... All of these are simply different methods used to focus and understand this practice. But yoga is only one, and it is accessed through these paths or routes that have emerged with the passing of time.

Yoga means "union." Its ultimate goal is to find the path that brings us to the union of the body and mind, of the individual spirit with the Universal Consciousness or the Supreme Spirit. In the West, the most popular methods for yoga are those that work on the physical body, such as Hatha Yoga. This is why it is necessary to know your body, and its anatomy, in order to perform the correct practice of these fundamental poses (asanas) and the respiratory techniques (pranayama).

This book is an explanation of yoga and the anatomy that is involved in the biological and energetic processes in the human body. It is divided into six chapters through which a reader can gain a solid idea of what yoga and its practices represent.

The first chapter, "Introduction to Yoga", is a brief history of yoga and its various paths. The primary characteristics of classical Patanjali Yoga are also described and an introductory explanation of the practice of this tradition is provided.

The second chapter deals with anatomy and physiology and describes all the systems that make up the human body and explains four of the most important ones for practicing yoga: the skeletal system, the muscular system, the nervous system, and the endocrine system.

The third chapter briefly explains what is included in the energetic anatomy of being human. This describes the three bodies of a being, the five koshas or layers, the nadis or energy channels and the chakras, which are the centers for energy in our natural body.

The fourth chapter shows 74 postures: 50 asanas and 24 variations. For each of these, the techniques are explained for their proper execution, the benefits they provide, and any possible risks, as well as some alternatives and anatomic considerations. All of these are accompanied with detailed images. At the end of the chapter, it describes the step-by-step process of all the poses that are included in a traditional Sun Salutation.

The fifth chapter is an introduction to the anatomy and biomechanics of the respiratory system, as well as the respiratory techniques used in yoga: pranayama. It also mentions the bhandas, which make it possible to control and channel our inner energy.

The book concludes with a final chapter dedicated to relaxation, the mudras, and meditation, all of which are necessary to advance along your inner path to discovering the true nature of being human.

**Mireia Patiño Coll**
Professor of Yoga for IYTA (International Yoga Teachers Association)
Masters in Cross-Denominational, Ecumenical, and Cultural Dialogue from Ramon Llull University

*"It is said that for a wise man who wishes to reach Yoga, action is his path; but once Yoga is achieved, his path is only stillness."*
(Bhagavad Gita; VI, 3)

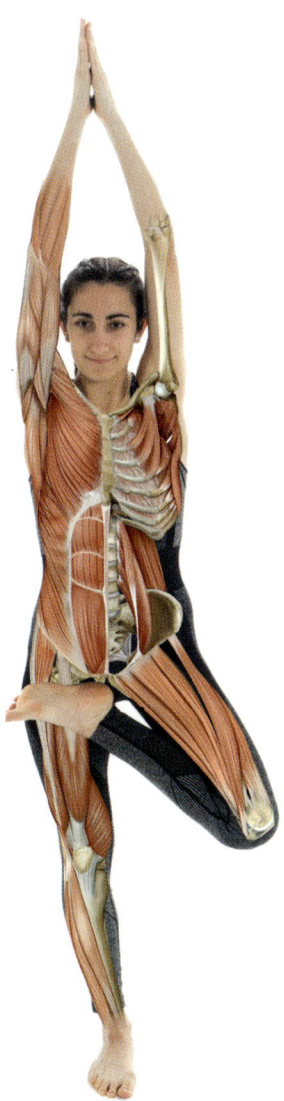

# Summary

| | | | |
|---|---|---|---|
| How to use this book | 6 | **ASANAS** | **44** |
| **INTRODUCTION TO YOGA** | **8** | INTRODUCTION | |
| | | The asanas of yoga | 46 |
| History of yoga | 10 | | |
| The paths of yoga | 12 | STARTING ASANAS | |
| Patanjali and the Yoga-sûtra | 14 | Tadasana | 48 |
| The practice of yoga | 16 | Dandasana | 50 |
| | | Savasana | 52 |
| **ANATOMY AND PHYSIOLOGY** | **18** | BASIC ASANAS | |
| | | Apanasana | 54 |
| The systems of the body | 20 | Marjariasana | 56 |
| | | Adho Muka Svanasana | 58 |
| SKELETAL SYSTEM | | Virabhadrasana I and II | 60 |
| The skeletal system | 22 | Virabhadrasana III | 62 |
| The bones of the human body | 24 | Malasana | 64 |
| The spinal column | 26 | Utkatasana | 66 |
| MUSCULAR SYSTEM | | ASANAS OF STRENGTH | |
| The muscular system | | Navasana | 68 |
| The muscles of the body | 30 | Vasishtasana | 70 |
| Planes, sections, and body movements | 32 | Chaturanga Dandasana | 72 |
| OTHER SYSTEMS | | ASANAS OF BALANCE | |
| The nervous system | 34 | Vriksasana | 74 |
| The endocrine system | 35 | Garudasana | 76 |
| | | ASANAS OF LATERAL FLEXING | |
| **ENERGETIC ANATOMY** | | AND TRIKONAS | |
| **OF BEING HUMAN** | **36** | Parigasana | 78 |
| | | Utthita Trikonasana | 80 |
| The three bodies of being human | 38 | Utthita Parsva Konasana | 82 |
| The five koshas or layers | 39 | | |
| | | ASANAS OF EXTENSION | |
| NADIS | | Setu-Bandhasana | 84 |
| The nadis or channels of energy | 40 | Purvottanasana | 86 |
| | | Bhujangasana | 88 |
| CHAKRAS | | Matsyasana | 90 |
| The chakras | 41 | | |
| Essential elements of the chakras | 42 | | |

# Summary

## CLOSED OR FORWARD-FLEXING ASANAS
Parsvottanasana 92
Paschimottanasana 94
Balasana 96
Kurmasana 98

## TWISTING ASANAS
Ardha Matsyendrasana 100
Jatara Parivartanasana 102

## SEMI-INVERTED AND INVERTED ASANAS
Prasarita Padottanasana 104
Sasangasana 106
Salamba Sarvangasana 108
Halasana 110
Salamba Sirsasana 112

Suryanamaskar, the Sun Salutation 114

## PRANAYAMA AND BHANDAS 118

### PRANAYAMA
The respiratory system 120
Basic types of respiration 122
The practice of pranayama 124
Starting pranayama 126
Basic techniques of pranayama 128

### BHANDAS
Bhandas and energy keys 130

## RELAXATION, MUDRAS, MEDITATION 132

Relaxation 134
Hasta Mudras 136
Meditation 138
The inner silence 140

Glossary 143
Bibliography 144

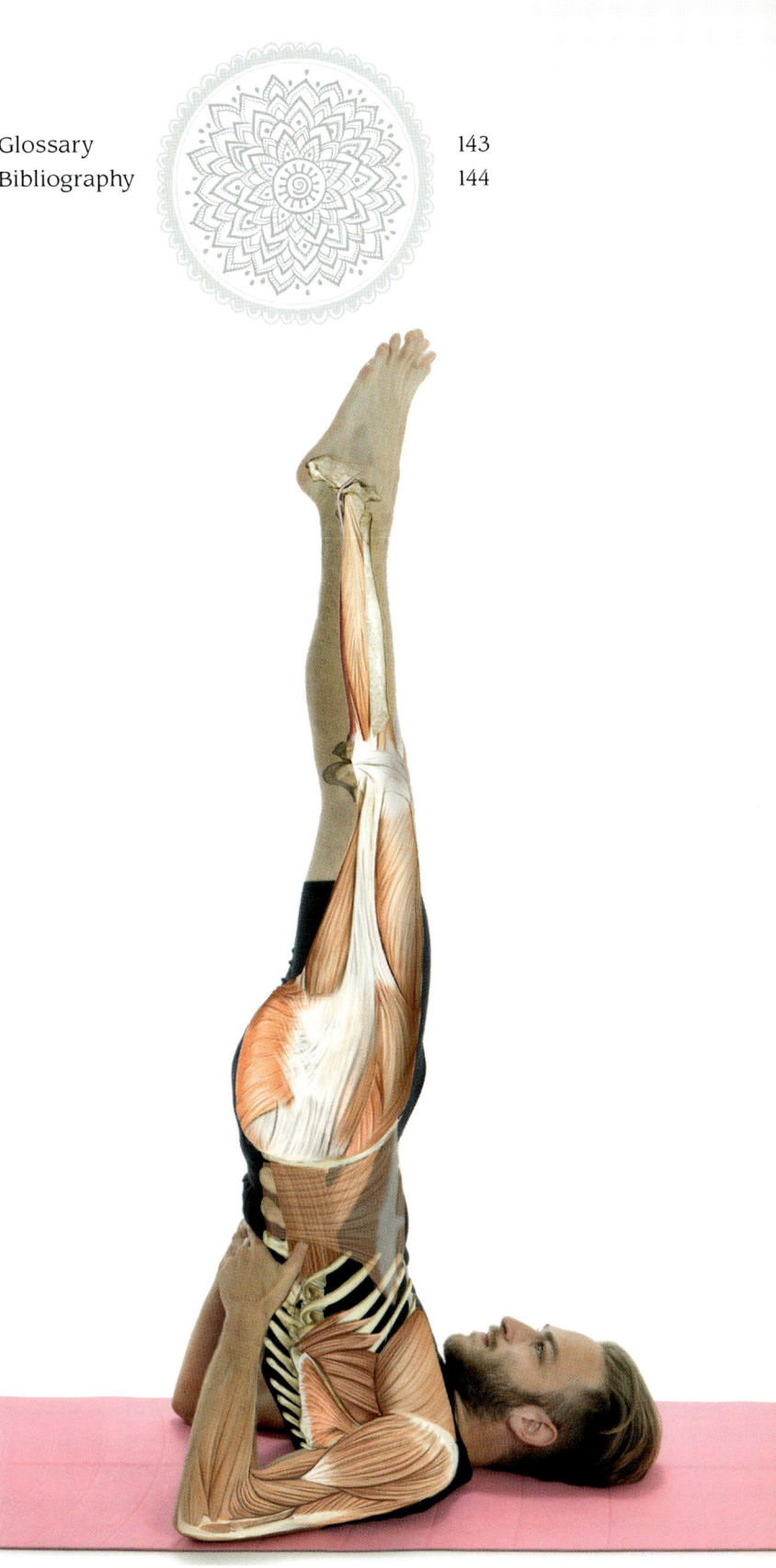

# How to use this book

## INTERPRETING THE ASANAS

Benefits and risks

Group of asanas

Name of the asana

Meaning of the name

You can view a video of the asana

Asana

Energetic anatomy

64

Asanas

BASIC ASANAS

## Malasana

*Mala* means "wreath." This is the wreath pose, since your arms make a crown that seems to hang on your neck. This asana creates an offering to your inner self; it is also a good way to prepare for meditation.

BENEFITS

- Tones the abdominal muscles, stimulates digestion, and relieves constipation.
- Relieves back pain.
- Encourages stretching of the lower back, pelvis, and pelvic floor. Since the feet are separated, it is very appropriate for pregnant women.
- Calms the nervous system.

WARNINGS

- Problems of hips, knees and shoulders.

**CLASSIFICATION**
Basic squatting pose, symmetrical.

**TECHNIQUE**
We start from the squatting position, the feet are together and flat on the floor. We raise the buttocks, maintaining our balance. Separate your legs and move your core forward, until the armpits pass your knees. Take the back part of your ankles in your hands, while your head lowers until you support your forehead on the floor. Hold this position for a few minutes. To release this pose, place your hands on the floor, under your shoulders, and exhale while you lift your head little by little.

**RELATED ASANA**
Upavesasana is an asana related to Malasana. To perform this, squat with your feet separated and your elbows resting on the inside part of your knees, your hands are together in *namasté*. Lightly press outward with your elbows that are on your knees, in this way you will open your hip. This is a very appropriate pose for pregnant women.
If you have a tight Achilles tendon, you can place a support under your heel.

BASIC ASANAS: Malasana 65

Malasana affects and stimulates the opening of the Muladhara Chakra and invigorates the Svadisthana Chakra. It offers us inner stability, balance, and safety.



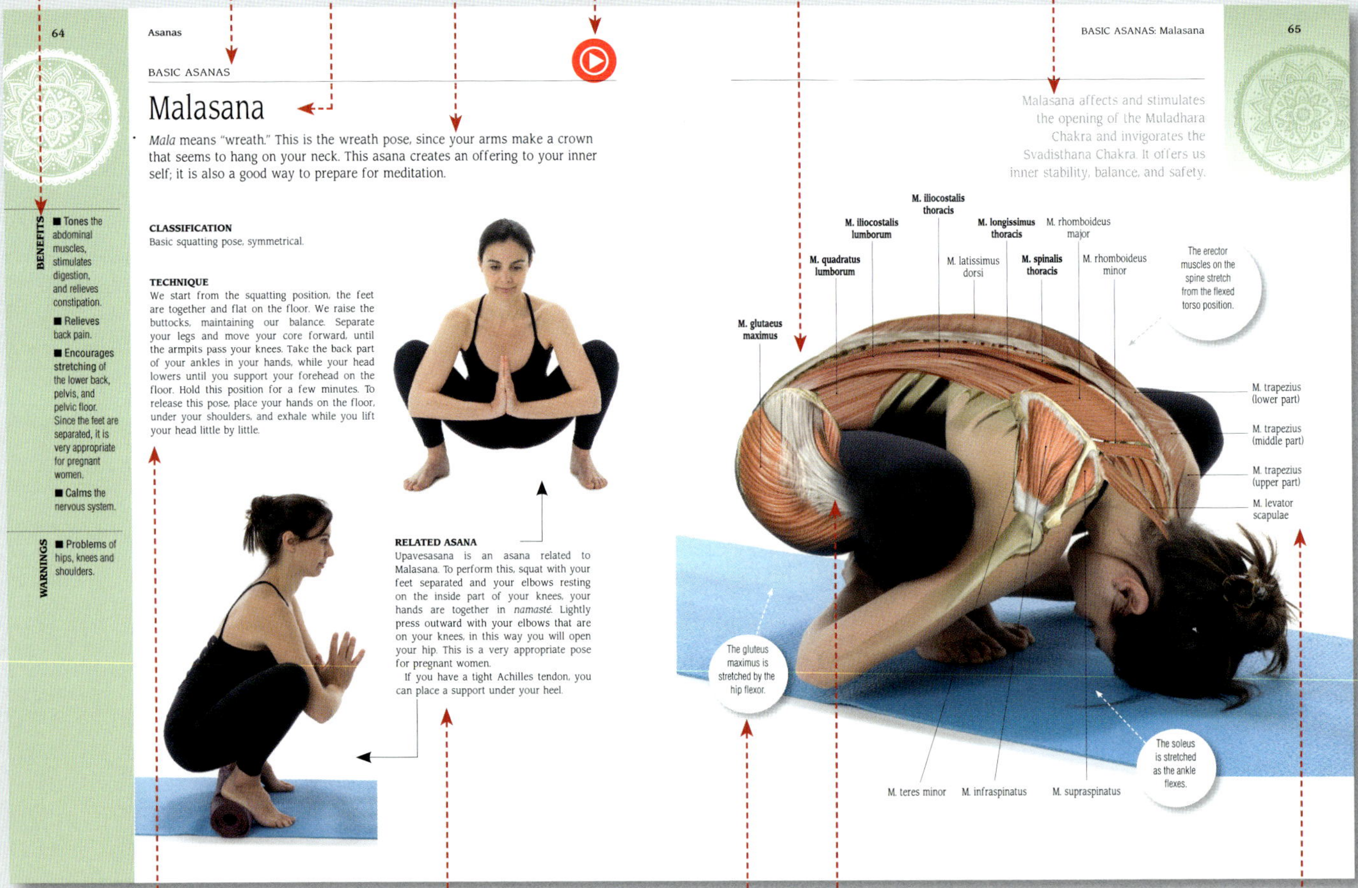

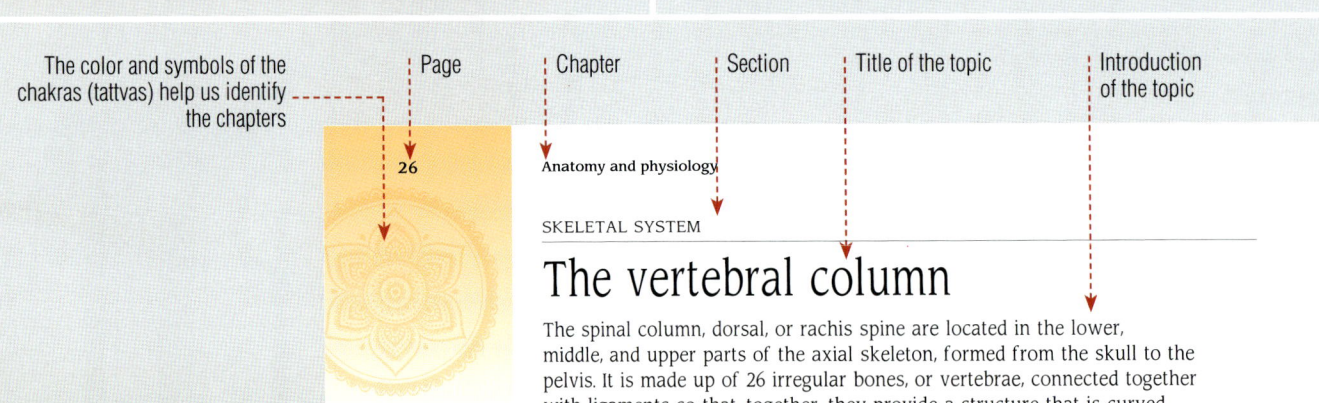

Description of the technique

Related asanas or variations

Drawing of the involved anatomy

Primary muscles involved

Actions highlighting some of the muscles involved in the pose

## CLASSIFICATION OF THE BOOK

The color and symbols of the chakras (tattvas) help us identify the chapters

Page

Chapter

Section

Title of the topic

Introduction of the topic

26

Anatomy and physiology

SKELETAL SYSTEM

## The vertebral column

The spinal column, dorsal, or rachis spine are located in the lower, middle, and upper parts of the axial skeleton, formed from the skull to the pelvis. It is made up of 26 irregular bones, or vertebrae, connected together with ligaments so that, together, they provide a structure that is curved,

How to use this book/How to access additional content

# How to use the additional content

In addition to the content published in the pages of this book, **Anatomy and Yoga** includes additional content with 50 tutorial videos.

## FROM A WEB PAGE

Register the page for free at:
**books2ar.com/pai**
by inserting the following code:

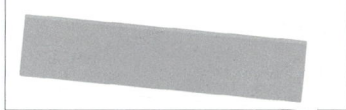

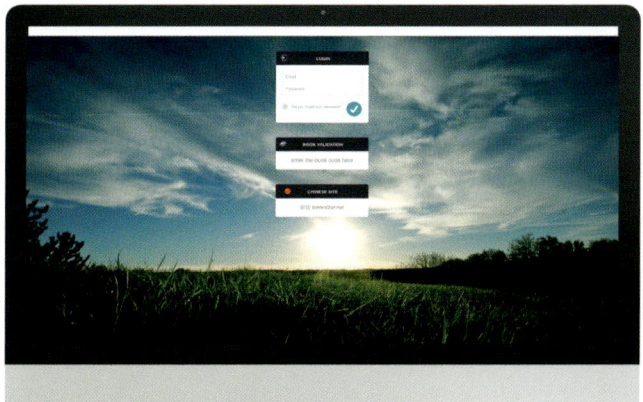

### THREE SIMPLE STEPS

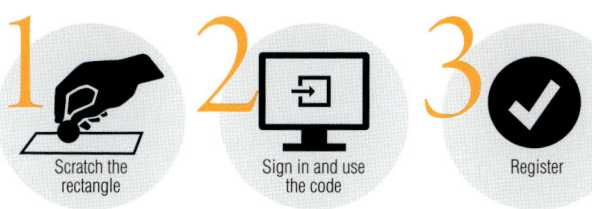

1. Scratch the rectangle
2. Sign in and use the code
3. Register

## THROUGH AUGMENTED REALITY

**1.** Download the application from AR at:
■ **books2ar.com/pai**
■ Scan one of these codes:

QR for iOS      QR for Android

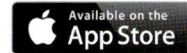 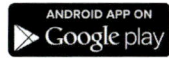

■ search for ANATOMY AND YOGA AR in the official store for your device, Android or iOs

**2.** Use the app to scan the page where this icon appears:

**3.** Discover additional content.

### THREE SIMPLE STEPS

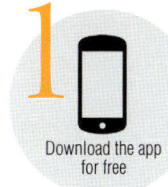 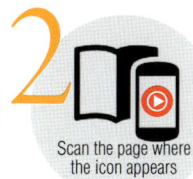 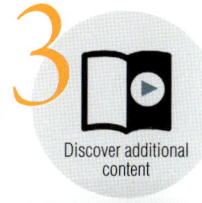

1. Download the app for free
2. Scan the page where the icon appears
3. Discover additional content

**INCLUDES TUTORIAL VIDEOS**

Accessible on all the pages where this icon appears

The app requires an internet connection to access the multimedia content.

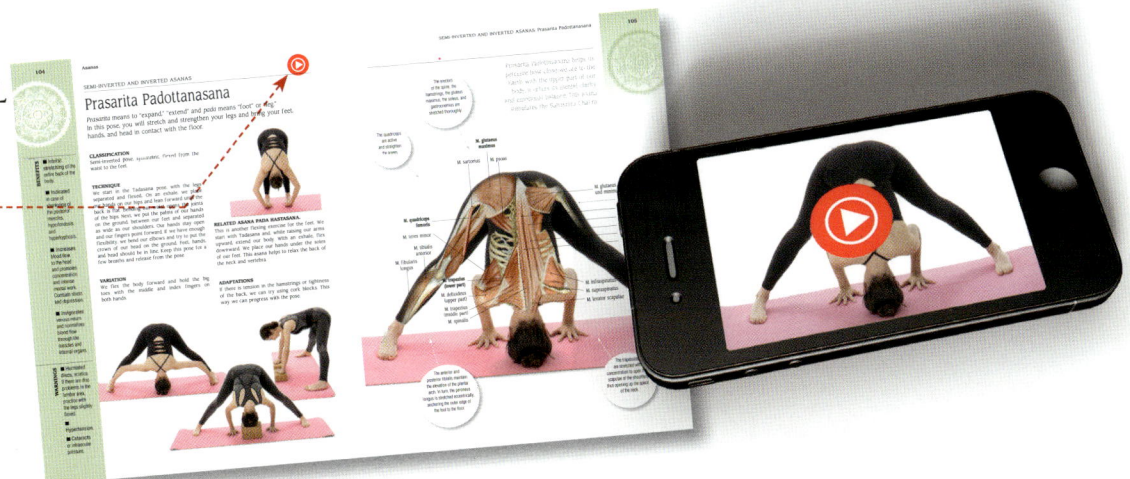

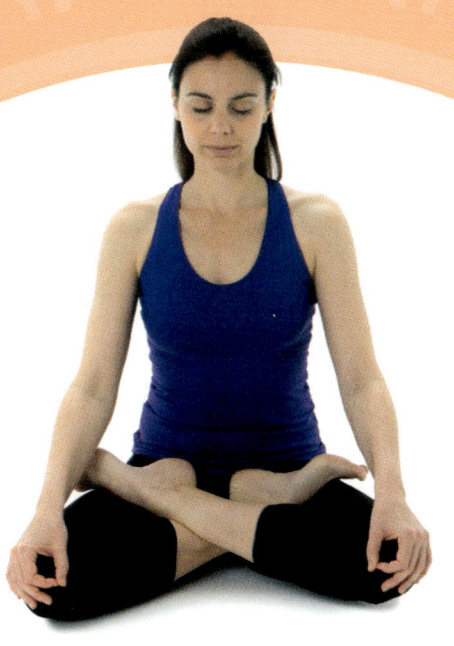

# INTRODUCTION TO YOGA

Yoga is one of the oldest techniques used to achieve serenity, whose practice involves the body, mind, and spirit. Originating from India, it has expanded greatly and in recent centuries has spread to Western culture. Through this praxis, we can reach a state of union, which is one of full consciousness, peace, and happiness. In addition, yoga offers huge health benefits at all levels. This chapter offers a brief history of yoga and its various paths, as well as an introduction to its practice.

# History of yoga

The word *yoga* comes from the root *yuj*, which means "unite," "concentrate," or "join". It may also have a different connotation, which is to subject yourself to a method of teaching. Therefore, yoga can be defined as a deep state of serenity, mental concentration, and unity that can be taught or mastered through a series of disciplined practices.

Old map of India.

Yoga is a union, but it is also a method and a discipline that are one and the same. Its practice puts us on a path to liberation, introspection, health, full consciousness, integrating the body-mind-spirit, and, in the end, a union of the most material aspects with the spiritual, with the Absolute (like a drop of water in an immense ocean).

It is also a state that we can access via different paths. From psycho-physical practices, up to the point that you realize your own self through knowledge or selfless action, we find a wide range of techniques, paths, and ways that are very diverse and have emerged throughout history.

Yoga was born in India and its history remains full of Hindu spirituality. Its origins come from the earliest stages of spirituality, from very old times. Although this is only an approximation, since all the stages are interconnected, it is possible to outline the history of yoga into six general periods.

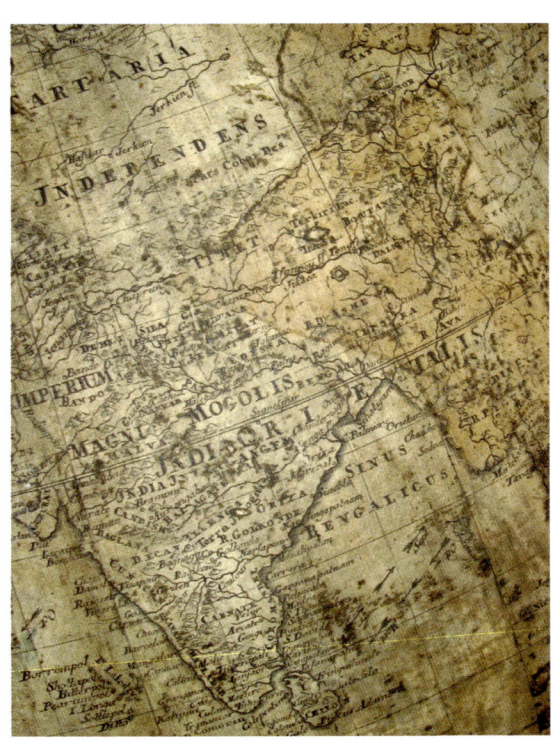

Bronze statue of the Shiva Dance

### ANCIENT YOGA, PRE-VEDIC

Agricultural communities established in the Indus Valley during the Neolithic periods (7000-6000 B.C.E.) evolved into a single urban civilization located in the watershed of the river there, which is called the Indus Valley Civilization. Terracotta figures in various poses have been found in this area, which evoke some poses from yoga meditation. This is the first sign, although inconclusive, of the possible first appearance of this discipline.

On the other hand, in primitive Dravidic towns, primarily located in the south of India, a spirituality of mysticism and emotions emerged. The spirituality of yoga seems to originate from this culture, although its practice is unknown.

### PRE-CLASSIC PERIOD

Classic texts are created from Hinduism, which started to describe yoga and its paths. In the *Upanishads*, or secret doctrines, the first reference to yoga appears as a path of salvation and consciousness (*Svetasvatara Upanishad*).

The *Bhagavad Gita* (V-II centuries B.C.E.), or the Lord's Song, a religious-philosophical poem and center of the extensive epic work of *Mahâbhârata*, explicitly defines three paths or ways to freedom: *Jñaña Yoga* (way of knowledge), *Karma Yoga* (way of selfless action), and *Bhakti Yoga* (way of spiritual devotion). Freedom assumes the work that involves guiding daily life toward the Supreme Being. The *Bhagavad Gita* integrated various methods of spiritual thought that were characteristic of Hinduism in that period, which reformulated various types of consciousness that move from Orthodox ritualism to *Upanishads*.

## CLASSIC PERIOD

The classic philosophical systems of the Hindu philosophy (III-VI centuries A.D.) are the *Darsanas*, six philosophical systems that hope to provide a vision or conception of our own world. These systems are: Vaisheshika, Nyaya, *Samkhya, Yoga, Mimansa,* and *Vedanta*. *Samkhya* is the oldest system, and at some point it was combined with yoga. In fact, yoga would come to represent the practical aspect or the discipline that would apply the Samkhya system. The need for freedom is ultimately provided by practicing the discipline of the body and the mind, which yoga provides. Classic yoga is coded in the *Yoga-sûtra* of Patanjali (the exact date of its creation is unknown), which gathers and organizes the antique doctrines of this discipline and its practice.

## POST-CLASSIC PERIOD

This coincides with the Middle Ages of western civilizations. Large religious currents from Hinduism appear (Sivaism, Vaishnavism, and Shaktism), along with various schools of spirituality, among which Sankara (IX century) should be mentioned. Sankara was the largest exponent of the Advaita Vedanta doctrine. Classic yoga maintained dualist meta-physics (which means it differentiated between material and spiritual); however, many other post-classic systems of yoga sustained a non-dual philosophy (advaita). During this period, there is a full development of Bhakti Yoga, of which one of its most supreme models was Sri Caitanya (XVI century). Towards the XV century, the oldest manual appeared, which is known as Hatha Yoga: *Hatha-Yoga-Pradipika*, written by Suami Suatmarama.

## MODERN PERIOD

Some authors call this the "dark age," due to the practice of Hatha Yoga being limited to specific castes, different from the previous period, during which it was accessible to the whole world. Two important texts of Hatha Yoga appeared in this period: the *Gheranda Samhita* (XVII century) and the *Shiva-Samhita* (XVIII century). The first presents a series of techniques that would later make up the basis of contemporary yoga.

## CONTEMPORARY PERIOD

The contemporary period is one of expansion and diffusion, of yoga spreading to the West. The doctrines of many masters moved across the world and went on to create different schools of yoga everywhere. Some of the masters that are worth mentioning are: Râmakrishna (1836-1886), Tirumalai Krishnamacharya (1888-1989), Swami Sivananda (1887-1963), Paramahansa Yogananda (1893-1952), and Sri Aurobindo (1872-1950). It is also possible to talk about the post-contemporary period of the XX century, whose principal representatives would be: Iyengar, Desikachar, Svami Visnudevananda, and Yogi Bhajan.

Sanskrit text of *Bhagavad Gita*.

Sacred city of Varanasi, in the north of India.

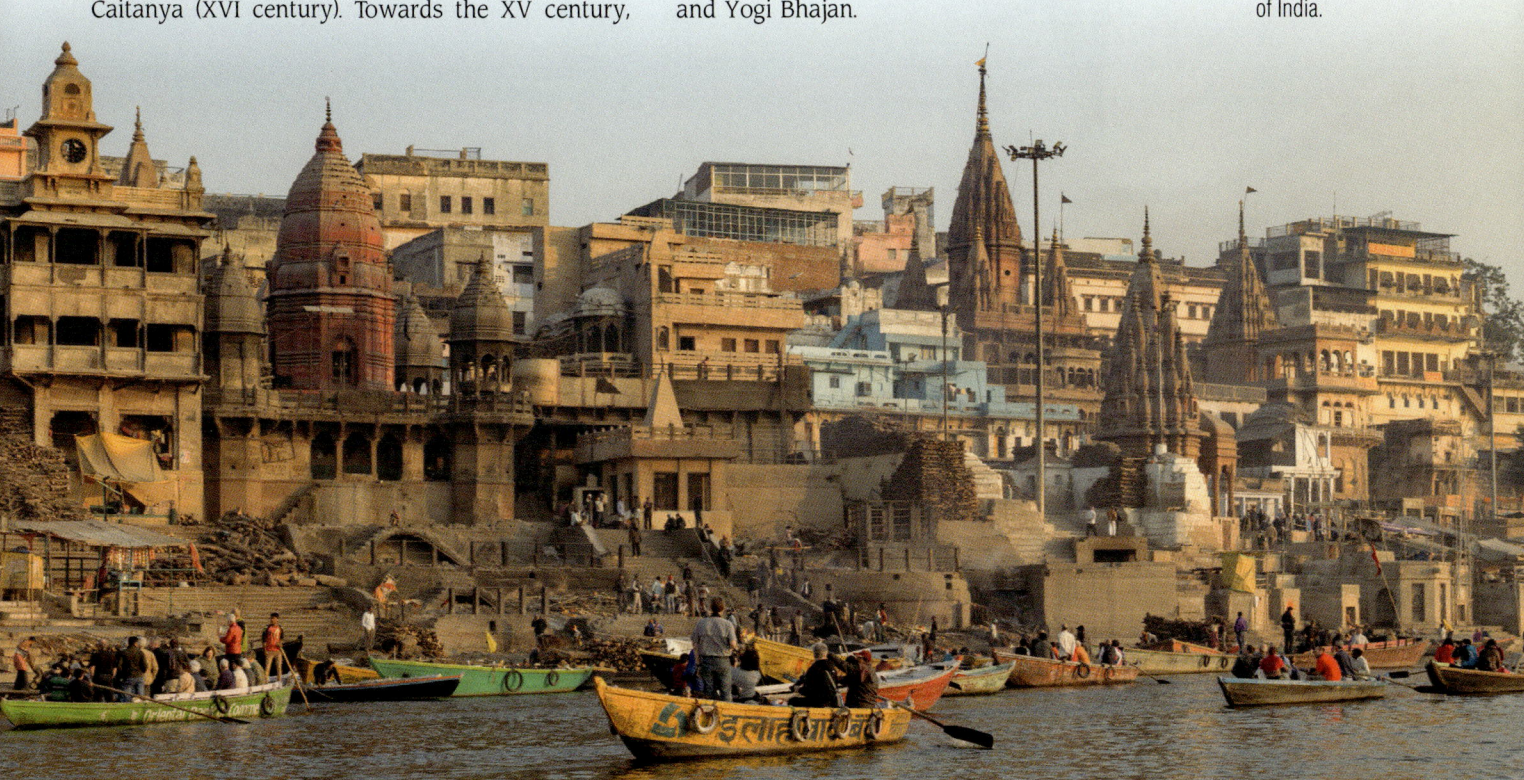

# The paths of yoga

Within yoga there are various paths that bring us to the union of the body-mind-spirit. As well as the fact that every person is different, yoga is also different as a technique for transcendent knowledge; it offers us various methods from which we can choose according to our personality or temperament.

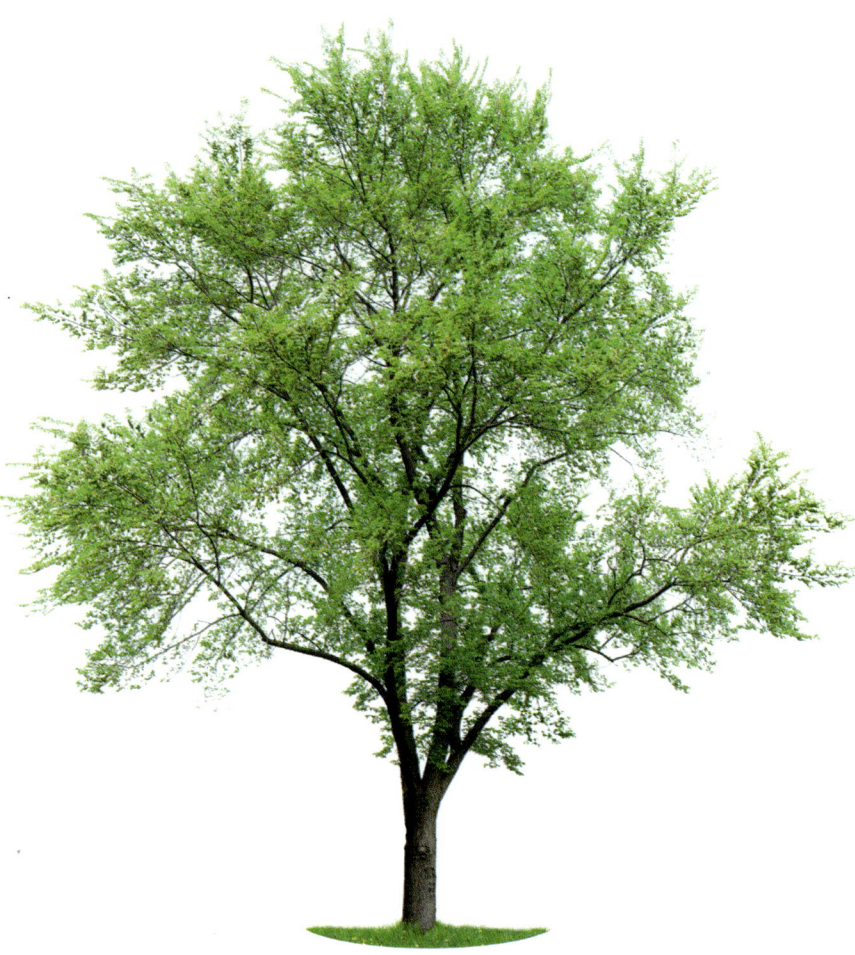

Yoga, like a tree, splits off into various branches.

These techniques have been appearing throughout history. *Bhagavad Gita* (V-II centuries A.D.) tells us about the three types of yoga as a path to freedom: Jñaña Yoga, Karma Yoga, and Bhakti Yoga. Patanjali, in his work *Yoga-sûtra* outlines Raja Yoga. As for Hatha Yoga, it was already mentioned in an *Upanishad* and in the *Puranas*, although its practice is believed to be much older.

In these different methods of praticing yoga, we find the most mental, spiritual yogas and even those that focus on physical tasks and the awareness of the body. It doesn't matter which path we choose, all of them are a source of freedom; they take us to a place to overcome the ego, find rest and mental peace, wake up our consciousness, increase our energy and inner happiness, and finally find the union of the body-mind-spirit.

Although there are dozens of yogas, these can be summarized in five important branches: Karma Yoga (path of action), Jñaña Yoga (path of wisdom), Bhakti Yoga (path of love and devotion), Hatha Yoga (path of vital and mental strength), and Raja Yoga (path of introspection).

### KARMA YOGA

This is the yoga of selfless action, although it was not always like this. In ancient Vedic literature, action was understood as the ritual action of sacrifices, which was characterized by accuracy and exactness when it came time to carry out a ritual; it was an external action. India, little by little, became free of this Vedic ritualism in a way that transformed this external action into a selfless act through deeds.

Human beings are, in fact, responsible for every thought and action that they create, and this will create a consequence within the law of karma, which is the moral law of cause and effect. Therefore, within the action of yoga, the attitude of life is characterized by any deed or service that is selfless. Someone practicing Karma Yoga will let go of being the hero of the action and turn into an instrument of the action. This action, service, or task is done through selfless implication and delivery.

### JÑAÑA YOGA

This is the path of consciousness, of wisdom. Jñaña does not refer to an intellectual knowledge, but to supreme wisdom, which is acquired through reflection and meditation. It consists of two basic stages. The first stage is reflection, where we use our rational mind to analyze that which we wish to understand, for example, by using questions.

One of the most common questions is: Who am I? The second stage is that of meditation, where we abandon the rational mind and a vast wisdom appears that springs forth from our personal experience. Through this continued practice, prejudice, obsession, and preconceived ideas are destroyed, while an experiential understanding is acquired that allows us to discover the ultimate reality of things. As mentioned in the fourth chapter of *Bhagavad Gita*, it eliminates the bad and doubts and a supreme peace is finally achieved.

## BHAKTI YOGA

This is the yoga of devotion, of pure love. Someone practicing this yoga is committed to the motive of devotion, which can be a Divinity, the Absolute, or any other devotional purpose. Just like Karma Yoga, love of a devout practitioner is unconditional, it does not expect anything in return. It is an attitude of dedication and of total abandon to the divine will.

A practitioner or *bhakta* should be a person who is not very attached to the desires of feeling and who has a high moral value. This path of yoga could very well be combined with other practices of yoga and incorporated into daily life.

## HATHA YOGA

This is the path of bodily and mental strength. Its meaning comes from the name *Ha* which means "moon" and *Tha* which means "sun", and they represent these strengths, of the body and the mind. When the strength unite, Kundalini appears, a spiritual strength. Hatha Yoga is one of the most practiced yoga forms in the West because its initial practice focuses on the physical body: with its *asanas* (poses), and *shatkarmas* (purification exercises), and *pranayama* (controlled and regulated breathing). These practices provide a physical balance and a control of the body, which allow energy to flow within, thus purifying and regulating our physiological activity. In addition, Hatha Yoga is done with *mudras* (psychic gestures) and *bandhas* (energetic keys) which induce concentration and meditation.

## RAJA YOGA

This is Real Yoga, although it is known as Mental Yoga. This is the path of introspection, of a shrinking of our senses, where our focus is directed to the interior in order to transcend the physical plane and reach a much deeper level of meditation. A practitioner reaches a state of consciousness (super-consciousness) where the Real is discovered along with the true nature of self.

The path of Raja Yoga includes other branches of yoga, such as Patanjala Yoga (based on *Yoga-sûtra* of Patanjali), Kundalini Yoga, Kriya Yoga, Mantra Yoga, and Dhyana Yoga.

Various paths of practicing yoga lead toward unity.
Path in Fatehpur, Rajasthan, India.

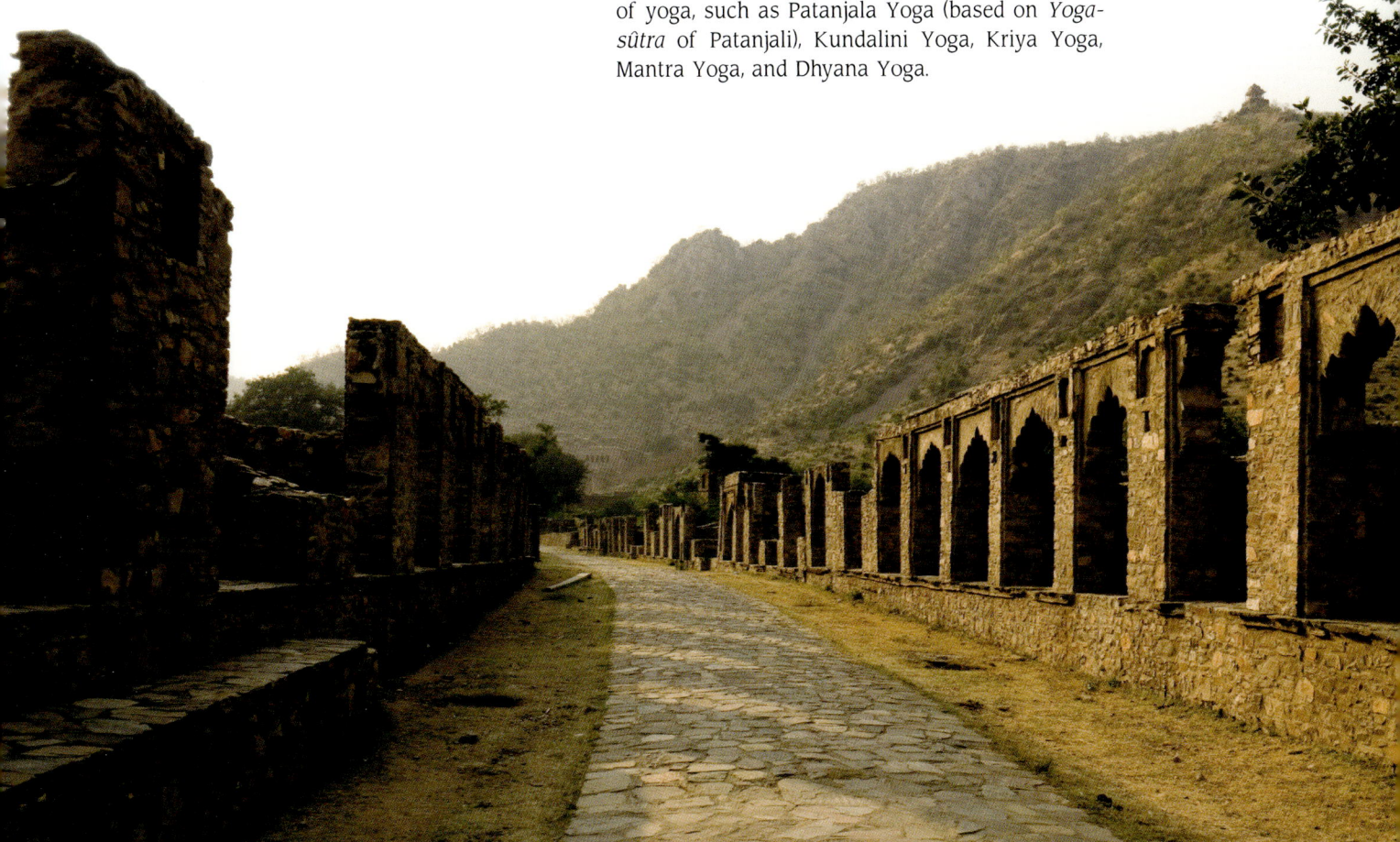

# Patanjali and the Yoga-sûtra

*Yoga-sûtra* is considered to be one of the most important texts in classical yoga. This work represents the first systematic approach that concretely describes the rules for practicing yoga. The exact period that it appeared is unknown, but it is believed to have been produced in the year 200 B.C.E., although some authors date it to later times.

Pranava mantra. The sacred syllable "OM," (pronounced "AUM,") represents the sacred triad of Brahma (the Creator), Vishnu (the Preserver), and Shiva (the Destroyer). "The repetition and thought of the meaning of Pranava leads us to Samâdhi."
*Sutra*, 28

The text is comprised of 195 sutras or aphorisms, written in Sanskrit, and it is divided into four chapters: "Concentration" (Samâdhi Pada), "Practice" (Sadhana Pada), "Experiences" (Vibhuti Pada), and "Absolute freedom" (Kaivalya Pada). *Sûtra* means "to link or connect." The sutras summarize a large amount of meaning using few words.

## CALM YOUR MIND

At the beginning of his declaration, Patanjali reveals to us what yoga is: "Yoga is the control of the states of the mind", and can be used to stop the fluctuations of the mind."

If we observe our mind for a few moments, we see that it does not stop; we are constantly thinking about something, continuously, and we jump from one thought to the next without stopping. This leads us to act in an unorganized way at times, where we cannot concentrate in the present, thus living separated from the here and now. According to Patanjali, the patterns of thought can be controlled through the persistent and constant practice of concentration, without any interruptions, and the disregard for material things. This is the way to calm the mind and achieve an appropriate perception of the real world, transforming yourself in order to obtain happiness and absolute peace.

## OBSTACLES TO INNER PEACE

According to *Yoga-sûtra*, there are five primary obstacles that prevent us from reaching tranquility and inner peace. These five obstacles, which are the primary causes of the ego and suffering, are known as *kleshas*.

**Avidya.** Ignorance of false understanding with respect to the true nature of things.
**Asmita.** Egoism and the false appreciation of self.
**Raga.** Adherence or need for mental feelings or feelings toward objects.
**Dvesha.** Distaste for patterns of thought, connected to painful past experiences.
**Abhinivesha.** Instinctive adherence to life and the fear of death.

To progressively overcome the kleshas, we have to make ourselves aware of that which disturbs us. Remain in a state of alertness, and when we feel bad, we should stop for a moment and reflect on why. Once we achieve a clear consciousness and distinguish that which we feel, we will free ourselves from suffering.

# Patanjali and the Yoga-sûtra

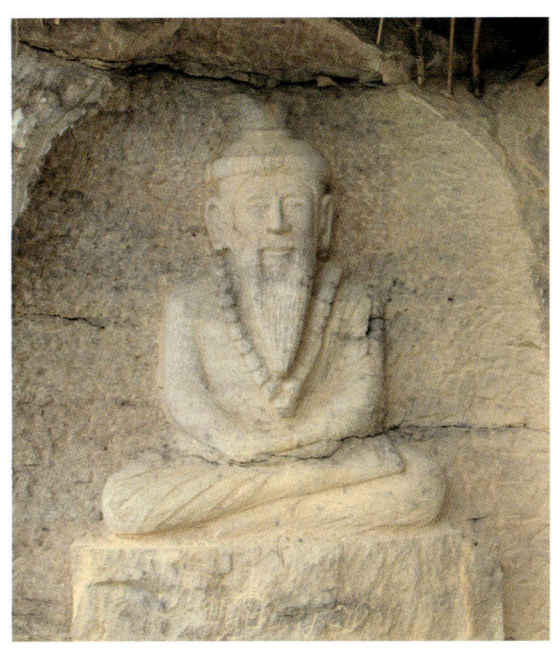

## ASHTANGA YOGA, THE EIGHT MEMBERS OF YOGA

In the second chapter of his work *Yoga-sûtra*, Patanjali explains the stages of practice, the necessary path for achieving yoga *(sadhana)*. In the path of yoga, known as *Ashtanga Yoga*, there are eight *angas* or members that correspond to the eight practices that must be completed to reach *Samâdhi*.

### External preparation: Bahyrangas

The eight practices of yoga move from the most external to the most internal. The first five steps, Bahyrangas, are considered an external preparation so that you can develop and purify your body and withdraw from external stimulation before moving deeper into the inner world.

**Yama.** These are the disciplines of ethics, the necessary and universal rules so that the world functions and avoids chaos. This addresses five fundamental rules: *ahimsa* (non-violence), *satya* (telling the truth), *asteya* (not robbing), *brahmacharya* (moderation) and *aparigraha* (not coveting, not hoarding).

**Niyama.** These are the five psychophysical disciplines of self-control *saucha* (purity, interior and exterior cleanliness), *santosa* (satisfaction, serenity), *tapas* (frugality, self-discipline), *svadyaya* (understanding of self), and *Isvara Pranidhana* (dedication, adoration of the Absolute).

**Asana.** This is the pose, the bodily position that is adopted while practicing yoga. It should be stable and pleasant, as well as easy to maintain for a certain period of time.

**Prânâyâma.** This is the conscious control of breathing, the prana or vital and vibrant energy. The prânâyâma combines prolonged inhaling and exhaling. Holding your breath in the lungs or emptying them is also a part of this discipline.

**Prâtyâhâra.** This means "to distance" and it includes retracting the organs of the senses in order to pacify them, moving them toward our inner self.

### Inner search: Antarangas

Once you have begun the practice of the first five external steps, you start the three-step process of *Samyama*, which means "balance". It starts when the mind is in a condition of moving its concentration toward a single point *(Ekagrata)*.

**Dhâranâ.** This means "control" or "concentration". The mind concentrates while keeping its attention focused on something, any object, which could be real or fictitious.

**Dhyâna.** This phase of meditation happens when prolonged concentration occurs in time and requires no effort. This creates a deep level of internalization and an important transformation of the consciousness.

**Samâdhi.** This is the complete culmination. The mind is engrossed and the practitioner identifies with the object of meditation. The consciousness of the mind is lost and a full consciousness (super-consciousness), peace, and supreme happiness come alive.

Bajorrelieve on a stone in Rishi (wisdom).

Walking up the Ganges River; for a Hindu, it is a source of life and spirituality, but also death, understood as freedom.

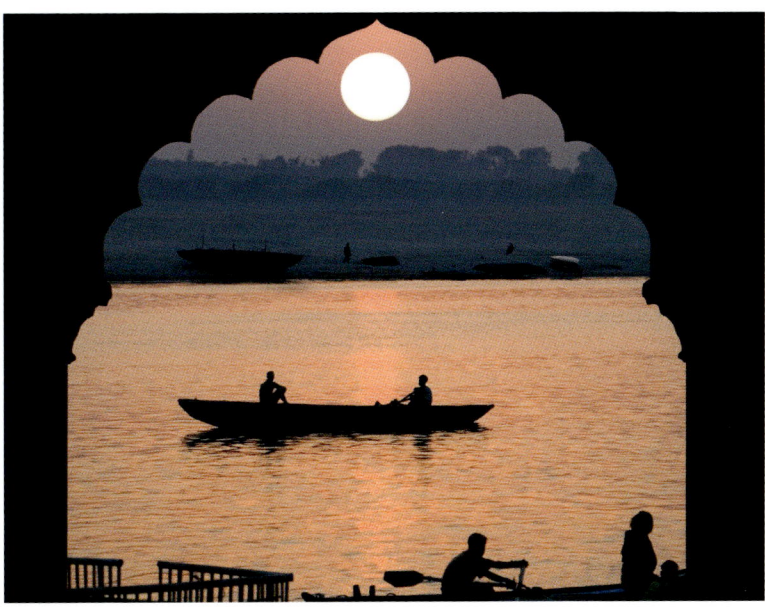

# The practice of Yoga

Yoga encompasses a wide range of physical, mental, and spiritual techniques that a practitioner will discover, and which prepare people to live a more intense life, accepting a greater detachment from material things, external events of life, and the internal states of the mind.

Through the practice of yoga, we develop a greater level of consciousness that allows us to be more aware of all that surrounds us. This expands our ability to perceive and helps us become aware of every action and thought that accompanies our daily life.

### YOGA VERSUS OTHER PHYSICAL TECHNIQUES

There are many methods and schools for practicing yoga, and each one of them instructs its own *sadhana* (practice) in order to guide a practitioner toward supreme freedom. They all have aspects in common that distinguish yoga from physical exercise and other psychophysical techniques. In fact, out of context, an *asana* (or pose) from yoga could be no different from a stretch from a fitness class. However, every practice of yoga brings together certain primary characteristics, which are essential for the self-fulfillment of being human in all its vastness.

Yoga is a discipline that is recommended for all ages.

The differences between yoga and physical exercise or other psychophysical techniques are summarized with the following points.

### DIFFERENCES BETWEEN YOGA AND OTHER PHYSICAL TECHNIQUES

**1. Awareness of the here and now.** With our full attention on everything that surrounds us, we create a space that allows us to live presently and with intensity.

**2. Centers attention on the physical body.** We can keep our focus on the position of the body, the movement from the beginning and end of a pose, muscles, and joints, which allow us to hold this pose.

**3. Breathing awareness.** This allows us to observe inhaling and exhaling, and will help us in the final pose or exercise. The way we breathe also tells us how our body is internally (physically and mental).

**4. Control of the body and breathing.** Control of our movement and our breath will only appear when we become aware of them. This represents a more advanced step in the practice of yoga.

**5. Mental control.** Paying attention to the processes of the mind allows us to be aware of our thoughts. In this way we become responsible for them and their influence on our physical and mental bodies.

**6. Spiritual training.** Yoga trains a person to find a spiritual path, which transcends the mundane.

**7. Increase energy.** At the end of practicing yoga, it is common to experience an increase in physical energy and inner happiness.

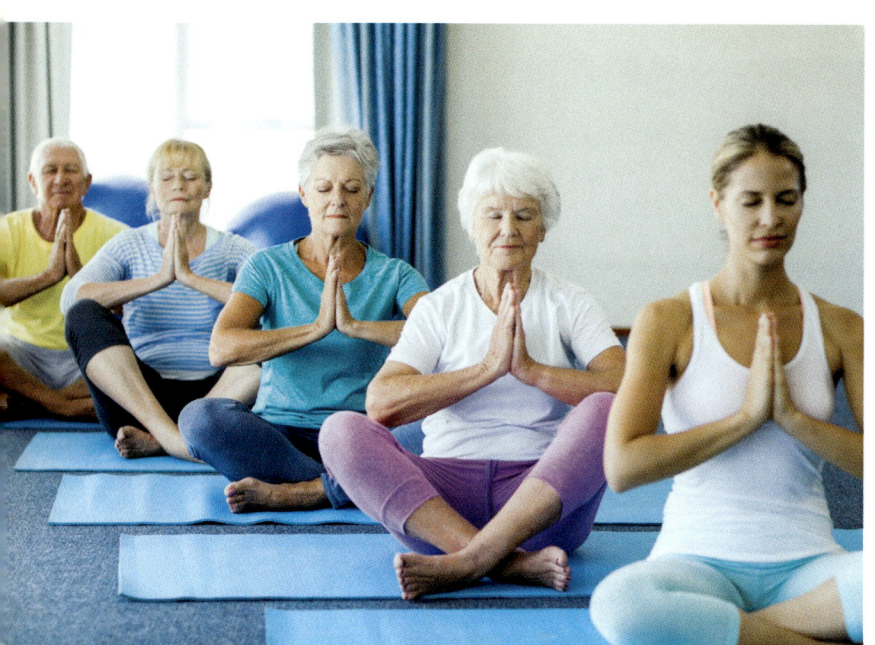

# The practice of Yoga

## BENEFITS OF YOGA

The goal of yoga is not to cure the body; instead its continued practice provides great benefits not only on a physical level, but also on mental, psychological, and spiritual levels. Yoga, as a source of health, boosts well-being and helps to prevent sicknesses by taking on an active role against them. It is also credited with great healing and therapeutic effects.

### PRIMARY BENEFITS

- **Re-trains** posture, in particular in the face of back problems. Improves flexibility, increases vitality and strength.
- **Tones** the body and keeps it healthy.
- **Expands** respiratory capacity.
- **Provides** psychological and mental balance, creating a positive state that translates into improved certainty and confidence in oneself.
- **Decreases** stress, calms the mind, and provides an inner peace.

Yoga offers a complete benefit to the body, as it has effects on all the systems and structures (primarily the muscular, skeletal, nervous, endocrine, cardiovascular, respiratory, and digestive systems).

In addition, through continued practice we see a healthy lifestyle and habits develop (body posture, consistent breathing, managing mental stress) which have an effect not only on our physical health, but also on the way that we see the world and experience an encounter with ourselves.

## PRECAUTIONS FOR PRACTICING

Yoga is a universal practice that is appropriate for all stages of life, from youth to old age. It is also used frequently for **therapeutic purposes**, as it helps to recover from difficult processes due to sickness, dealing with ailments or injuries, or fighting against stiffness in people with some type of limitation to their movement.

But, even though it is a practice that adapts to each individual, it is necessary to take certain precautions. Those who suffer from health problems must give extra effort to be careful when doing asanas and consider its warnings. If there is some underlying sickness or disease, prior to doing these exercises, you should consult with a doctor. In regards to meditation, those people who going through a process of psychological pain should abstain.

The following table shows the basic precautions that must be considered before starting to practice yoga.

### BASIC PRECAUTIONS

- While recovering from an illness, you must practice simple and basic poses which do not come with any warnings. Start gradually.
- If there are injuries or inflammation in the joints, problems with the back, bulging disks, severe injuries, or circulatory or cardiac problems, practicing yoga should be supervised by a health professional.
- Yoga may be beneficial during pregnancy as long as exercises are adapted to each stage of the pregnancy.
- During menstruation, women should pay attention to their bodies' signals. Inverted poses are not appropriate.
- Elder people who lack balance or are prone to injuries from falling should pay attention to poses that work on balance.
- In the event of an illness, always consult a health professional.

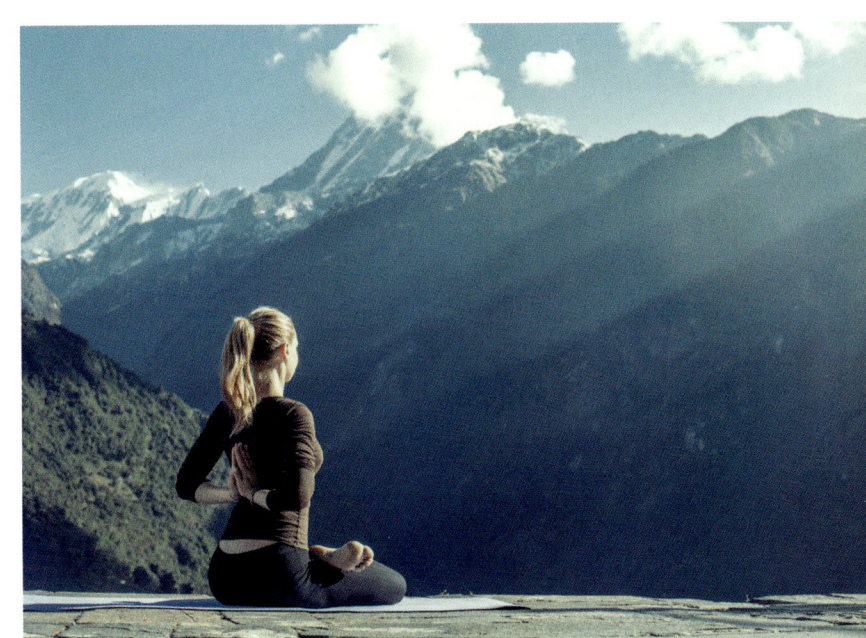

Practicing yoga in the open air offers huge benefits: we are in contact with nature, we enter the meditative states more quickly, and we soak up prana.

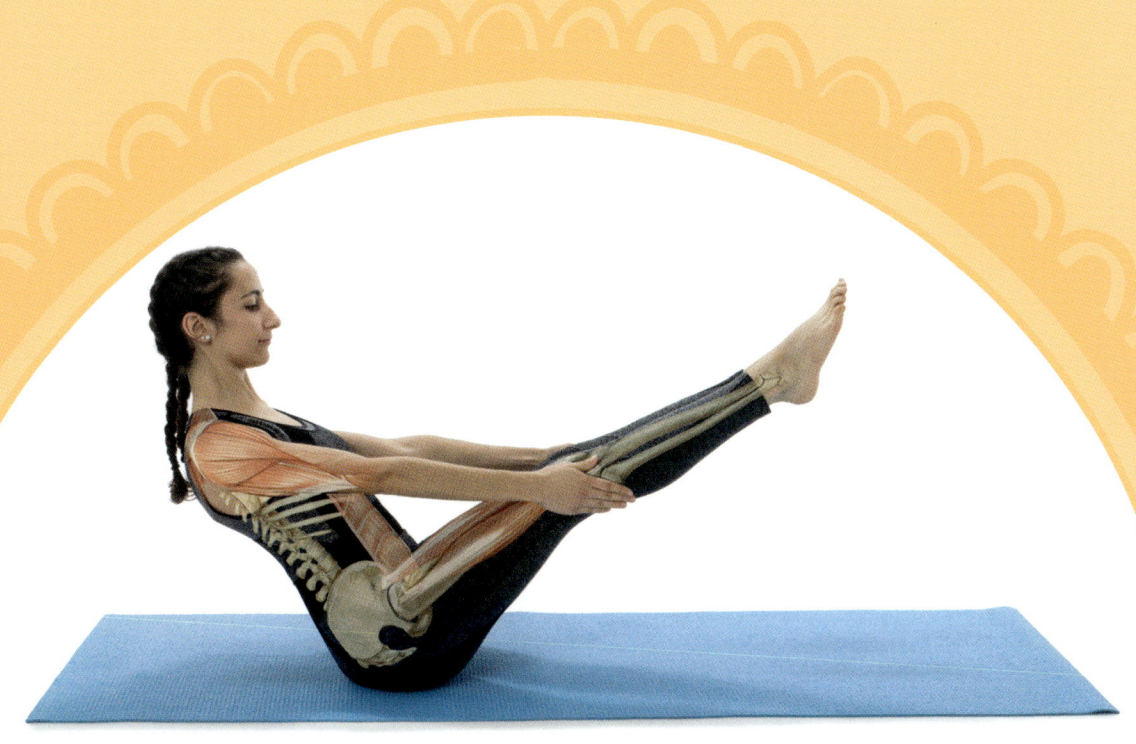

# ANATOMY AND PHYSIOLOGY

Anatomy is the study of the human body, its structure, its various parts, and the relationship between them. Since yoga is a technique that works at a physical level, it ends up being necessary to have a basic knowledge of physiology, or rather, the organ systems, and the movement general functions of the body. This chapter will explain the general concepts of the skeletal system, the muscular system, the nervous system, and the endocrine system. The continual practice of yoga will benefit all of these systems in one way or another.

# The systems of the body

We find various levels of organizational structure within the human body. The most complex group of systems are found in the body, and all of these together make up an organism or living being. Every system is built up of different organs, which themselves are made up of a combination of tissues. These tissues are a grouping of cells, which are the smallest pieces of our body that have life.

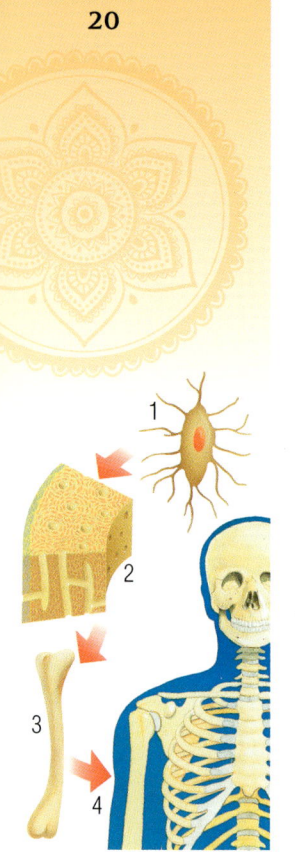

Four levels of organizational structure:
1. cellular level,
2. tissue level,
3. organ level, and
4. organ system level.

## ANATOMY AND LEVELS OF ORGANIZATION

Human anatomy is the study of the structures and parts of the human body, as well as the relationships that exist between them. General anatomy can be subdivided into two disciplines, depending on the field of study: macroscopic anatomy and microscopic anatomy.

Macroscopic anatomy is the study of large body structures, for example, bones and organs.

Microscopic anatomy is the study of very small body structures such as cells, fibers, and tissues.

In the human body, according to anatomic studies, we see six levels that are relevant to internal structural organization: atoms, cells, tissues, organs, systems, and, finally, the humans body.

## ATOMS AND CELLS

The first level of structural organization is chemical; atoms are combined together to make molecules (proteins, glucids, lipids). From the association of these molecules, cells appear. The human body is made up of billions of cells. These represent the smallest units that make up human beings and, in themselves, have the capacity to interact with the environment, metabolize, and reproduce. The vital functions of a human being depend on the state of its cells, and therefore, a healthy body will be made up of healthy cells.

## THE TISSUES

Groups of similar cells with a common function make up a tissue. The human body has four primary tissues: epithelial, muscular, nervous, and connective.

## THE ORGAN SYSTEMS BENEFIT THE MOST FROM YOGA

**Skeletal system.** Comprised of bones, cartilage, ligaments, and joints. These are the support of the body and the passive organs for movement. They also protect the delicate parts of the body (e.g., the skull). Also, blood cells are made and minerals are stored in the bones. Practicing yoga benefits the joints and tones the spinal column.

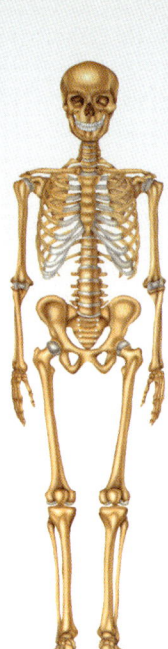

**Muscular system.** This is made up of the skeletal muscles, which are responsible for movement, since the skeleton is moved by means of its contractions. All muscles are connected to the bones, which make movement possible. To keep the muscles healthy, it is necessary to exercise them regularly, so that they don't atrophy. Yoga gives them strength and elasticity.

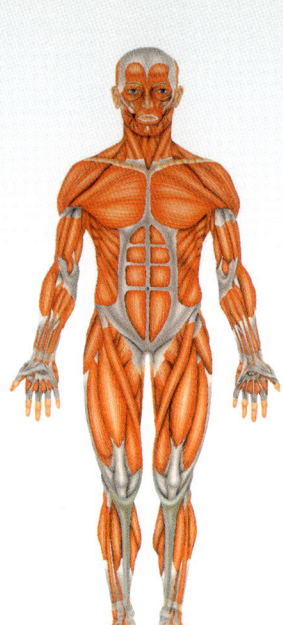

**Nervous system.** Comprised of the brain, the spinal cord, nerves, and sensor receptors. It controls the body's behavior, that is, when there are internal and external changes, it responds by activating the muscles or glands. The nervous system protects the tissues of the body by warning us with pain when an excessive stretch is caused. In general, yoga improves the function of the nervous system and brain function.

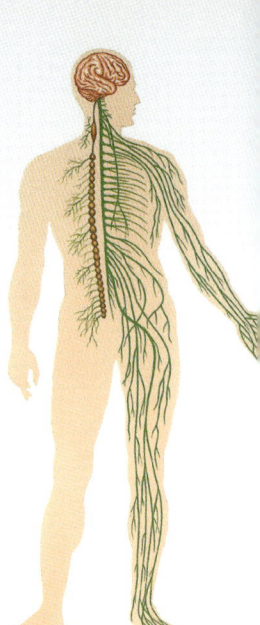

# The systems of the body

**Epithelial tissue.** This covers the largest part of internal organs, makes up all the glands, and produces some specific structures (e.g., hair, nails, gastric mucus, eye cornea).

**Muscular tissue.** Made up of muscular fibers that have the ability to contract. Its function is movement and support.

**Nervous tissue.** Responsible for transmitting information throughout the entire body through nervous impulses. It is made up of neurological cells and neurons.

**Connective tissue.** Wraps around other tissues, holding them in place, giving them shape, and controlling their movement. During a stretch, connective tissue is what establishes the maximum limits (e.g., fats, ligaments, tendons, bones, and cartilage).

## ORGANS

A group of tissues creates organs, with each one of them performing a specific function in the body (e.g., the eyes, the heart, the liver, the intestines). At the same time, organs can coordinate and work together and execute complex functions, making up organ systems.

## ORGAN SYSTEMS

Our body is made up of eleven organ systems: integumentary system, skeletal system, muscular system, nervous system, endocrine system, cardiovascular system, lymphatic system, respiratory system, digestive system, urinary system, and the reproductive system.

Practicing yoga influences, in one way or another, all systems, but in particular it has wide benefits to the skeletal, muscular, nervous, endocrine, respiratory, and cardiovascular systems.

## HUMAN BODY

The grouping of these eleven organ systems make up the highest level of structural organization: the human body. The balanced collaboration and relationships of all these systems contribute to the proper functioning of our body.

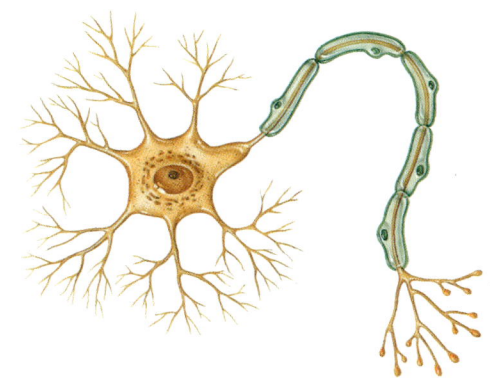

Neuron: a cell from the nervous system with the capacity to receive and transmit nervous impulses from one part of the body to another.

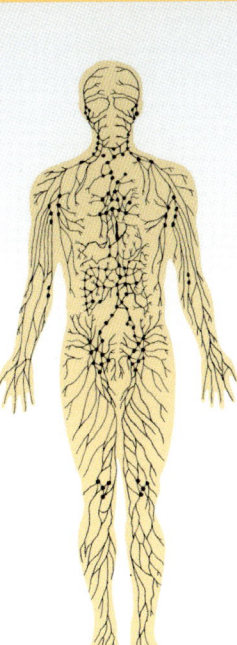

Endocrine system. Made up of the following endocrine glands: hypothalamus, thyroid and parathyroid, adrenal, thymus, pancreas, pineal gland, ovaries, and testicles. These glands produce hormones that regulate and control body functions. Yoga decreases the levels of the hormone cortisol (which is secreted in response to stress).

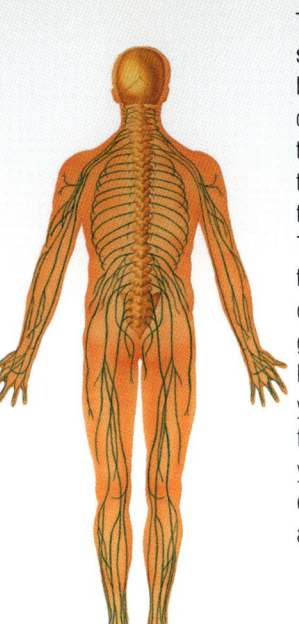

Cardiovascular system. Its primary organs are the heart and blood vessels. The heart is responsible for pumping blood and transporting it through the blood vessels to all the tissues of the body. Yoga improves venous return, increases blood flow to peripheral parts of the body (hands and feet), and improves aerobic capacity.

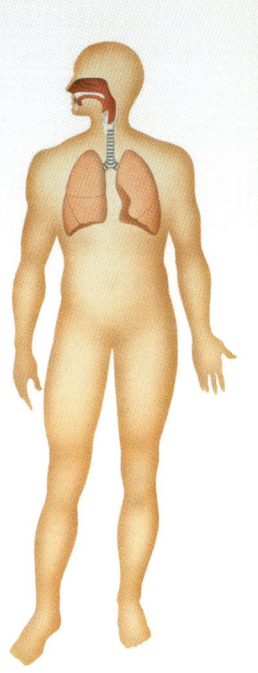

The respiratory system. Made up of the nasal cavities, the larynx, the pharynx, the trachea, the bronchial tubes, and the lungs. The alveolus are in the lungs, which carry out the exchange of gasses within the blood. Practicing yoga improves lung function and helps you to breathe more consistently, slower, and deeper.

## SKELETAL SYSTEM

# The skeletal system

The skeletal system is the organized grouping of bony structures that have the role of protecting and supporting the organs of the body. Along with the muscular system, it provides movement. Blood cells are made and minerals are stored inside the bones. This system is made up of bones, joints, cartilage, and ligaments.

There are three primary types of bony cells: the osteoblasts (cells that make up the bones), osteoclasts (those that destroy the bone and free calcium ions in the blood), and osteocytes (mature bony cells, which are inside the bony matrix).

**THE BONES**

They make up the internal structure of the body. Along with the skeletal muscles, they allow body movement and operation. In addition to supporting the body's weight, they protect the organs and soft tissues from any impact that comes from outside of the body: the skull protects the brain, the vertebrae in the spine surround the spinal cord, and the bony thorax protects the lungs and heart.

Minerals that are essential for life are stored in the bones, such as calcium and phosphorus, and inside some of them blood cells are made.

The human body is made up of 206 bones, which are classified into four major groups according to their shape and size:
• large bones (the femur, the humerus),
• short bones (the kneecap),
• flat bones (the skull, sternum, and ribs), and
• irregular bones (vertebrae).

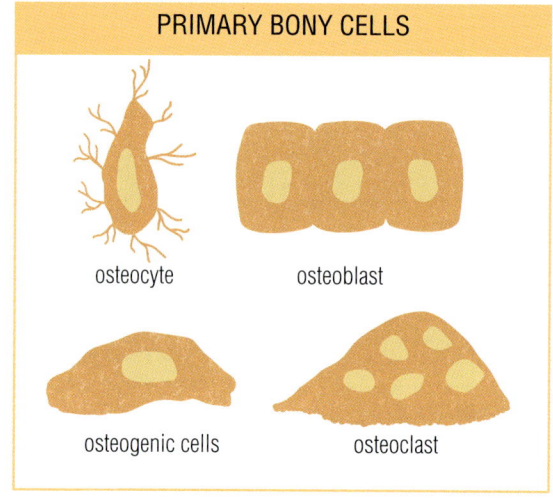

PRIMARY BONY CELLS: osteocyte, osteoblast, osteogenic cells, osteoclast

The structure of a large bone has two epiphysis or extremes, which is where the bone ends. These are covered by joint cartilage, and they are the areas that connect one bone to another. The diaphysis is the cylindrical area, comprised of compact bony tissue, which is covered by a membrane, the periosteum. The bone contains spongy and fatty tissue inside its internal cavities, which is yellow bone marrow.

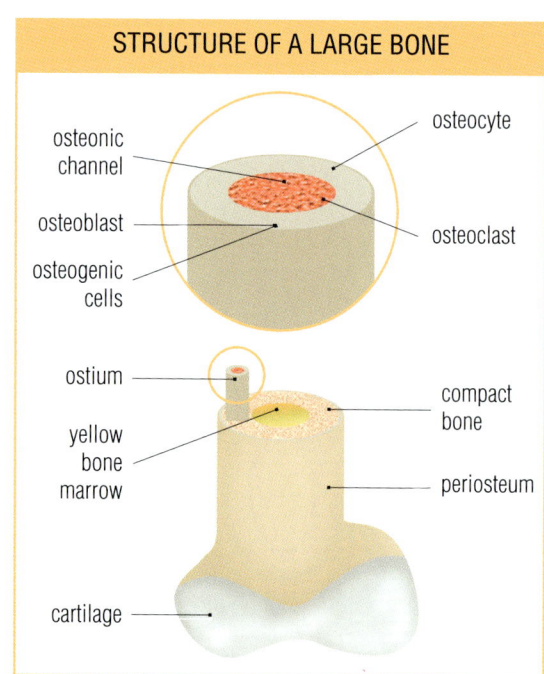

STRUCTURE OF A LARGE BONE: osteonic channel, osteoblast, osteogenic cells, osteocyte, osteoclast, ostium, yellow bone marrow, compact bone, periosteum, cartilage

**THE JOINTS**

These are the parts of the body where two or more bones are found. Their role is to connect the bones and provide mobility to the body. They are classified according to their level of movement and their structure.

According to the amount of movement that the joint allows, they are classified into:
• synarthrosis: these are rigid joints, such as those of the skull.
• amphiarthrosis: these allow for light movements, such as the vertebral bodies.
• diarthrosis: these are completely mobile joints: like the or the knee, humerus with the scapula.

Another classification is structural, since it depends on the tissue and the way in which the bony structures are connected together:
• by a fibrous tissue (fibrous joints),
• by cartilage (cartilage joints), or
• by a joint capsule (synovial joints). These joints correspond to the diarthrosis, which are more numerous in the skeleton and allow us to complete various movements. The bones are directly connected to them, but they are separated by a joint capsule or synovial joint (which contains synovial liquid).

# The skeletal system

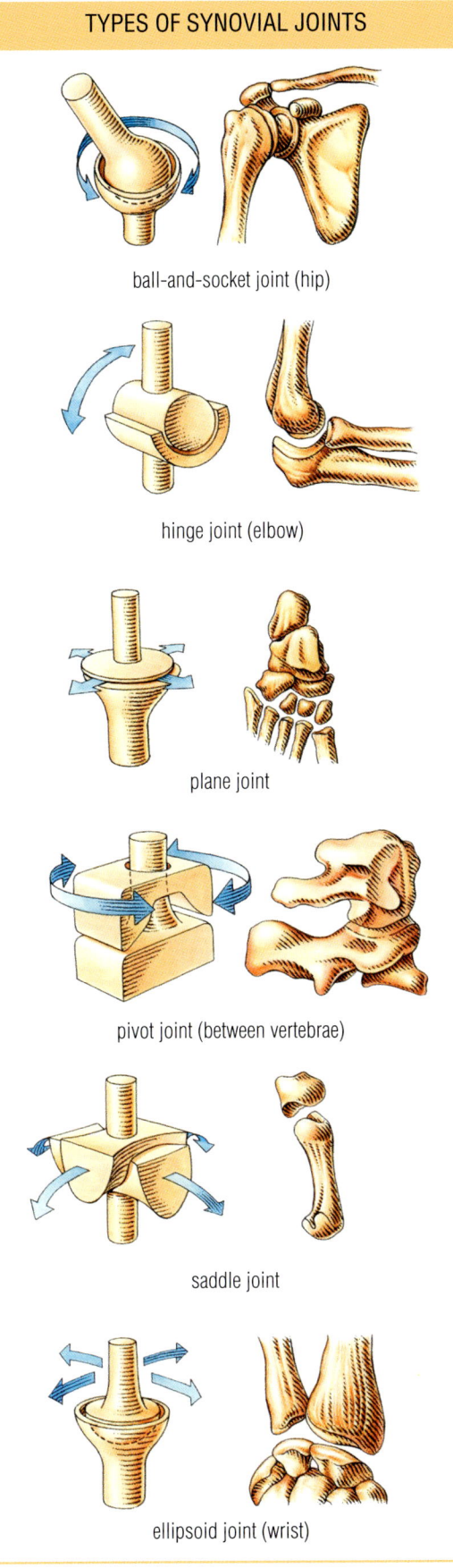

**TYPES OF SYNOVIAL JOINTS**

ball-and-socket joint (hip)

hinge joint (elbow)

plane joint

pivot joint (between vertebrae)

saddle joint

ellipsoid joint (wrist)

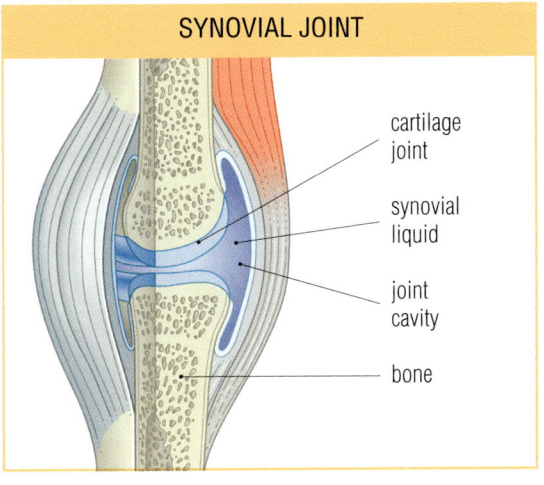

**SYNOVIAL JOINT**

- cartilage joint
- synovial liquid
- joint cavity
- bone

## CARTILAGE

There are three types of cartilage: hyaline cartilage, fibro-cartilage, and elastic cartilage. Hyaline cartilage is the most abundant type in the body; it covers the ends of many bones and joins the ribs to the sternum. Fibro-cartilage is found in the vertebral discs. Elastic cartilage is, for example, what is found in the ears.

## LIGAMENTS

These are fibrous tissues that join two adjacent bones together; normally they are found between bones and cartilage. Ligaments have a proprioceptive sensitivity, which means, they perceive (thanks to their sensitive nervous receptors) the position of any movement and its speed, which allows us to carry out an anatomically natural movement and, at the same time, restrict any abnormal movement and prevent injury.

The most common **injuries** in the ligaments are those sprains that are caused by an excessive movement of the joint. Not all ligaments join two bones together, some connect internal organs.

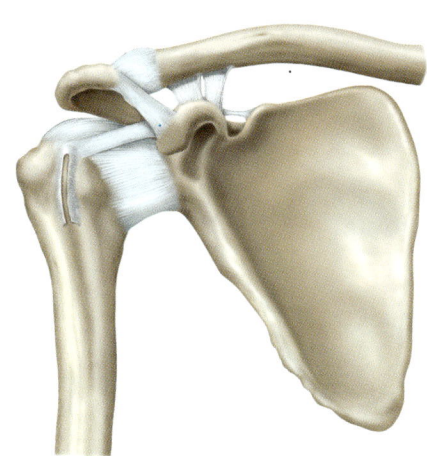

The ligaments of the shoulder.

Anatomy and physiology

SKELETAL SYSTEM

# The bones of the human body

To make this study easier, we divided the human body into parts that are well distinguished: the axial skeleton and the appendicular skeleton.

skull

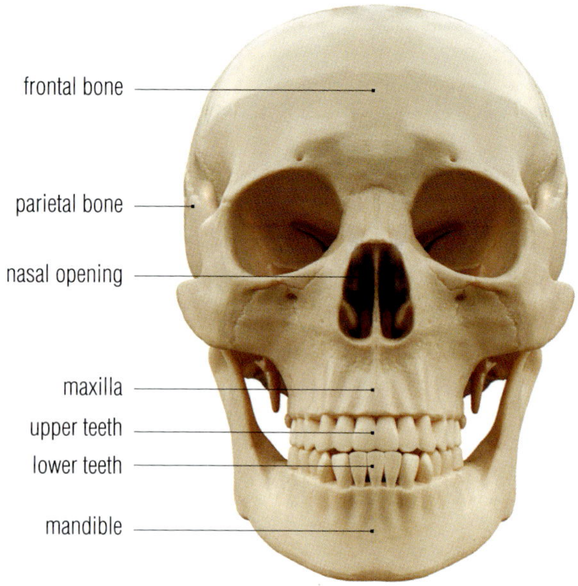

- frontal bone
- parietal bone
- nasal opening
- maxilla
- upper teeth
- lower teeth
- mandible

skeleton (front view)

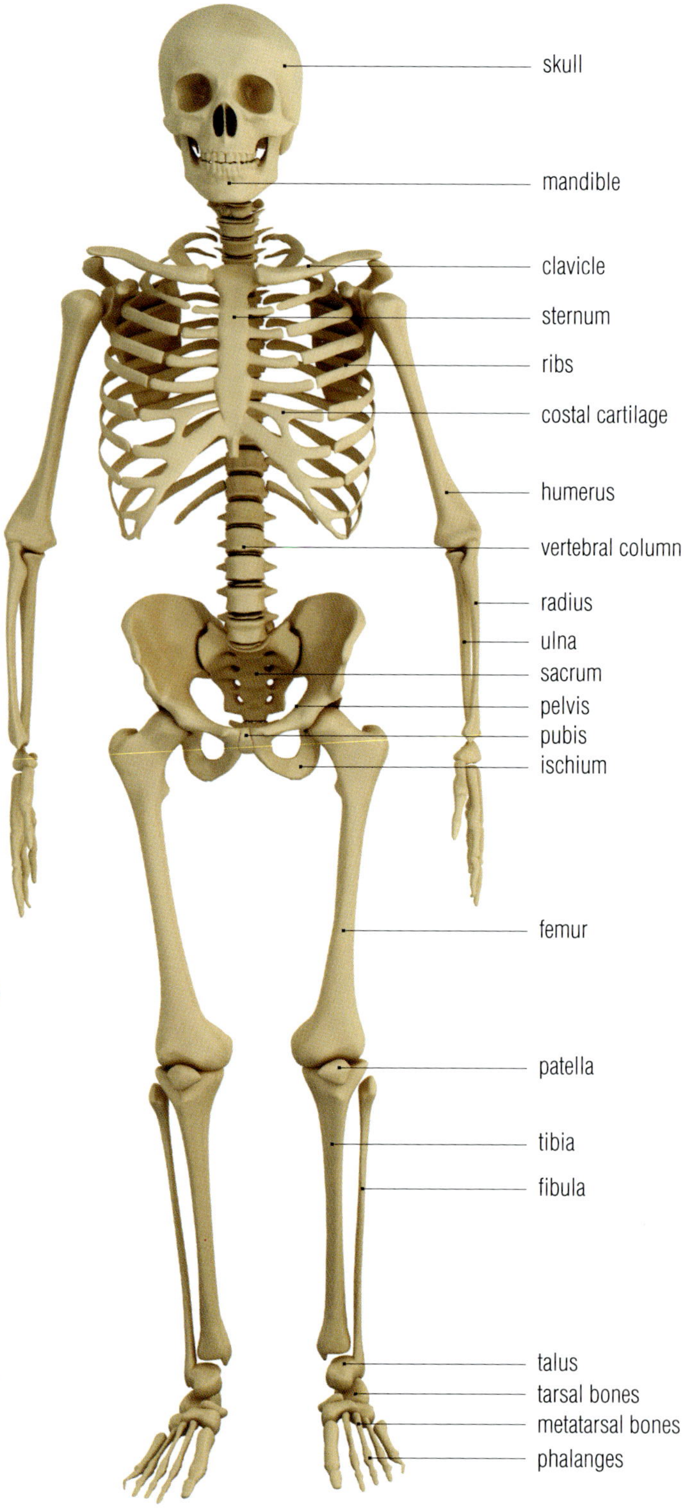

- skull
- mandible
- clavicle
- sternum
- ribs
- costal cartilage
- humerus
- vertebral column
- radius
- ulna
- sacrum
- pelvis
- pubis
- ischium
- femur
- patella
- tibia
- fibula
- talus
- tarsal bones
- metatarsal bones
- phalanges

mandible

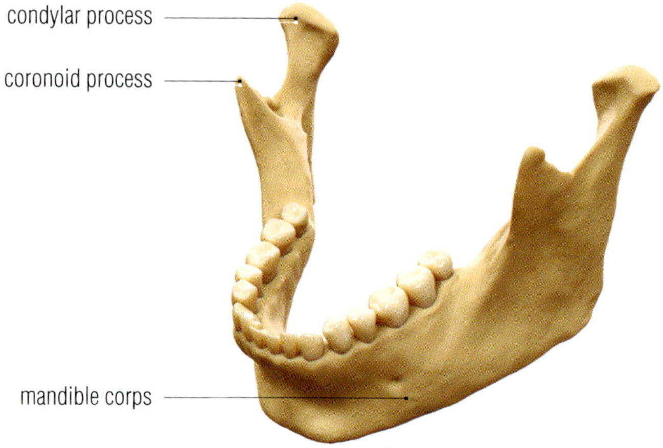

- condylar process
- coronoid process
- mandible corps

The bones of the human body  25

**AXIAL SKELETON**
This makes up the longitudinal axis of the human body, and includes the bones that are found close to or on the central axis. The appendicular skeleton is going to the axial skeleton. It is comprised of three parts: skull, bony thorax, and vertebral column.

**APPENDICULAR SKELETON**
Made from the bones of the lower and upper parts of the body and the bones in the pelvis.

skeleton (rear view)
- cervical vertebrae
- clavicle
- acromion
- scapula
- thoracic vertebrae
- humerus
- floating ribs
- lumbar vertebrae
- sacrum
- coccyx
- iliac crest
- femur
- tibia
- fibula
- calcaneus
- talus

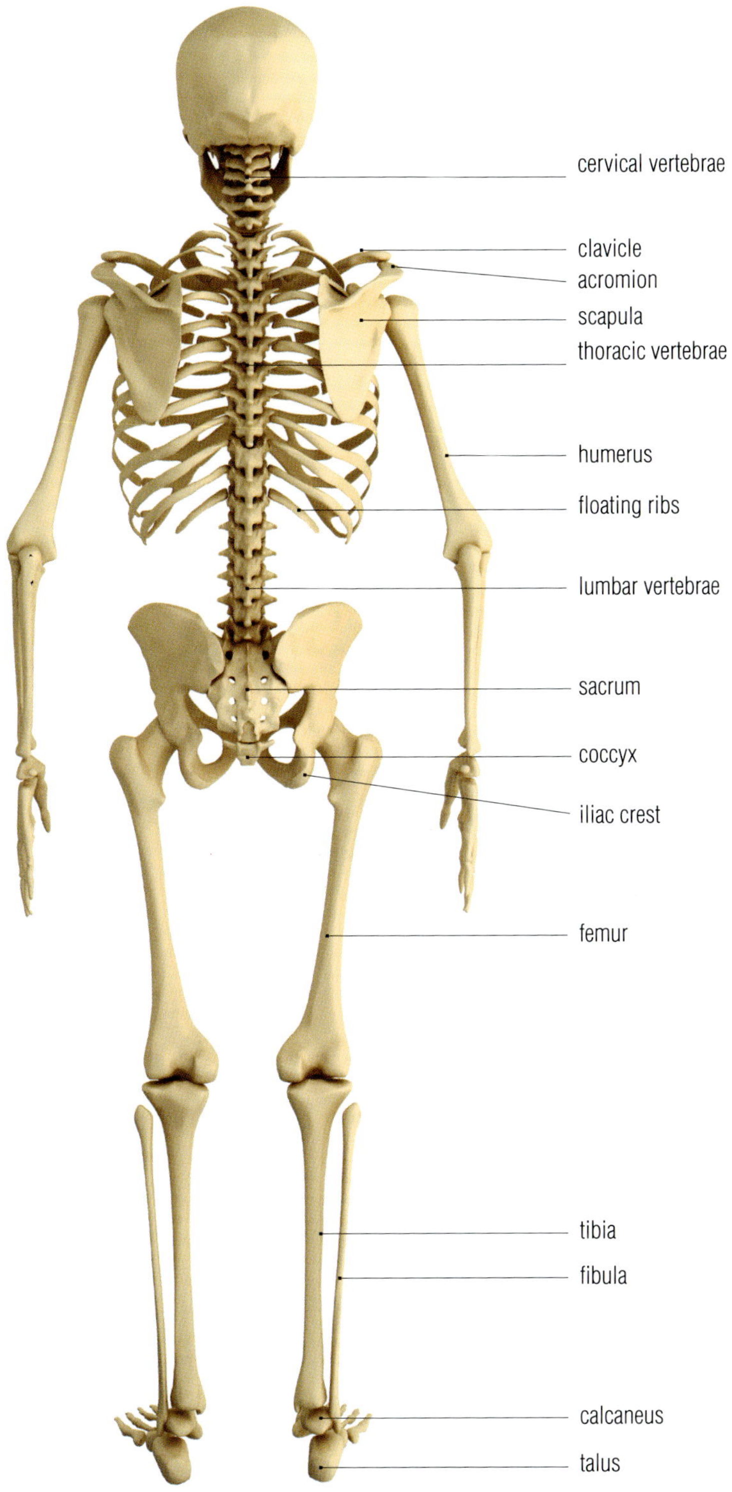

skeleton (side view)
- skull
- sternum
- spinous process
- radius
- ulna
- femoral head
- phalanges
- femur
- patella
- tibia
- fibula
- ischium
- calcaneus
- talus
- matatarsal bones

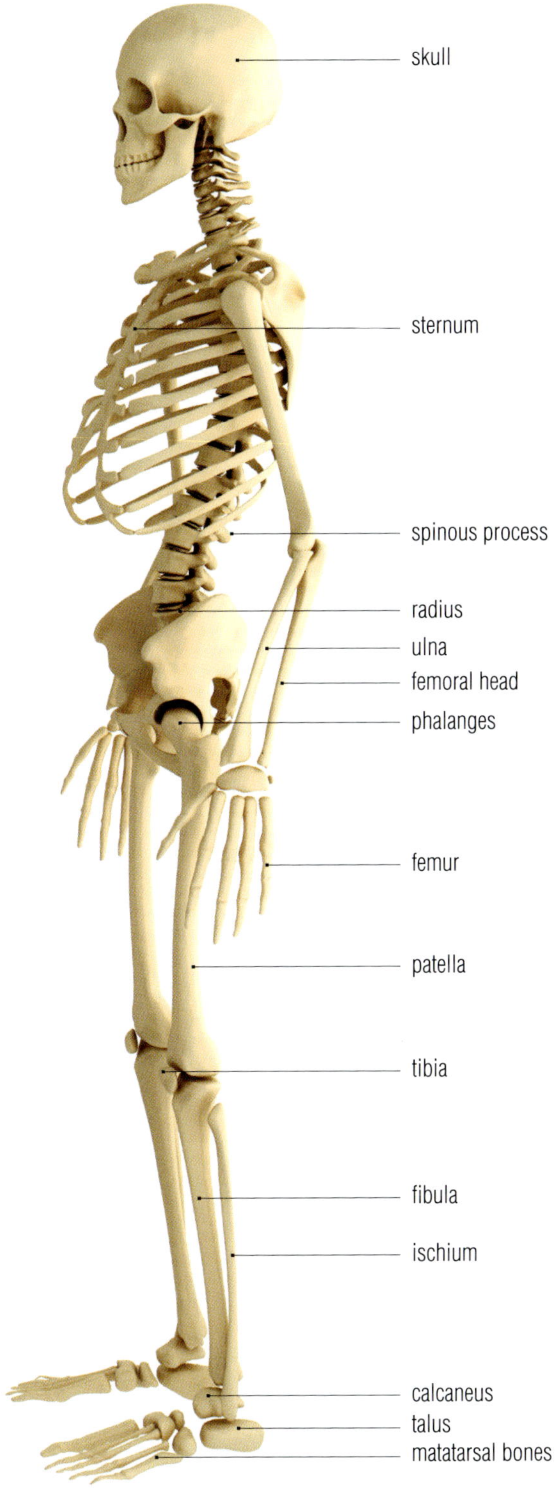

SKELETAL SYSTEM

# The vertebral column

The spinal column, dorsal, or rachis spine are located in the lower, middle, and upper parts of the axial skeleton, formed from the skull to the pelvis. It is made up of 26 irregular bones, or vertebrae, connected together with ligaments so that, together, they provide a structure that is curved, joined, flexible, and resistant.

Rear view and left side view of the vertebral column.

**THE VERTEBRAE**
Before we are born, we have 33 vertebrae, 9 of which fuse together to form the sacrum and the coccyx, which means that an adult vertebral column has 26 vertebrae. They are classified into five regions according to their common characteristics.

**Cervical curve.** Made up of seven vertebrae (C1-C7) that are responsible for making the head turn. The first cervical vertebra, the highest (C1), allows us to nod affirmatively with the head, and its joint along the axis (C2) makes it possible to made negative motion with the head. The cervical vertebrae are the smallest and lightest.

**Thoracic curve.** Comprised of 12 vertebrae (T1-T12) to which the ribs are connected, this is the largest section of the cervical vertebrae.

**Lumbar curve.** This curve is made up of five vertebrae which are the largest (L1-L5). They are large in size and the strongest, since they are responsible for holding up the weight of the body.

**Sacral curve.** This is made up of vertebrae that are fused together and make up the sacrum. The top of it is joined with the L5. The sides are joined with the bones of the hips (sacro-iliac joints).

**Coccyx.** A bone made up of the union of four fused vertebrae, also known as the tail bone.

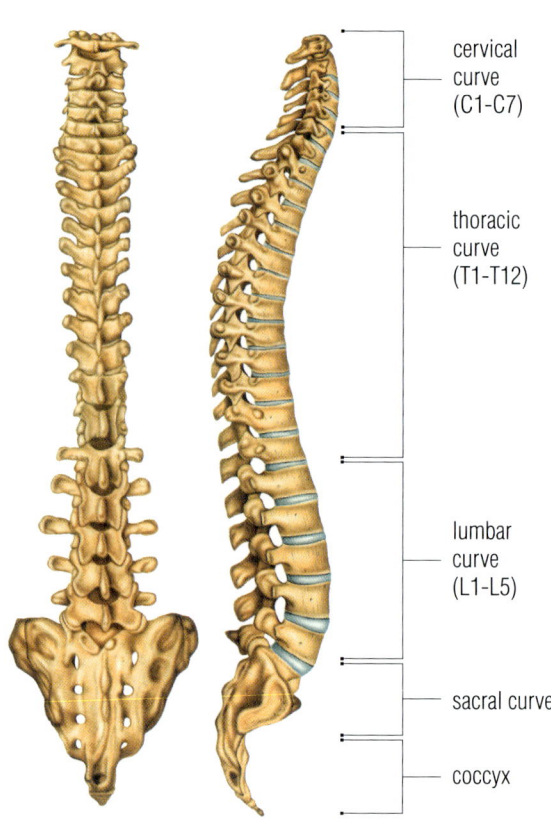

cervical curve (C1-C7)

thoracic curve (T1-T12)

lumbar curve (L1-L5)

sacral curve

coccyx

**THE INTERVERTEBRAL DISKS**
There are intervertebral or spinal disks between the vertebrae. These are made up of fibrocartilage cushions that are resistant to compression, absorb impacts, and, at the same time, provide flexibility to the vertebral column.

Their thickness depends on the area where they are located in the column. The intervertebral disks are thickest in the lumbar region (9 mm), then the thoracic (5 mm), and finally the cervical (3 mm). The relationship between the thickness of a disk and the height of the vertebral body (disk/body) determines the specific mobility of each part of the column.

As time passes, the intervertebral disks lose hydration and become less spongy and

Top view of a lumbar vertebra

## LUMBAR VERTEBRAE

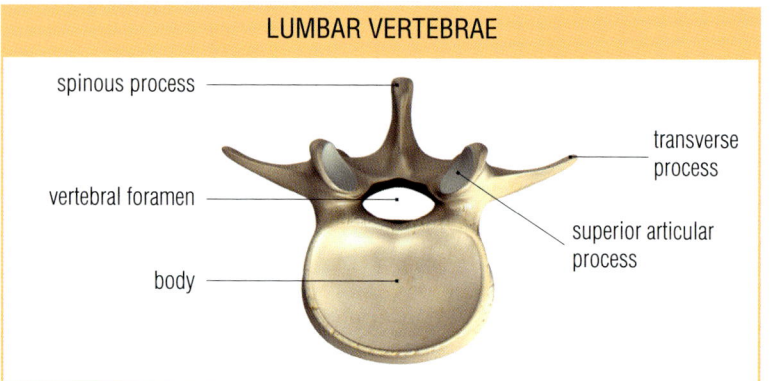

spinous process

vertebral foramen

body

transverse process

superior articular process

# The vertebral column

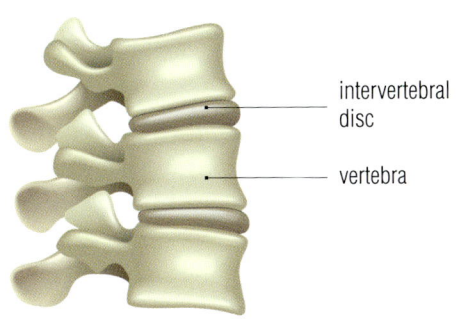

intervertebral disc

vertebra

compressible. With age, the drier the disks become, and weaker ligaments can cause hernias.

## GLOBAL MOVEMENTS OF THE VERTEBRAE COLUMN

The vertebrae column has the mobility to complete four movements: flexing (forward), flexing back or extending, lateral flexing, and rotation. The scope of these movements will vary depending on the region of the column and depending on different factors such as the shape of the vertebrae, the relationship between the thickness and height of the vertebral body, and the presence of ribs.

We use the term **hinge** when two vertebrae meet and a change in mobility occurs; you must pay attention to movement in these locations, and at times stop moving to avoid injury.

### Flexing (forward)

This movement, just like extension, is produced on the sagittal plane. The cervical region has a thick disk, which is why hypermobility occurs when flexing. You must consider the change in mobility in the cervical-thoracic hinge (C7-T1). The thoracic region is limited in its flexibility due to the ribs, and there is also a thin intervertebral disk there. There is great mobility in the lumbar region as well.

### Extending or flexing backward

This is the shifting of the body backward on the sagittal plane. While extending, the cervical region shows hypermobility between vertebrae C2 and C6, due to the short processes. The thoracic column has limited mobility due to the thin disk, the long spinous processes, and the bony thorax. The lumbar column does have good mobility thanks to the thick intervertebral disk and the short spinous processes. In these poses, you must be careful of the sacro-lumbar hinge and the T12-L1 hinge.

### Lateral flexing

This is the movement of the column on the frontal plane. In the cervical area, mobility is limited due to the wide transversal processes and the rectangular shape of the vertebral bodies. In the upper thoracic area, the ribs limit mobility, thus allowing for a greater range of mobility in the lower thoracic column. The lumbar column, due to the thickness of the disks related to the height of the vertebral body, has high mobility. You must pay attention to the thoracic-lumbar hinge (T12-L1).

### Rotation

This movement is produced on the transversal plane. There is good mobility in the entire cervical column; between the atlas and the axis where there is hypermobility, hinge C1-C2. The thoracic column has good mobility when rotating, since the articular processes make this possible. The orientation of these processes and the articular surfaces represent an osseous limit that stops the twisting of the lumbar area. You must pay attention to the hinge rotation T11-T12.

*The vertebrae are separated from one another by intervertebral disks. The disks located between the lumbar vertebrae are the thickest, provide flexibility, and, at the same time, absorb the shock of the weight and compression of the body.*

## MOVEMENTS OF THE VERTEBRAL COLUMN

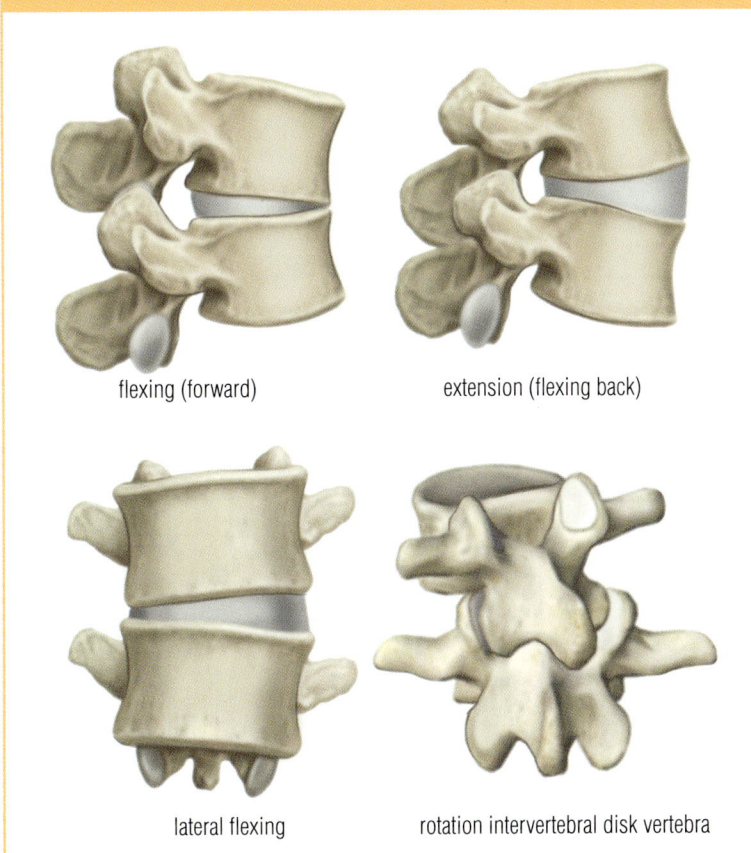

flexing (forward)　　extension (flexing back)

lateral flexing　　rotation intervertebral disk vertebra

MUSCULAR SYSTEM

# The muscular system

This is what enables all of the movements of the body and provides heat. It is made up of muscles whose sole function, different from tissues, is to contract or shorten, moving with the bones and the internal organs.

According to its cellular structure, we can see a difference between three types of muscles: skeletal muscles, cardiac muscles, and smooth muscles.

**SKELETAL MUSCLES**
These are muscles that make up the muscular system. They are inserted in the bones and are responsible for moving the skeleton. The cells that they are made from are long and stretch-marked. They are also called striated muscles and voluntary muscles, since we can control them consciously. Apart from providing movement, they maintain body posture and create heat.

**The strength** of a muscle is due to the muscle fibers being connected together and wrapped with connective tissue and then grouped together to form a bundle, called a fascicle. Many bundles are wrapped in an epimysium, which serves to support the entire muscle, and this is connected to the tendons, which at the same time are anchored to the bones.

**Movement** is produced by the muscles contracting. Contractions may mean a change in the length of a muscle (isotonic contraction), or it may be caused by a tensing that forces the muscle to keep the same length (isometric contraction). Isotonic contractions may be concentric (the muscle shortens, producing movement) or eccentric (the muscle lengthens and stops movement).

**RESPONSIBLE FOR MOVEMENT**
Muscles have the ability to create many diverse movements, combining actions of various muscles at the same time. The **primary muscle** is the one responsible for the movement, while the **antagonistic muscles** resist it or keep it tense in order to limit it. When the primary muscle is contracting, its antagonist is relaxed or stretched. As for the **synergetic muscles**, they help the primary muscle with its action, supporting the same movement or avoiding undesired movements. Within the synergetic muscles we find **stabilizer muscles**, which operate to keep the bone fixed or to stabilize the start of the primary muscle.

**The position** of the body is controlled thanks to the skeletal muscles. These adjust their position continuously so that we can remain upright, and they stabilize the joints. They also create body heat, which is the result of the muscle activity that, by contracting, frees energy in the form of heat.

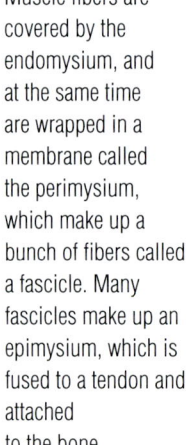

Muscle fibers are covered by the endomysium, and at the same time are wrapped in a membrane called the perimysium, which make up a bunch of fibers called a fascicle. Many fascicles make up an epimysium, which is fused to a tendon and attached to the bone.

## STRUCTURE OF SKELETAL MUSCLES

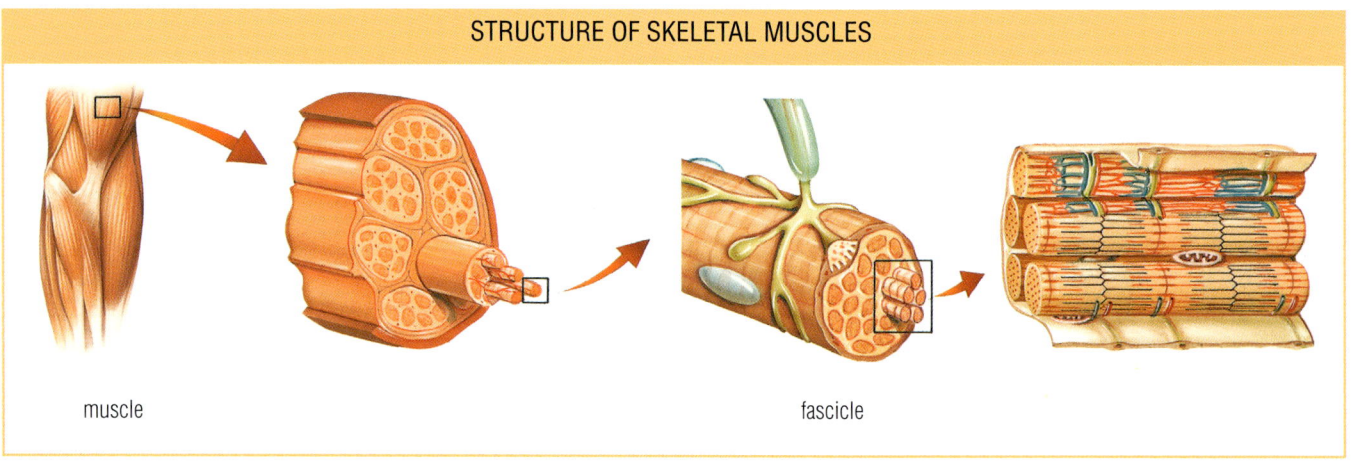

muscle          fascicle

# The muscular system

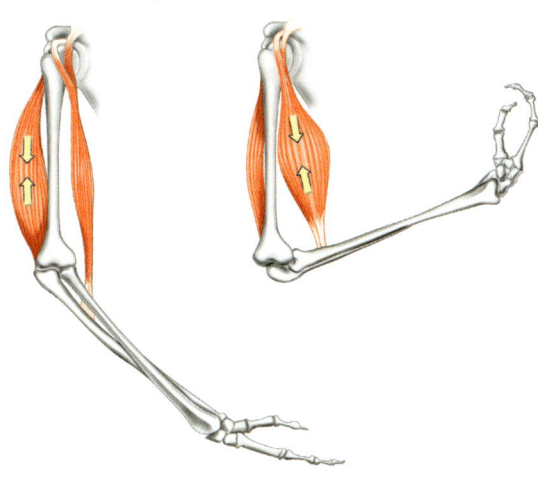

### CARDIAC MUSCLE
This is located on the walls of the heart, and it is myocardial. It is responsible for pushing the blood, via the blood vessels, through the entire body thanks to these contractions. Cardiac tissue is also stretched but involuntarily, which means that it is controlled by the autonomic nervous system.

**The job** of the cardiac muscle is constant and permanent, and it is able to perform strong and continuous contractions without tiring. Different than skeletal muscles, cardiac muscles cannot rest, even for a second.

### Blood circulation
When the heart contracts, its internal chambers (ventricles) become smaller and push the blood toward the arteries. From the right ventricle, blood is pushed to the pulmonary arteries and then to the lungs; there the blood that is poor in oxygen exchanges and becomes rich in oxygen. The blood that is rich in oxygen returns to the heart through the pulmonary veins to the left atrium, passing the left ventricle. From there, the blood leaves through the aorta to be sent out into the entire body; blood that is rich in oxygen will feed the cells (this occurs from the exchange of $O_2$ and $CO_2$ in the capillary veins). After, the blood that is poor in oxygen returns to the heart through large veins that enter into the right atrium. It passes the right ventricle and once again is sent to the lungs.

### SMOOTH MUSCLES
These are located on walls of the hollow organ (e.g., digestive track, blood vessels, urinary track). Different from previous muscles, smooth muscles do not have striations, and they are also involuntary, which means they cannot be controlled consciously. Their contractions are slow and regular and may be prolonged for a long time. One example of this function would be moving food through the digestive track.

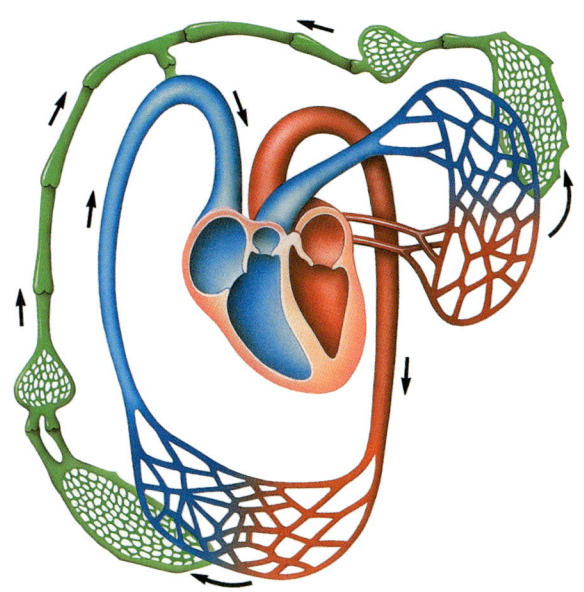

Chart of blood flow

For every contraction, there must be at least two anchoring points: the starting (adhered to the less mobile bone) and the insertion (attached to the mobile bone). When the primary muscle contracts, movement is produces by moving the insertion toward the origin.

## COMPARATIVE CHART FOR SKELETAL, CARDIAC, AND SMOOTH MUSCLES

| Characteristic | Skeletal Muscles | Cardiac Muscles | Smooth Muscles |
| --- | --- | --- | --- |
| Location | Attached to primary bones | On the walls of the heart (myocardial) | Walls of hollow viscous organs |
| Contracting | Voluntary. Regulated through the nervous system | Involuntary. Regulated by the nervous system and some hormones | Involuntary. Regulated by the nervous system and some hormones |
| Type and speed of contraction | Variable contraction, from slow to fast | Rhythmic contraction, slow | At times, rhythmic contraction are very slow |

MUSCULAR SYSTEM

# The muscles of the body

The muscular system allows our skeleton to move and keep its stability. In the following, we detail the muscles that are most relevant to practicing yoga.

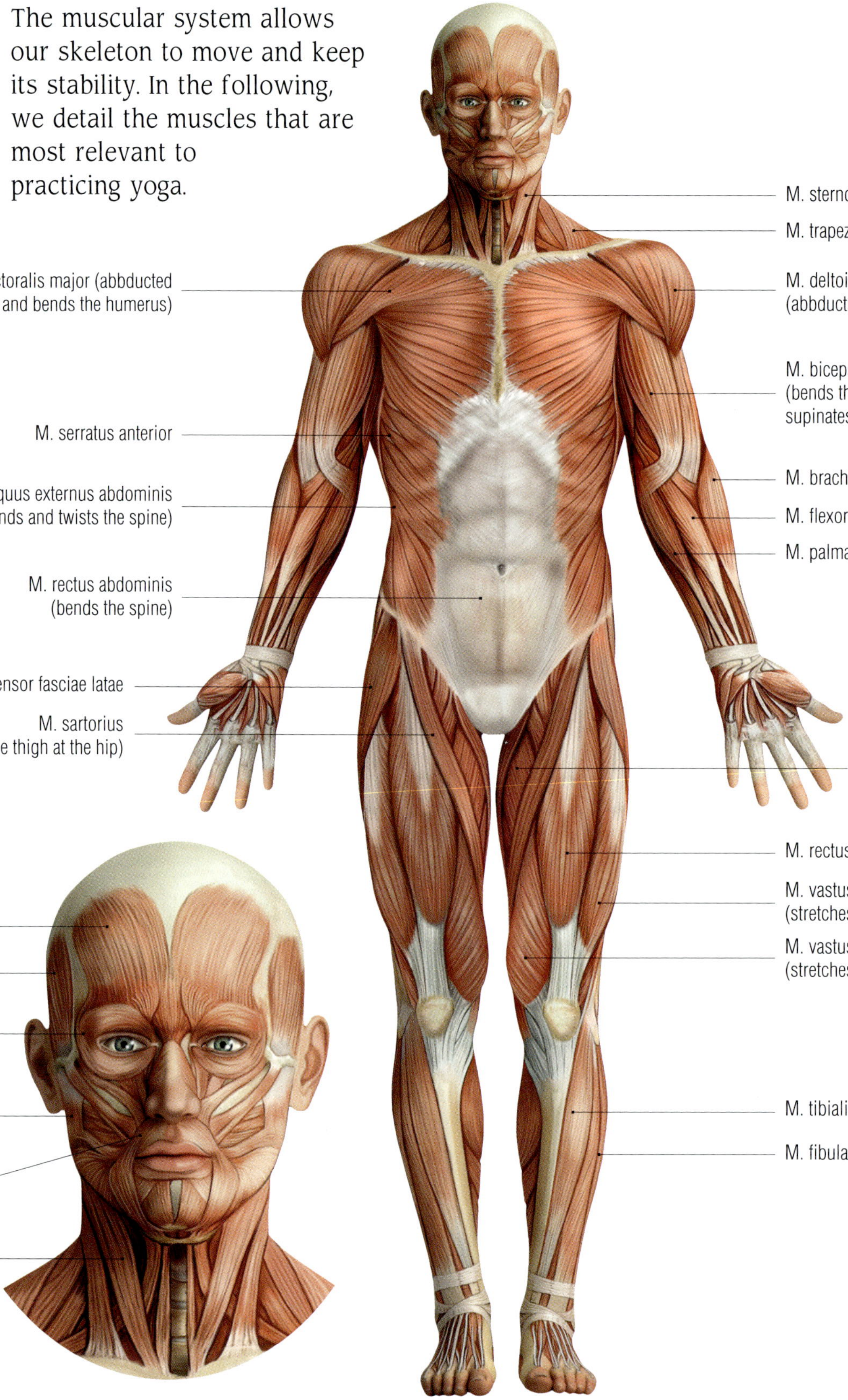

- M. pectoralis major (abbducted and bends the humerus)
- M. serratus anterior
- M. obliquus externus abdominis (bends and twists the spine)
- M. rectus abdominis (bends the spine)
- M. tensor fasciae latae
- M. sartorius (bends the thigh at the hip)

- M. frontalis
- M. temporalis
- M. orbicularis oculi (closes the eyes)
- M. masseter (closes the jaw)
- M. orbicularis oris
- M. sternocleidomastoideus (bends the neck, turns the head)

- M. sternocleidomastoideus
- M. trapezius
- M. deltoideus (abbducts the arm)
- M. biceps brachii (bends the elbow, supinates the forearm)
- M. brachioradialis
- M. flexor carpi radialis
- M. palmaris longus
- M. adductor longus (adducts the thighs)
- M. rectus femoris
- M. vastus lateralis (stretches the knee)
- M. vastus medialis (stretches the knee)
- M. tibialis anterior
- M. fibularis longus

# The muscles of the body

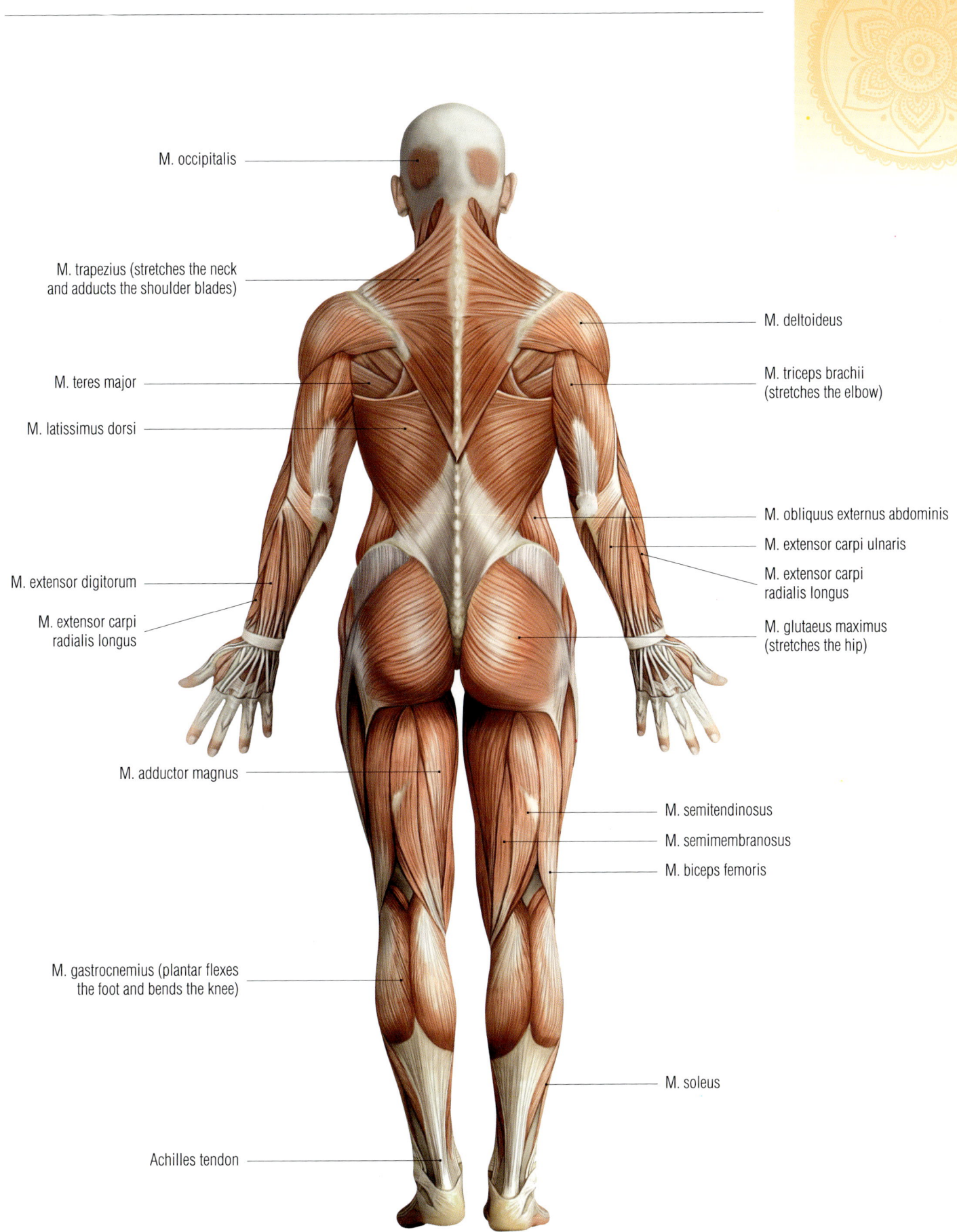

Anatomy and physiology

MUSCULAR SYSTEM

# Planes, sections, and body movements

The various body movements occur in three different sections or planes, which are the frontal plane, the sagittal plane, and the transverse plane. Each of these planes corresponds to a specific group of movements, as we will see in the images.

**MOVEMENT PLANS**
The human body is three-dimensional, such that it makes reference to three planes that form a right angle to each other and that divide the body into two halves.
**Frontal plane.** Longitudinal section that divides the body into a back half, or ventral part, and a posterior half, or dorsal part. Also called a coronal section. Movements that are visible from the front are done on this plane (abduction, adduction, lateral flexing, inversion, and eversion).
**Sagittal plane.** A longitudinal cut that divides the body into a right and left half. This is also called the medial plane or sagittal half. Movements that are visible in profile are performed on this plane (flexion, extension, antepulsion, retropulsion, dorsal flexion, and plantar flexion).

**Transversal plane.** A cut on a horizontal plane that divides the body into upper and lower halves. Movements can be seen from above or from below on this plane (external rotation, internal rotation, pronation, and supination).

**BODY MOVEMENTS**
The most important body movements, from the point of view of yoga, are the following.
**Flexing.** Movement that normally takes place in the sagittal plane, flexing reduces the angle of a joint, for example, by bending the knee or elbow, bringing two bones closer together. In yoga, bending generally means bending the hip forward.

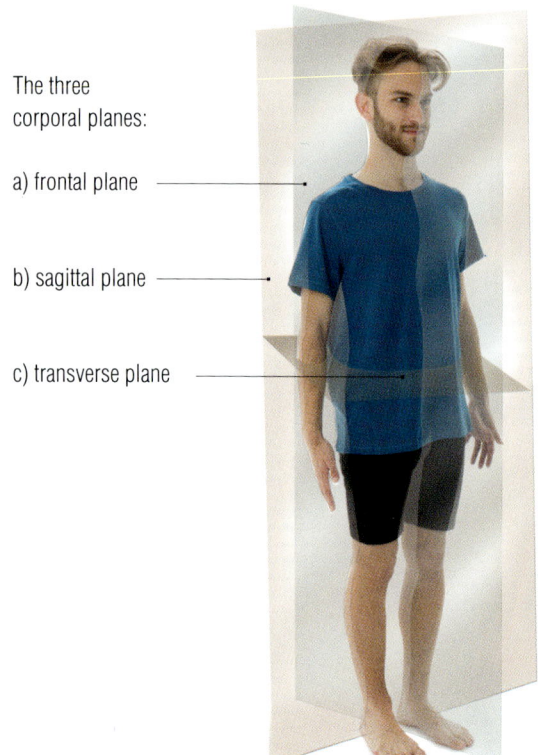

The three corporal planes:

a) frontal plane

b) sagittal plane

c) transverse plane

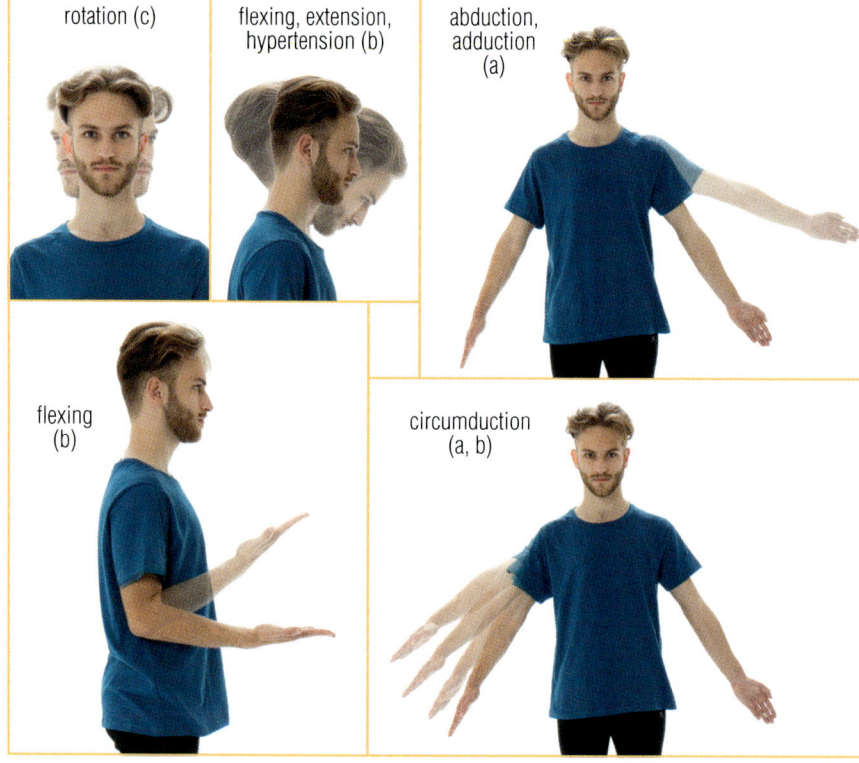

**Extension.** This is produced on the sagittal plane. Contrary to flexing, in an extension, the angle of the joint or distance between two parts of the body is increased. When 180º is passed, for example, by bringing the head back, it is known as hypertension.

**Rotation.** This is perceived on the transversal plane. It is the movement of a bone around its own longitudinal axis. If the rotation occurs outward, the rotation is external; when the turn is inward, the rotation is internal as, for example, when we say "no" with the head.

**Abduction.** Tis is movement from the frontal plane in which we move a limb away from the central line of the body (e.g., putting the arms into a cross). It also refers to the fan movement of the fingers, hands, or feet when moving outwards.

**Adduction.** It occurs in the frontal plane, inverse to abduction, when a limb is brought closer to the midline of the body (e.g., lowering the arms and crossing them).

**Circumduction.** This happens on the frontal and sagittal planes. It is the combination of movements of flexing, extension, abduction and adduction. It is a typical movement of the extremities, although we can also perform it on the hip. One end of the joint is stationary and the other, distal, moves in a circle.

## SPECIAL MOVEMENTS

Certain movements only occur in some joints; they are special movements, but no less important.

**On the foot and ankle.** Four movements occur in more than one plane: dorsiflexion, plantar flexing, inversion, and eversion. Dorsal flexing occurs when the foot is lifted upwards, and the plantar flexing when we lower the foot with the toes pointed down. Inversion turns of the sole of the foot inward, and eversion turns it laterally.

**On the forearm.** Two movements refer to the rotation produced between the radius and the ulna: supination and pronation. In supination, the forearm rotates until the palm of the hand faces up, and the radius and ulna are parallel. Pronation is the opposite movement: the arm rotates inward with the palm facing down or backwards; in this case, the radius crosses the ulna and the bones form an x.

**Opposition.** Opposition of the fingers of the hand occurs thanks to the articulation between the metacarpal and the trapezius bone of the carpus, which allows the opposition of the thumb, which can thus touch the tips of the other fingers.

**Antepulsion and retropulsion.** These are the movements that are equivalent to flexing and extending the shoulder, respectively.

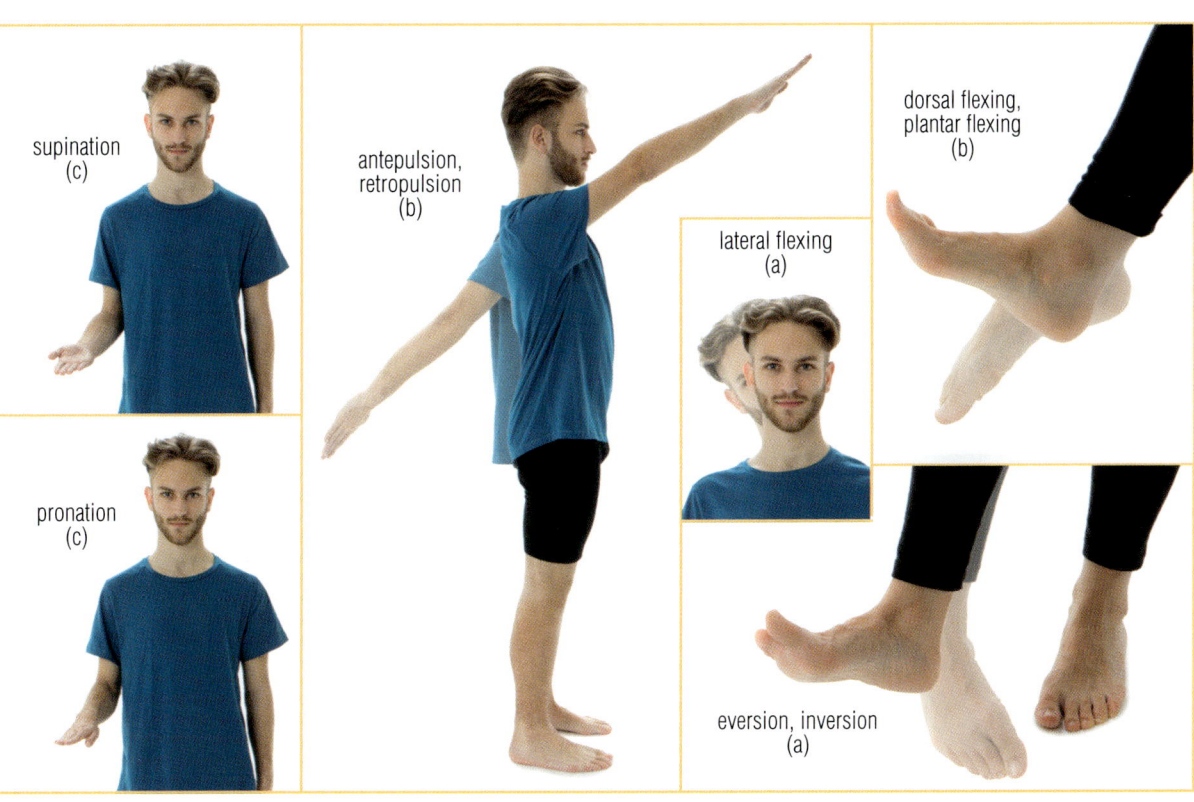

## OTHER SYSTEMS

# The nervous system

The coordination and organization of vital activities in our body is controlled by the nervous system. This includes a complex cell network that almost instantaneously communicates electric impulses to all the cells of the body.

The nervous system is organized, into two systems: nervous system central (CNS), composed of the brain and spinal cord, and the peripheral nervous system (PNS), composed of nerves and ganglia.

**PRIMARY FUNCTIONS**
The nervous system controls and coordinates the other organs thanks to its high specialization of three essential functions.
**1. Receiving information.** Through its sensitive receptors, the nervous system gathers information from our body and the changing exterior or environment (stimulus). This information that is gathered is known as sensory input.
**2. Integration.** The brain processes the information that was obtained, processes the most efficient action, and decides what to do in the face of any situation.
**3. Responding.** A response is sent quickly and adequately through the motor responses.

**STRUCTURAL CLASSIFICATION**
A group of organs are involved in the activity of the nervous system. There are two large sub-divisions: the central nervous system and the peripheral nervous system.

**The central nervous system (SNC)**
This is made up by the brain and the spinal cord. The brain is located within the skull and the spinal cord is inside the duct of the vertebrae in the vertebral column. This is where the information from the sensors is gathered and instructions are sent to the body.

**The peripheral nervous system (PNS)**
This is a network of cables that communicate with the body and the SNC, transporting impulses from the sensory receptors to the spinal cord and the brain and, from there, up to the glands and effector muscles. These are spinal nerves and the cranial nerves, respectfully. Therefore, the peripheral nervous system has a functional classification with two sub-divisions.
■ **Sensitive or afferent division.** This is made up of the nerves that transfer nervous impulses to the central system, keeping it informed of everything that happens inside and outside of the body.

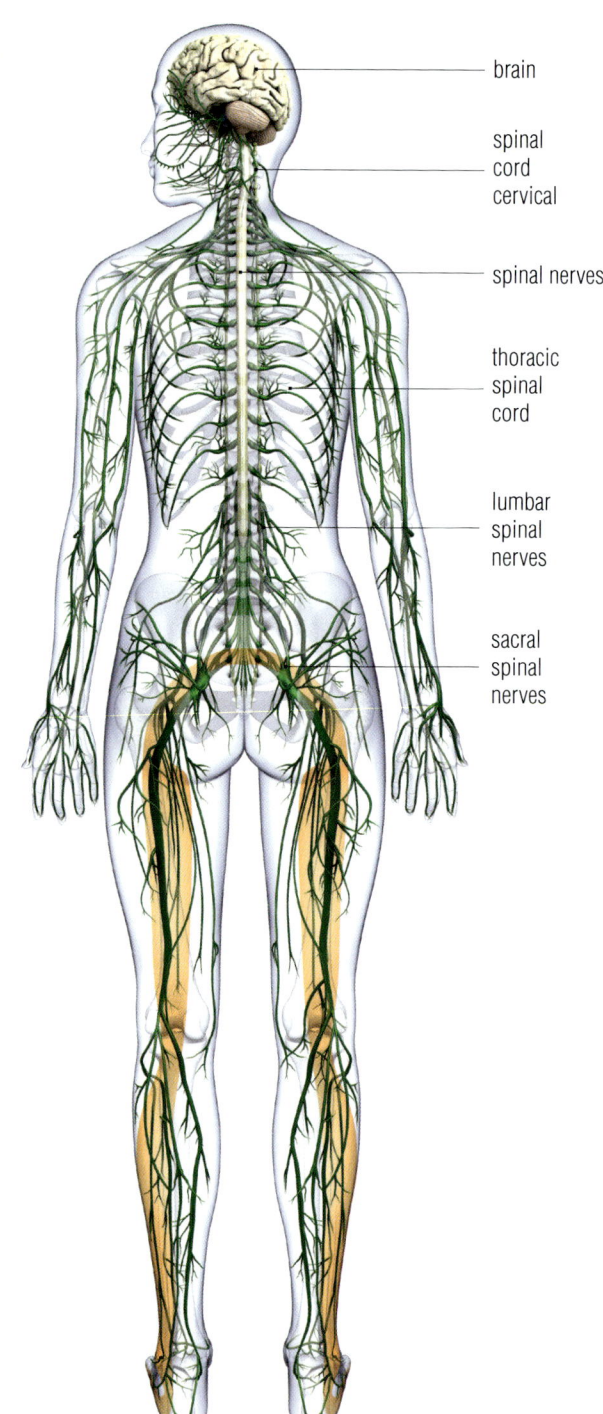

■ **Motor or efferent division.** It transports impulses from the central system to the muscles and glands. At the same time, it is divided into:

**Somantic or voluntary nervous system.** This allows us to control muscular activity consciously, as well as let us feel sensations, such as touch, pressure, hearing, or pain.

**Autonomic or involuntary nervous system.** It regulates physiological functions automatically and independently of our will, such as movements of the intestine and heart. This automatic system is also made up of two parts: *the sympathetic nervous system and the parasympathetic nervous system*. The first prepares the body in the face of any threat or emergency (fight or flight), activating the cardiac frequency and arterial pressure. The second controls homeostasis (digestion, elimination) and the functions of internal organs (reducing cardiac and respiratory frequency, increasing stomach secretion). If the autonomic nervous system appears to function outside of our own will, by practicing yoga you can influence it consciously through respiration.

# The endocrine system

This system continuously combines with the nervous system to control body actions. This is achieved through the glands, small organs, which are separated and distributed by the body and whose primary purpose is to produce hormones. Hormones are responsible for stimulating slow processes such as growth, metabolism, body defenses, and reproduction.

**SUPRARENAL GLAND**

Spread out throughout the body, there are various endocrine organs: the hypophysis (anterior and posterior), the pineal gland, the thyroid gland, the parathyroid glands, the pancreas, the suprarenal glands, and the gonads (male and female). There are also other organs in the body with endocrine activity (e.g., the hypothalamus). In regard to yoga, the importance of the suprarenal gland stands out.

The response to stress creates a fight-or-flight response from the sympathetic nervous system, which will stimulate the **suprarenal gland**. This organ is made up of two pyramid-shaped glands located in the upper part of the kidneys. These glands have glandular sections on the suprarenal cortex, and parts of nervous tissue, the suprarenal medulla. The **suprarenal cortex** creates two hormones that give a response to stress over the long term, such as increasing sugar in the blood, retaining sodium and water in the kidneys, increasing blood pressure, and suppressing the immune system. The suprarenal medulla is stimulated when it receives an exterior threat, pumping the catecholamine hormones (adrenaline, noradrenaline) to the blood. This produces a shortterm response: faster heartbeat, increase in blood pressure, and dilation of the bronchioles, and the liver frees glucose into the blood and increases the metabolic rhythm.

Yoga helps the body to manage situations of stress, which we have seen can create a complex hormonal response. Ongoing stress over time can seriously damage the body, making it more prone to contract all types of illnesses and weaken the immune system.

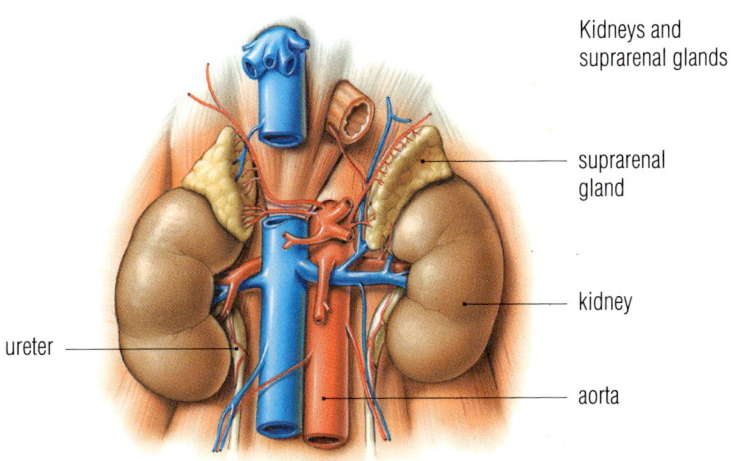

Kidneys and suprarenal glands

- suprarenal gland
- kidney
- ureter
- aorta

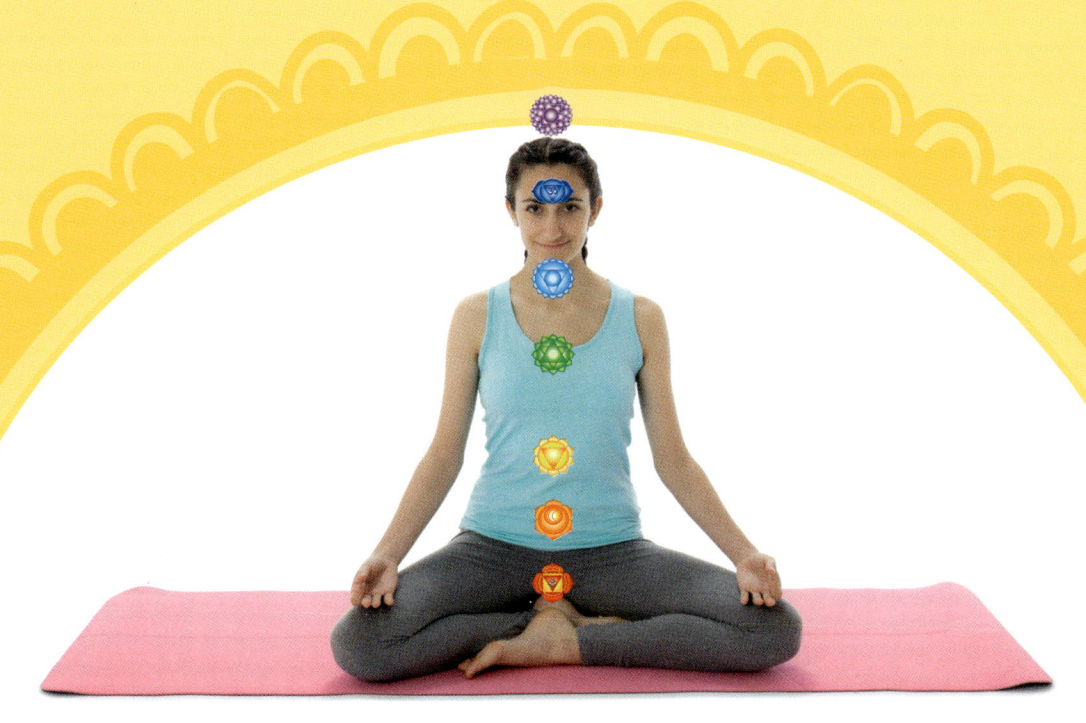

# ENERGETIC ANATOMY OF A HUMAN BEING

The study of the energetic anatomy of the human body from the perspective of the various energetic bodies, channels, centers and coverings that are found in the body. Practicing yoga not only works at a physical level, but also activates the energetic and subtle body. Without this practice, yoga would only be a mere physical exercise. This chapter will describe the three bodies of a being, the five *koshas* or layers, the *nadis* or energy channels and the *chakras*, which are the centers for bodily and psychic energy of our natural body.

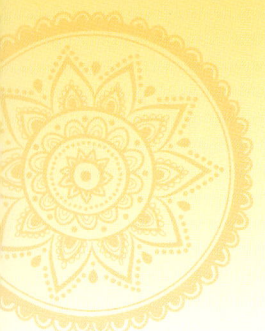

## SHARIRAS

# The three bodies of the human being

From the perspective of yoga, the human being is something more than a physical body composed of different organic systems; it is also formed by other more subtle bodies, invisible to the human eye.
While practicing yoga, the various bodies work together, a complete task without which this discipline would be mere physical exercise.

We find a dual classification. One of them refers to the three bodies of a human being, which are interrelated: *Sthula Sharira, Sukshma Sharira,* and *Karana Sharira.* The other classification, more precisely, agrees with the previous category and understands the human being as a body with five layers or *koshas: Annamaya Kosha, Pranamaya Kosha, Manomaya Kosha, Vijnanamaya Kosha,* and *Anandamaya Kosha.* There is link between the three bodies, the koshas, and the states of consciousness.

### STHULA SHARIRA

This first body corresponds to the physical body, in other words, a multi-cellular organism that functions as a perfect complex machine. This is the body that is studied in human anatomy, made up of different organic systems. This is comprised of material that is transformed and restructured into new material. According to an old philosophy, this would be comprised of five elements or *tattvas*: land, water, air, fire, and ether.

### SUKSHMA SHARIRA

This is the subtle or astral body. This encompasses all emotional, mental, and physical facets of a human being. It is not visible, however, we experience it every day. It is interconnected with the physical body by means of a cord (etheric double) where the vital current passes. It is believed that this body can survive for some time after death before it also stops existing. It is made up of 19 elements:

- five vital airs *(pancha pranas),*
- five subtle organs of action *(karmendriyas),*
- five organs of consciousness *(gñanendriyas),* and
- four mental abilities *(antah karana)* of the individual mind: *buddhi* (the intellect), *ahamkara* (ego), *manas* (thought), and *chitta* (memory).

**The gunas.** The mental abilities will be influenced by the three gunas. These are the basic qualities that permeate everything that exists and are inseparably found in all the cosmic creation: sattva (representing purity, enlightenment, and perfection), rajas (the active, tough aspect) and tamas (the inert, dark aspect).

When the intellect or buddhi is influenced by sattva, it becomes discriminative consciousness (and the result is wisdom, purity, and humility). Otherwise, if it is influenced by tamas, confusion and ignorance (advidya) appear.

The same thing happens with the ego. When it is influenced by rajas and tamas, our most selfish tendencies are aroused, and when it is influenced by sattva, it forms a more spiritual consciousness of one's own being.

### KARANA SHARIRA

This is also called causal body. It is the essence of the human being, the cause and origin of the other two bodies. Found beyond the mind and mental processes, it corresponds to the Spirit, the purest essence of the human being. In this body resides the Being or Atman (soul or supreme consciousness). It can be experienced through meditation.

| BODY | KOSHA |
|---|---|
| **STHULA SHARIRA** (physical body, dense) | Annamaya Kosha (layer of matter) |
| **SUKSHMA SHARIRA** (astral body) | Pranamaya Kosha (layer of vital air) |
| | Manomaya Kosha (layer of the mind) |
| | Vijnanamaya Kosha (layer of consciousness) |
| **KARANA SHARIRA** (causal body) | Anandamaya Kosha (layer of happiness) |

KOSHAS

# The five koshas or layers

The *koshas* or five layers are surrounded by the pure spirit, the Being. As has been presented in many mystic writings, within the interior of our being is the true I, the enduring spirit.

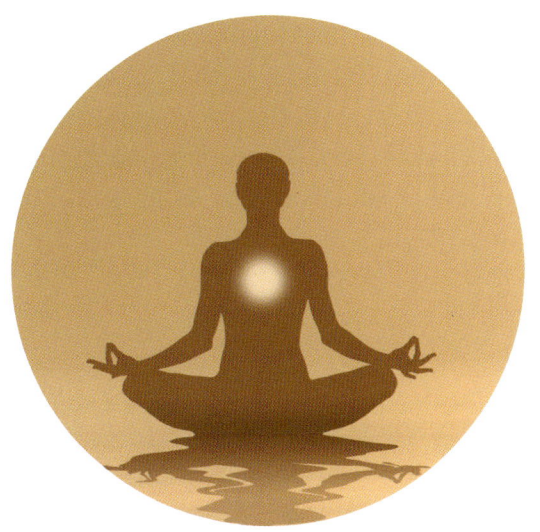

*[...] in the center of the Brahman castle (our body) there is a tabernacle in the shape of a lotus flower that has a small space. We should find who dwells in it and we should know it [...] The Spirit that resides in the body that does not grow or die ... this is the true castle of Brahman, in which all the love of the universe lives.*
Chandonga Upanishad 8,1

"...I dwell in the heart of every being."
*Bhagavad Gita*, XV, 15

**ANNAMAYA KOSHA**
This is the layer where all others are found. It is the dense physical body, with which we can manifest ourselves in the terrestrial plane. It is constituted by food and by the five elements. It coincides with *Sthula Sharira*.

**PRANAMAYA KOSHA**
This is the energy layer, composed of five vital pranas *(prana, apana, samana, udana,* and *vyana)* and five secondary pranas. Prana is the vital energy that is found everywhere; we can capture it, mainly through breathing. The function of this layer is to absorb Prana and distribute it throughout the body; it also acts as an intermediary between the physical body and the astral body. *Pranamaya Kosha* is a replica of the physical body, subsisting a few days after death.

**MANOMAYA KOSHA**
This is the mental body, composed of the conscious mind and the subconscious, the five organs of perception (*jñanaindriyas:* hearing, touch, sight, taste, and smell) and the five organs of action (*karmendriyas:* organs of movement, manipulation, excretion, procreation, and speech). This kosha uses the organs of the senses and past experiences to, on the one hand, transmit the information to the higher mental body and, on the other, put the two higher koshas in communication with the two lower ones.

**VIJNANAMAYA KOSHA**
This is the mental or intuitive layer of the consciousness that understands without reasoning. Only through intuition can the consciousness experience the "I" as an individual being. It is comprised of a *buddhi* (intellect that can discern and make decisions). The higher faculties of the mind (beauty, wisdom, and inspiration, as well as all creative process) are in this layer.

**ANANDAMAYA KOSHA**
This is the layer of happiness or bliss. In this kosha, you experience the transcendence of the human being, without consciousness or mental experience. Space, time, and individual being disappear, and liberation and union emerge. In the interior of this layer resides the Being or Atman, whose nature is *SAT-CHIT-ANANDA*, that is, Existence, Pure Consciousness, and Bliss, respectively.

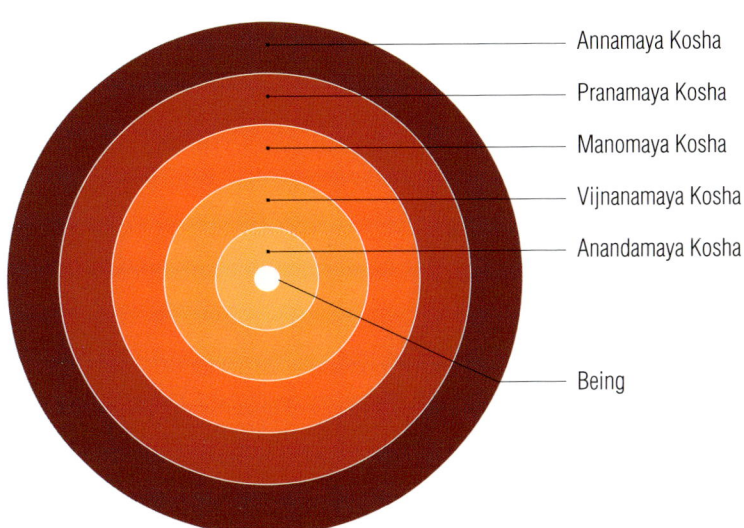

Chart of the five koshas or layers.

- Annamaya Kosha
- Pranamaya Kosha
- Manomaya Kosha
- Vijnanamaya Kosha
- Anandamaya Kosha
- Being

## NADIS

# Nadis or energy channels

The nadis are nerves or subtle channels that belong to the astral body. The word *nadi* comes from a Sanskrit root *nad*, which means "movement." Nadis are the paths where energy moves, or the channels that the flow of prana uses. Prana is the life energy of the universe and the body, which translates as strength, breath, life, vitality, energy, and respiration. The text *Hatha Yoga Pradipika* says that there are 72,000 nadis, which make up a huge interconnected network with all of the body's energy *(Pranamaya Kosha)*. It is subtle in nature, not physical.

As the nadis Ida and Pingala ascend, they are linked with the main chakras and Sushumna in an alternate and opposite manner.

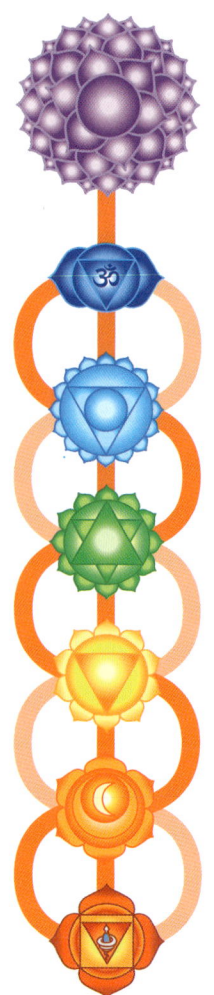

The ten main nadis are connected to the ten gates, or openings of the body, which are: *Sushumna* (fontanelle), *Ida* (left nostril), *Pingala* (right nostril), *Gandhari* (left eye), *Hastajihva* (right eye), *Yahasvini* (left ear), *Pusha* (right ear), *Alambusha* (mouth), *Kuhu* (male genitals), and *Shankhini* (female genitals). In acupuncture, there are some meridians that appear to correspond with these nadis.

Out of them all, there are three that are most important: Sushumna, Ida, and Pingala. All of the nadis are linked to Sushumna, which is the central nadi. When practicing yoga, you primarily work with these three channels.

### SUSHUMNA NADI

This is the central and most important channel. It starts from the perineum/cervix (Muladhara Chakra) and ascends through the inside of the spine until it reaches the crown of the head (Sahasrara Chakra). This nadi moves through all the intermediate chakras of the body. Within Sushumna, there are three other essential nadis that are concentrically locked within each other: *Vajrini, Chitrini,* and *Brahmanadi*. In this last one, the energy *Kundalini* (spiritual energy) ascends when it wakes up, traveling up all the central channel and moving through all the chakras until reaching the crown. Thousands of smaller nadis come out of Sushumna that move through the human body like a network. This nadi is linked to the central nervous system of the physical body.

### IDA NADI

This is the left channel. Through this channel moves mental strength or energy of thought *(manas shakti)*. It starts on the left side of the Muladhara Chakra and ascends in a semicircular pattern, passing through all the intermediate chakras and the left nostril, until they reach Ajna Chakra. This controls the left side of the body and the right side of the brain in a way that it is the channel for the visual, creative, emotional, and intuitive nature. It is associated with lunar energy, which is why it is also called *Chandra Nadi* (lunar nadi). Its color is metallic or silver. It represents THA in Hatha. This channel is stimulated by breathing through the left nostril and is linked to the parasympathetic nervous system.

### PINGALA NADI

This is the right channel. This circulates life energy or physical strength *(prana shakti)*. It originates in the right side of the Muladhara Chakra and follows the opposite ascending track of Ida, passing the intermediate chakras and the right nostril to reach Ajna Chakra. It governs the right part of the body and the left side of the brain, which is what relates to the rational, logical, and verbal part of a being. It is associated with solar energy, which is why it is known as *Surya Nadi* (solar nadi). It represents HA in Hatha. Its color is gold. It is stimulated by breathing through the right nostril and is linked to the sympathetic nervous system.

CHAKRAS

# The chakras

The chakras are the centers of vital and mental strength of the subtle body. The word *chakra* means "circle" or "wheel." We can imagine them as energetic whirlpools in which each one vibrates differently, creating and accumulating energy.

They can capture cosmic energy, transmit it through all of Sushumna, and spread it throughout the network of nadis, in the form of prana. They are connection points between the physical body and the astral body; between *Annamaya Kosha* (layer of matter) and *Pranamaya Kosha* (layer of vital air); and between this last one and *Manomaya Kosha* (layer of the mind).

**CLASSIFICATION AND RELATIONSHIP OF THE CHAKRAS**

The most important chakras found in the human body are the seven that run through the central Sushumna canal; from bottom to top: *Muladhara Chakra*, *Svadhisthana Chakra*, *Manipura Chakra*, *Anahata Chakra*, *Vishuddha Chakra*, *Ajna Chakra*, and *Sahasrara Chakra*. Each one of them has a specific energy pattern that is not commonly represented with a symbolic drawing. It is also related with a different level of consciousness, with the lower (from the first to fourth chakra) being those that have a lower level and are coarse, and the upper ones (from fifth to seventh) with a much more subtle level.

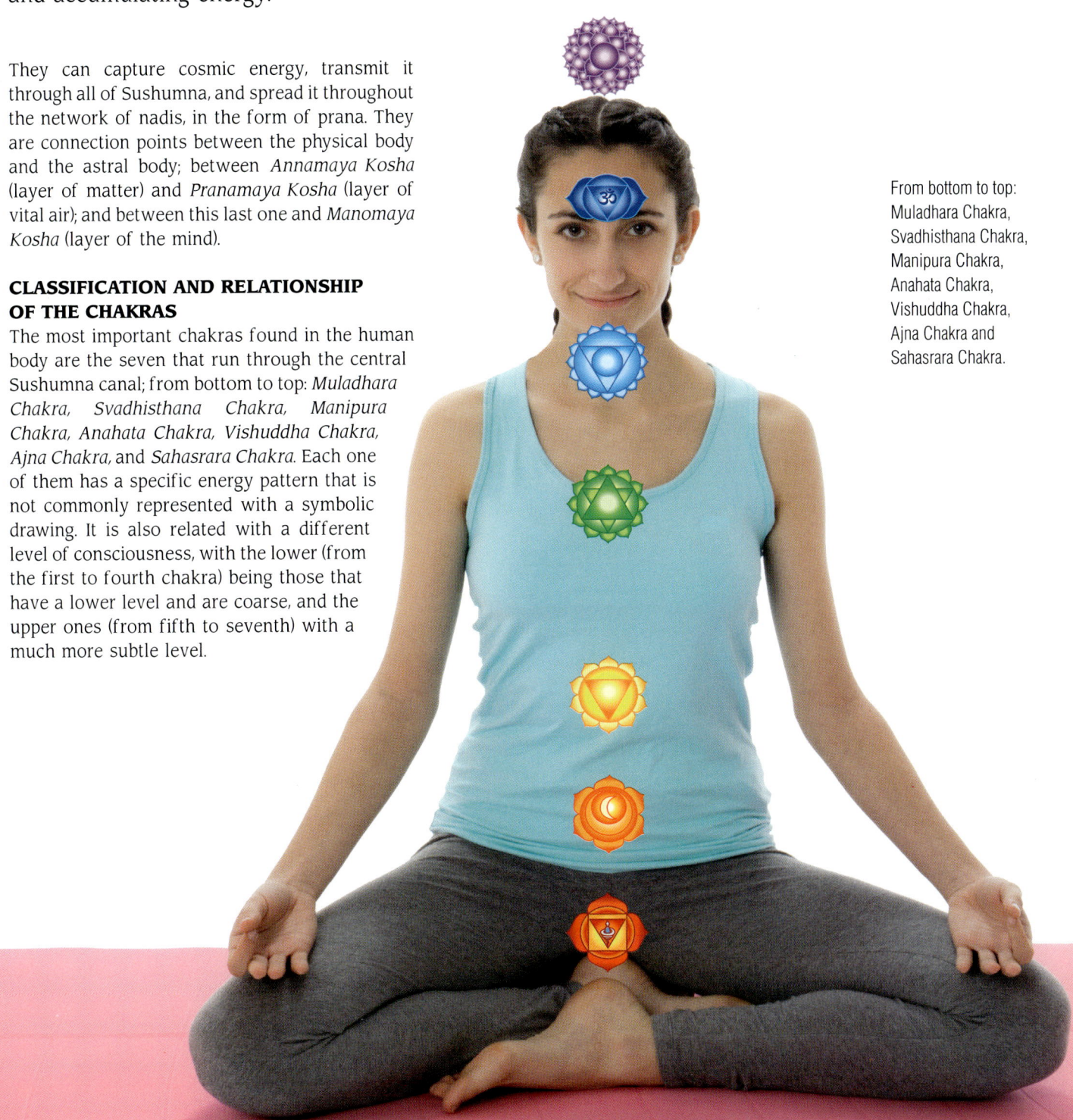

From bottom to top: Muladhara Chakra, Svadhisthana Chakra, Manipura Chakra, Anahata Chakra, Vishuddha Chakra, Ajna Chakra and Sahasrara Chakra.

## CHAKRAS

# Essential elements of the chakras

The chakras correspond to a physiological or psychological part of our body. When functioning at a low level, or if they are blocked, the energy does not flow properly and physical illnesses may appear. Some techniques in yoga are very effective in purifying and reducing any blockage of the chakras, for example, through visualization, pranayama, singing mantras, and meditation.

| NAME OF THE CHAKRA: **MULADHARA** Meaning: root, support, foundation 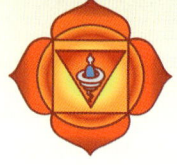 | **ESSENTIAL ELEMENTS**<br>■ Number of petals: 4<br>■ Tattva (element): earth<br>■ Color of tattva: red<br>■ Shape of tattva: square. The inside has a triangle with the point downwards, a seat of the vital force or Kundalini.<br>■ Bija-mantra: LAM<br>■ Devada (Deity): Bala Brahma (Brahma child)<br>■ Shakti: Dakini<br>■ Dominant planet: Mars | **PHYSIOLOGICAL CONNECTION**<br>■ Location: base of the spine, first three vertebrae<br>■ Gland: suprarenal<br>■ Nerve plexus: pelvic plexus, sacral coccyges<br>■ Sensory organ (Jñanaindriya): olfaction<br>■ Age of development/influence: from birth to seven.<br>■ Physical disorders due to malfunction: problems in the lower part of the body, feet, legs, hemorrhoids, and testicular dysfunction. | **PSYCHOLOGICAL AND ENERGY CONNECTION**<br>■ Energy in balance: strength, vitality, emotional balance, resistance.<br>■ Excess energy: insecurity, fear, violent behavior, selfishness.<br>■ Energy defect: distrust, lack of will, incoherence, indecision, low self-esteem, sadness, and depression. |

**BALANCING AND STIMULATING THE CHAKRA:** contact with the Earth. Practice Tadasana, Navasana, and Pranatasana.

| NAME OF THE CHAKRA: **SVADHISTHANA** Meaning: place where the being dwells  | **ESSENTIAL ELEMENTS**<br>■ Number of petals: 6<br>■ Tattva (element): water<br>■ Color tattva: orange<br>■ Shape of tattva: circle. Crescent Moon<br>■ Bija-mantra: VAM<br>■ Devada (Deity): Vishnu (the conservative)<br>■ Shakti: Rakini<br>■ Dominant planet: Mercury | **PHYSIOLOGICAL CONNECTION**<br>■ Location: pelvis<br>■ Gland: gonads<br>■ Nerve plexus: hypogastric plexus<br>■ Sensory organ (Jñanaindriya): taste<br>■ Age of development/influence: from eight to fourteen.<br>■ Physical disorders due to malfunction: urinary problems, kidney dysfunctions, problems of reproductive organs, poor circulation. | **PHYSIOLOGICAL AND ENERGY CONNECTION**<br>■ Energy in balance: conscious of your own desires and emotions, creativity.<br>■ Excess energy: uncontrolled emotions, addiction to pleasure, ambition.<br>■ Energy defect: lack of emotion, coldness, insensitivity, envy, jealousy, lack of creativity. |

**BALANCING AND STIMULATING THE CHAKRA:** visualize the setting sun close to the ocean or rivers. Practice Pachimottanasana.

| NAME OF THE CHAKRA: **MANIPURE** Meaning: city of the jewel  | **ESSENTIAL ELEMENTS**<br>■ Number of petals: 10<br>■ Tattva (element): fire<br>■ Color of tattva: yellow<br>■ Shape of tattva: triangle<br>■ Bija-mantra: RAN<br>■ Devada (Deity): Rue (destroyer)<br>■ Shakti: Lakini (goddess of plenty)<br>■ Dominant planet: Sun | **PHYSIOLOGICAL CONNECTION**<br>■ Location: navel<br>■ Gland: pancreas<br>■ Nerve plexus: solar or epigastric plexus<br>■ Sensory organ (Jñanaindriya): sight<br>Age of development/influence: fifteen to twenty-one.<br>■ Physical disorders due to malfunction: digestive disorders, diabetes, hypoglycaemia, liver problems, nervous tension, chronic fatigue. | **PSYCHOLOGICAL AND ENERGY CONNECTION**<br>■ Energy in balance: vitality, motivation, respect toward oneself and toward others, will.<br>■ Excess energy: egocentricity, pride, resentment, perfectionism, irritation, anger, impatience, nervousness, uneasiness, ambition.<br>■ Energy defect: insecurity, lack of self-confidence, doubt, apathy. |

**BALANCING AND STIMULATING THE CHAKRA:** sunbathing. Walking through a field of sunflowers. Practice Setu-Bandhasana and Purvottanasana.

Essential elements of the chakras

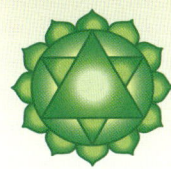

| NAME OF THE CHAKRA: **ANAHATA** Meaning: sound not emitted | **ESSENTIAL ELEMENTS**<br>■ Number of petals: 12<br>■ Tattva (element): air<br>■ Color of tattva: green<br>■ Shape of tattva: hexagon. The six-pointed star symbolizes the element of air.<br>■ Bija-mantra: YAM<br>■ Devada (Deity): Ishana Rudra Shiva<br>■ Shakti: Kakini<br>■ Dominant planet: Venus | **PHYSIOLOGICAL CONNECTION**<br>■ Location: heart<br>■ Gland: thymus<br>■ Nerve plexus: cardiac<br>■ Sensory organ (Jñanaindriya): touch<br>■ Age of development/influence: from twenty-two to twenty-eight.<br>■ Physical disorders due to malfunction: pulmonary and cardiac problems, hypertension. | **PSYCHOLOGICAL AND ENERGY CORRESPONDENCE**<br>■ Energy in balance: compassion, unconditional love, balance, serenity.<br>■ Excess energy: anxiety, excessive generosity, attachment to people, demands, and criticism towards others.<br>■ Energy defect: loneliness, depression, fear of rejection, disappointment, remorse. |

**BALANCING AND STIMULATING THE CHAKRA:** walking through fields or meadows. Practice Virabhadrasana and Trikonasanas.

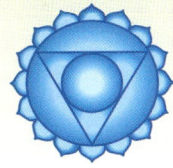

| NAME OF THE CHAKRA: **VISHUDDHA** Meaning: purity center | **ESSENTIAL ELEMENTS**<br>■ Number of petals: 16<br>■ Tattva (element): ether<br>■ Color of tattva: blue<br>■ Shape of tattva: circle<br>■ Bija-mantra: HAM<br>■ Devada (Deity): Panchavaktra<br>■ Shiva Shakti: Shakini (embodiment of purity)<br>■ Dominant planet: Jupiter | **PHYSIOLOGICAL CONNECTION**<br>■ Location: Throat<br>■ Gland: Thyroid<br>■ Nervous plexus: carotid, laryngeal-pharyngeal<br>■ Sensory organ (Jñanaindriya): sound<br>■ Age of development/influence: from twenty-nine to thirty-five.<br>■ Physical disorders due to malfunction: exhaustion, thyroid problems, weight problems, throat infections. | **PSYCHOLOGICAL AND ENERGY CONNECTION**<br>■ Energy in balance: communication, inspiration, joy, creativity.<br>■ Excess energy: arrogance, tendency to verbiage, rigidity and dogmatism, lies, screams.<br>■ Energy defect: shyness, manipulation of others, introversion, creative block, lack of communication. |

**BALANCING AND STIMULATING THE CHAKRA:** moving through high mountains, visualizing blue skies. Practice Halasana and Salamba Sarvangasana.

| NAME OF THE CHAKRA: **AJNA** Meaning: authority, command | **ESSENTIAL ELEMENTS**<br>■ Number of petals: 2<br>■ Tattva (element): Maha tattva (all elements are represented); Manas (mental abilities)<br>■ Color of tattva: indigo blue, luminescent blue<br>■ Shape of tattva: circle<br>■ Bija-mantra: AUM<br>■ Devada (Deity): Shiva-Shakti (half man, half woman)<br>■ Shakti: Hakini<br>■ Dominant planet: Saturn | **PHYSIOLOGICAL CONNECTION**<br>■ Location: glabella<br>■ Gland: pituitary<br>■ Nervous plexus: cavernous<br>■ Sensory organ: (none)<br>■ Age of development/influence: its awakening creates a high state of consciousness in the human being.<br>■ Physical disorders due to malfunction: headaches, insomnia, nightmares. | **PSYCHOLOGICAL AND ENERGY CONNECTION**<br>■ Energy in balance: high state of consciousness, perception, intuition, detachment, discernment, openness of mind.<br>■ Excess energy: mental confusion, hallucinations, schizophrenia.<br>■ Energy defect: lack of understanding, lack of assertiveness, lack of concentration, closed mind. |

**BALANCING AND STIMULATING THE CHAKRA:** silent meditation and observing night skies. Practice Balasana and Garudasanaj.

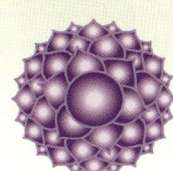

| NAME OF THE CHAKRA: **SAHASRARA** Meaning: one thousand petals | **ESSENTIAL ELEMENTS**<br>■ Number of petals: 1,000 (infinite)<br>■ Tattva (element): superior intuition<br>■ Color of tattva: white<br>■ Form of tattva: (has no form)<br>■ Bija-mantra: all sounds<br>■ Devada (Deity): the Absolute<br>■ Shakti: Chaitanya<br>■ Dominant Planet: Moon | **PHYSIOLOGICAL CONNECTION**<br>■ Location: upper part of the brain.<br>■ Gland: pineal<br>■ Nervous plexus: cerebral<br>■ Sensory organ: (none)<br>■ Age of development/influence: final goal of the human being. State of higher consciousness, Samadhi, Moksa.<br>■ Physical disorders due to malfunction: psychological problems. | **PSYCHOLOGICAL AND ENERGY CORRESPONDENCE**<br>■ Energy in balance: openness to the divine plane, full access to the conscious and unconscious mind, understanding, enlightenment.<br>■ Excess energy: psychic problems.<br>■ Energy defect: ignorance, dissociation. |

**BALANCING AND STIMULATING THE CHAKRA:** walking in nature while meditating. Practice Salamba Sirsasana.

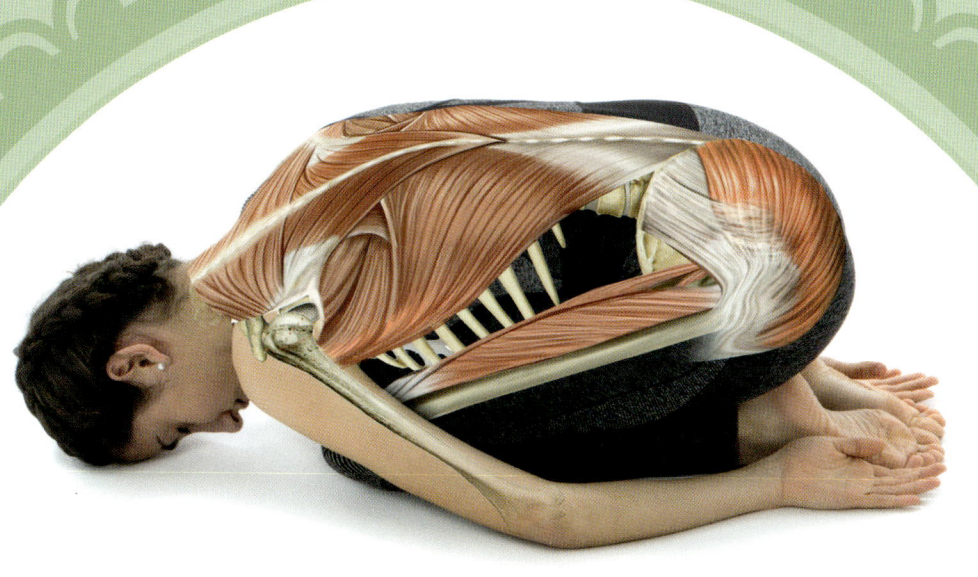

# ASANAS

Asanas are the poses that our body adopts in the physical practice of yoga. Its execution is indicated for most people, although some of the asanas may come with a warning in the case of pre-existing disease or illness. In this chapter, 34 asanas are described and classified according to the movement it creates for the spinal column. The different techniques used to execute each one of them is explained, as well as their benefits and warnings, alternatives and anatomic considerations. At the end of the chapter, it describes the step-by-step process of all the poses that are included in a traditional Sun Salutation.

# Asanas

## INTRODUCTION

# The asanas of yoga

Asanas are the physical poses that we adopt in the practice of yoga and that allow us to integrate body and mind. These are comfortable poses, which we can maintain for a time with a moderate effort and without losing concentration.

**CLASSIFICATION OF ASANAS**

To start practicing asanas, the most important thing is not to have flexibility and strength to carry out the poses but to learn to be aware of your body, the pose, and your breathing. This is an essential aspect of an asana, an aware mind that, with a full consciousness, observes everything that is happening to the physical body and breathing. Yoga is presence, full attention, living the moment; in other words, it is the "here and now." Putting our full attention on what we are doing will help us to move from the physical task to internalize it at a mental and psychic level.

We divide the asanas into different groups, according to their movement in connection with what is being worked and also in relation to the general movement of the trunk. It is a general classification, not definitive, to associate the positions. We organize the groups of asanas according to the sequence that we establish in the course of a yoga session:

- basic asanas,
- strength and balance,
- lateral flexing and trikonas,
- extension or bending back,
- forward flexing,
- twisting and
- inverted.

**EXTERNAL PREMISES FOR PRACTICE**

> "It's worth a gram more than a ton of theory."
> SWAMI VISHNUDEVANANDA

We need to have adequate space and conditions, enough time and a few accessories to practice the asanas. We can make a weekly plan, in which we mark the time we are going to dedicate to yoga (every day or alternate days, in the morning, in the afternoon). It is better to start with an easy and realistic goal and meet it.

**The location.** It should be a quiet place, with and a pleasant temperature, warm enough but not too cold during the relaxation. A slight penumbra helps the nervous system to relax.

**Time.** It is important to find a space of your own time, which is only for you, without interruptions; and resist the temptation to answer the phone or other distractions.

Yoga is a full, living experience of the present moment.

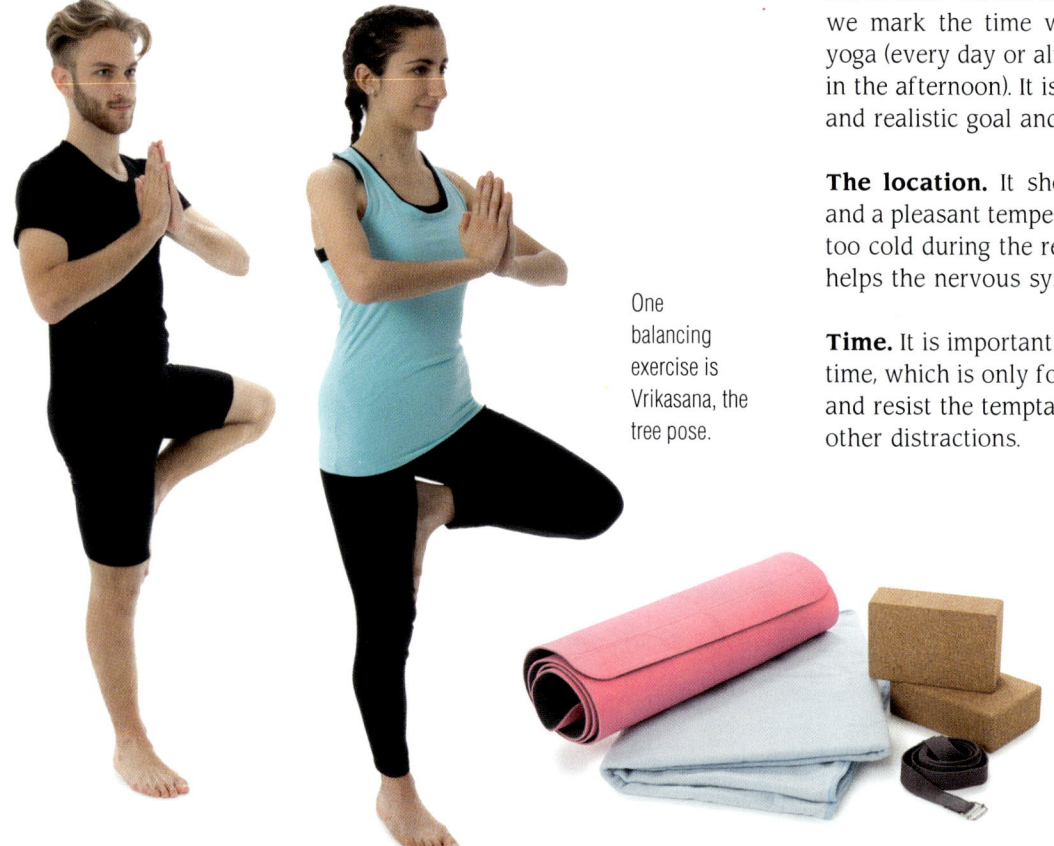

One balancing exercise is Vrikasana, the tree pose.

# The asanas of yoga

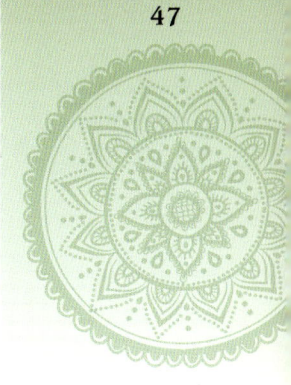

**The basic material.** We need a non-slip mat to perform the asanas without risk of slipping. It may be helpful to use a pillow or doubled-up blanket to support your head or sit on. A blanket will also serve to cover us a little when we are relaxing or meditating. Lastly, a cork block and a rope will help to advance with more difficult poses.

**Clothing.** It's preferred to use material with natural fibers. Some leggings and a cotton t-shirt that is slightly tight may be appropriate, as they allow us to see the positioning of our body and detect, for example, if a leg is in line or not. Loose clothing is also appropriate if you feel comfortable. If the temperature of the room is comfortable, it is recommended not to wear socks, since we can better feel more subtle sensations with a bare foot and observe the pose better.

## INTERNAL PREMISES: BODY PREPARATION

Every time we start a practice it is necessary to prepare the body with easy and simple movements. We can perform the basic asanas (such as Marjariasana or Apanasana), or also start the session with the Sun Salutation. Once these movements are finished, we can start the session. To perform an asana, we follow four fundamental steps:

1. We hold the starting pose.
2. We complete the movements to form the asana.
3. We hold the asana and stay for some time.
4. We exit the asana pose.

**The movements.** They should be slow, paused, and when it comes time to execute the asana, it can last from a few seconds to a few minutes or more, according to the criteria of the practitioner and their evolution.

**The pose.** It has to be comfortable and firm. When an asana is complete, take a brief rest, which could be a Savasana, Advasana, or even Pranatasana. Some poses are intense and have a specific impact on some part of the body, in a way that after we may hold a counter-pose, which counters the excessive effect that was experienced. For example an intense pose of extension may be followed by a counter-pose, soft one that implies flexing forward.

**Breathing.** Finally, once we have practiced a specific pose well enough, we will be aware of not only our physical body, but also the breathing that comes with it. We can direct our consciousness toward our interior, observe our thoughts and let them go, and calm ourselves, making ourselves fully aware of our body, mind, and breathing. In this way, the entire asana becomes a meditative union and experience in itself.

### CONSIDERATIONS FOR PRACTICE

- Practice them in a ventilated place with a pleasant temperature.
- Avoid practicing on a full stomach.
- Wear comfortable clothing (if possible, cotton).
- Perform a small warm-up before each session (for example, Sun Salutation or its variations).
- Enter and leave the asanas slowly and with full awareness.
- After each asana, take a short break.
- Work *ahimsa* (nonviolence) with our body, so we never get to a place of pain.
- Practice without forcing, without stress, and without demanding too much of the body.
- It is necessary to control the position and movement to avoid injuries.
- Respect our rhythm and observe any warnings for each position.
- Be constant and patient. It is better to work a little each day.
- See the box on page 17 about precautions in practice.

### SUGGESTED YOGA SESSION

- Be aware of the body (basic asanas 1)
- Unlock or warm-up (basic asanas 2 or Sun Salutation)
- Asana of balance
- Lateral flexing asanas and trikonas
- Asanas of extension
- Asana forward bending
- Twisting asanas
- Inverted asanas
- Pranayama
- Relaxation
- Meditation

Asanas

STARTING ASANAS

# Tadasana

*Tadasana* comes from the word *tada* meaning "mountain", so it would be translated as "mountain pose." Practicing this asana develops stability, soundness, and strength.

**BENEFITS**
- Eliminates bad posture and perform the correct alignment of the skeleton.
- It allows us to become aware of the proper distribution of body weight, thus facilitating the flexibility of the spine and rest of the pelvis and lower back.

**WARNINGS**
- Avoid if you have very low blood pressure.
- Avoid doing it after being stretched or sitting for a long time. First complete some movement exercise that increase blood circulation.

**CLASSIFICATION**
Basic pose, standing, symmetric.

**TECHNIQUE**
We stand with our feet together (if there is not much stability, at the beginning they can be separated slightly, without exceeding the width of the hips). We distribute our weight on both feet, on the entire surface of the feet, not pointed too far inward or out.

We imagine a vertical line that divides the body into two identical halves, which starts from the center of the feet and goes up to the crown of the head. The spine is upright, the chest is gently lifted, and the cervicals are stretched a little. The palms are together in front of the chest. We maintain the pose by observing the breath and being aware of the body, which remains calm in its natural balance.

**VARIATIONS**
Samasthiti. *Sama* means "right", or "equal", and *sthiti* means "quite" and "balance." This variation is done with the feet separated, so that we have a wider base of support. It is the starting point of other standing asanas.

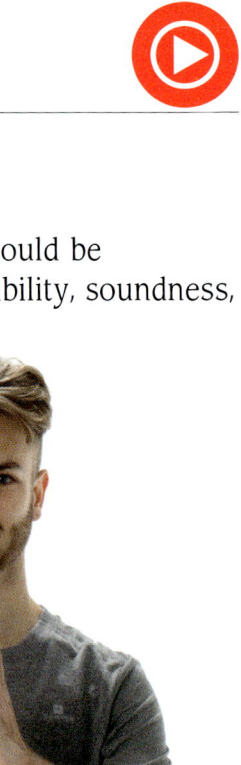

Hold the hands with the palms together at the height of the sternum. The fingers may be a little apart.

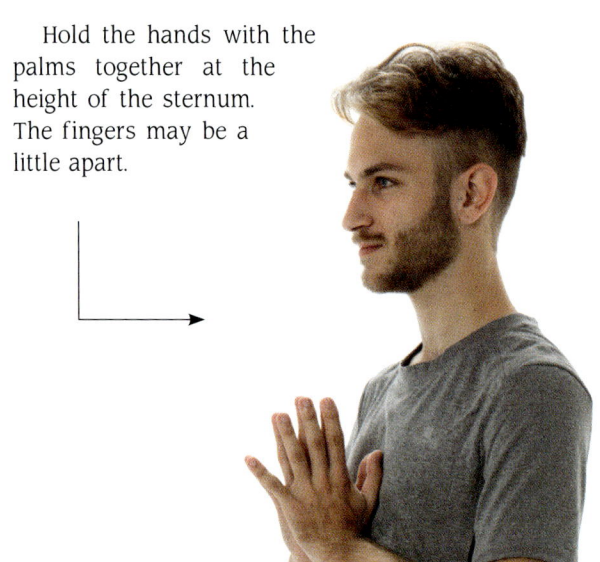

STARTING ASANAS: Tadasana  49

This pose connects us to the ground as we establish an important base for raising ourselves toward the sky, just like a mountain summit. This teaches us to remain calm on our feet, providing stability and soundness at a physical and mental level.

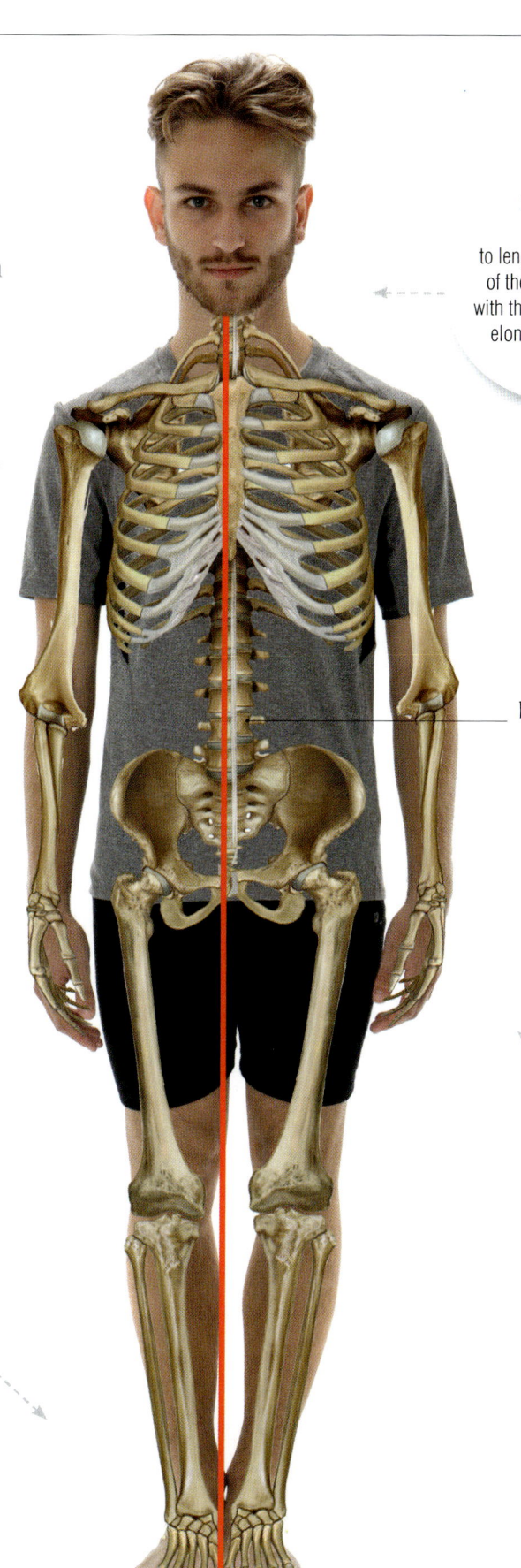

Stretching attempts to lengthen the crown of the head upward, with the chin tucked, to elongate the entire column.

backbone

The pelvis is slightly retroverted.

The feet remain together and firm on the ground.

Asanas

STARTING ASANAS

# Dandasana

*Danda* means "cane," "stick," or "rod." In this pose the backbone is held upright like a cane. It is a basic asana, a position where other poses start.

**BENEFITS**
- Strengthens the muscles of the back, abdomen and legs.
- Encourages stretching of the hamstrings.
- Raises the awareness of the aligned posture of the spine in a sitting position.

**WARNINGS**
- Avoid if you have spinal injuries.

**CLASSIFICATION**
Basic pose, seated, symmetric.

**TECHNIQUE**
Begin seated on the ground with legs crossed, the trunk upright, and hands resting on the ground. We put out until we feel the ischium bones come into contact with the the floor.

We stretch the legs, which should form a 90º with the trunk. We raise and tilt the thorax forward. We throw the shoulders back, with the hands resting on the floor, pressing down. We perform abdominal breathing. For a more advanced position, you can join the palms of the hands in front of the chest in *namaste* (by way of greeting).

To release the pose, we bend our legs again, keeping our feet on the ground, and wrap our arms around our legs and rest our heads on the knees.

**ADAPTATIONS**
If there are tensions in the back or lack of flexibility in the hamstrings, practice sitting on a cushion or blanket.

**VARIATION**
Starting from the initial position, we raise our hands from the ground and place them in namasté. This is an advanced variation that requires back strength.

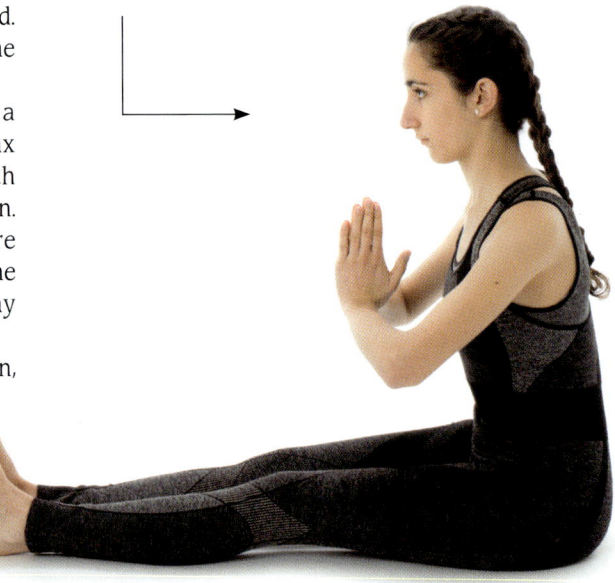

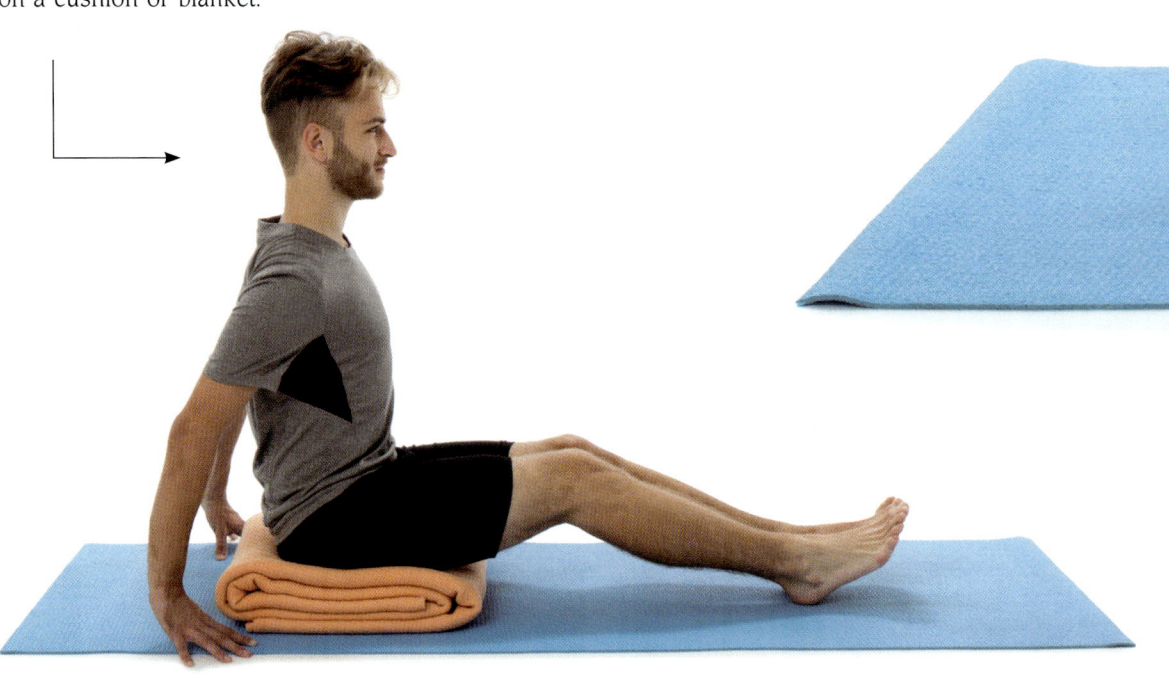

STARTING ASANAS: Dandasana    51

Dandasana offers us concentration and solidity. The Muladhara Chakra is used in this pose.

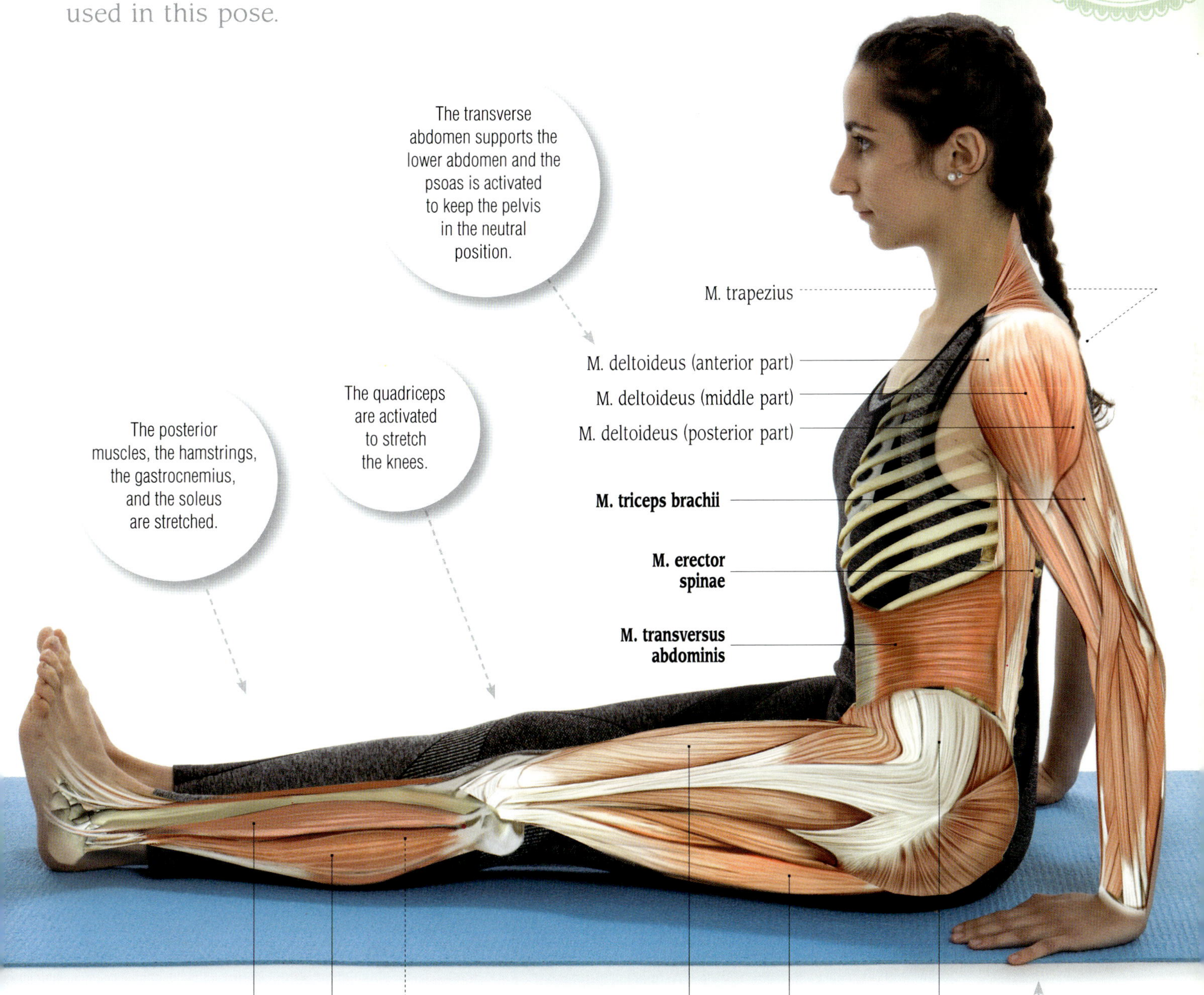

The transverse abdomen supports the lower abdomen and the psoas is activated to keep the pelvis in the neutral position.

The posterior muscles, the hamstrings, the gastrocnemius, and the soleus are stretched.

The quadriceps are activated to stretch the knees.

M. trapezius
M. deltoideus (anterior part)
M. deltoideus (middle part)
M. deltoideus (posterior part)
**M. triceps brachii**
**M. erector spinae**
**M. transversus abdominis**

M. gastrocnemius
M. soleus
M. fibularis longus
**M. quadriceps femoris**
M. biceps femoris
Pelvis

The triceps are activated by pressing the hands against the ground. The inferior fibers of both trapeziums descend down the scapulae and move away from the ears.

Asanas

STARTING ASANAS

# Savasana

*Sava* means "corpse." This pose imitates a corpse, due to its lack of mobility. It is also called the pose of death or *Mrtasana*. In this asana, the body remains still and the mind works to keep it calm.

**BENEFITS**
- Eliminates fatigue.
- Calms the body, calm, the mind.

**WARNINGS**
- Advanced management.
- If you have pain in your back, place a rolled-up towel or a cushion under your legs. If you have bronchitis or cardiac problems, place a cushion under the head.
- If you have low blood pressure, rotate to the left side before starting the position again to increase blood flow.

**CLASSIFICATION**
Basic pose, face-up position, symmetric.

**TECHNIQUE**
Lie on the ground, on your back, with your arms slightly separated from your body, and your hands up. Legs should be slightly apart; let the feet fall sideways. We check if there are tensions in the body and we are loosening them. We also relax any tension in the face; we drop the jaw and rest the eyes. We breathe softly, slowly, and deeply. If we have lumbar problems, we can place a folded blanket under the legs, even a cushion under the head. To release the pose, we take a few deep breaths and we stand slowly.

**ADAPTATION**
If the pose is uncomfortable, put thick blankets under the legs, or a pillow under the head. You may also try bending the legs or placing the arms on the chest.

**RELATED ASANAS**
Advasana is a related asana in prone position. Lying face down, we put the tips of our feet together and let the heels fall sideways. We extend our arms and place our cheeks on the ground.

This is the same position as in the previous one, but the forearms rest on both sides of the head. It can also be done with the arms stretched along the body and the palms of the hands turned upwards.

It is a variation of Advasana. It can be performed as a relaxation after an intense pose. We bend an arm and a leg, while the arm and the opposite leg remain stretched. We support the cheek on the floor.

*Savasana offers us harmony, an inner calm, peace, and rest.*

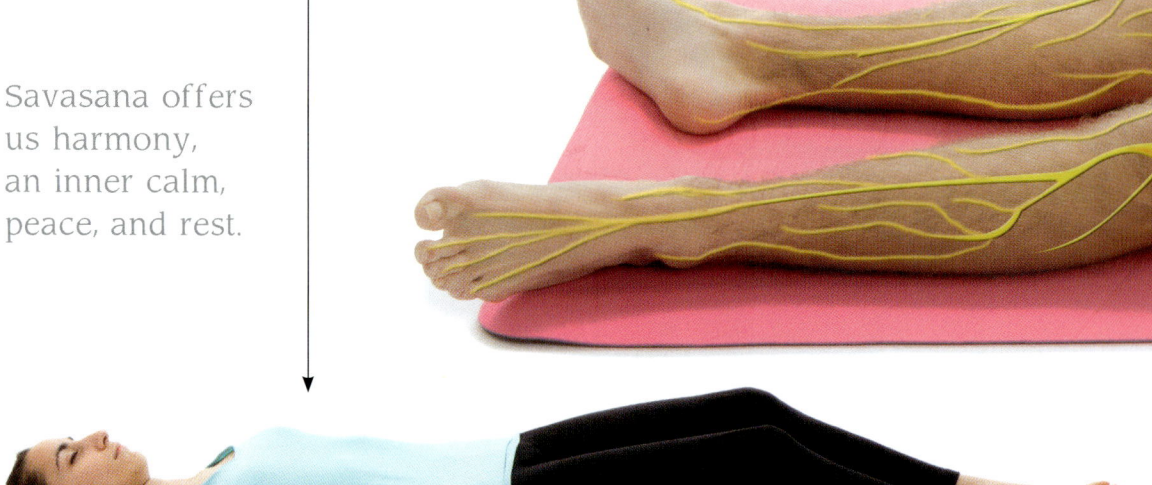

STARTING ASANAS: Savasana 53

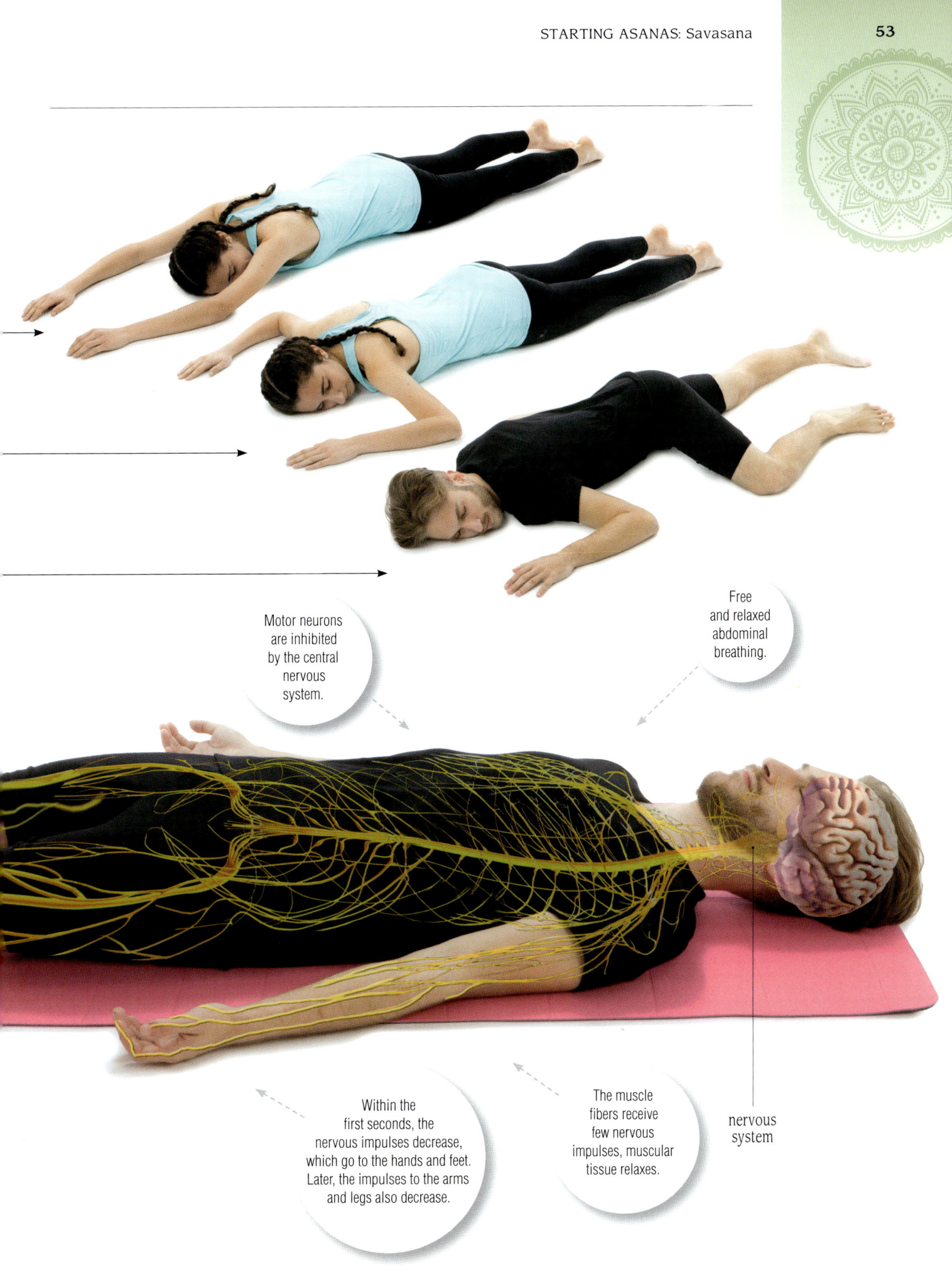

BASIC ASANAS

# Apanasana

*Apana* is the vital air. The pose is basic and it is a simple movement coordinated with the breath to perform. It allows us to aerate our body well and activate it to start the yoga session.

**BENEFITS**
- Eliminates tension in the lower part of the back.
- Increases the eliminating of toxins from the body.

**WARNINGS**
- High blood pressure.
- Inflammation of abdominal organs.

### CLASSIFICATION
Symmetric flexed position of the trunk in a face-up position.

### TECHNIQUE
Starting from the Savasana position, we bend the legs and place the feet on the ground. For a second, we become aware of our breathing. We lift our feet off the floor and place each hand on their corresponding knee. As we exhale, we bring the legs close to the body. While breathing, we push them away, and so on.

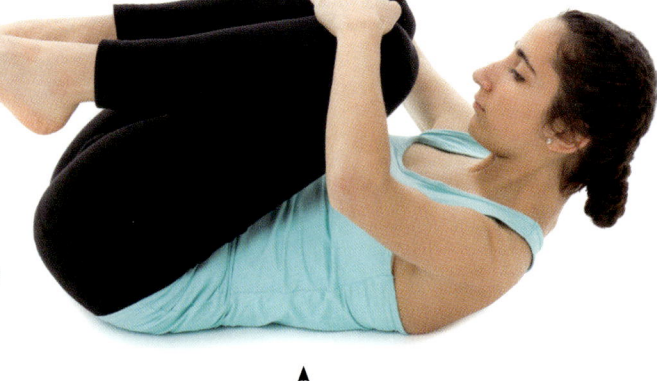

### RELATED ASANAS
Pavana Muktasana.

Preparation of Pavana Muktasana. We bend the right leg, while the left remains stretched. We take the knee with both hands and, with a breath, we carry this toward the thorax, pressing with a full breath. Exhale and return the leg to its original position. We repeat three times with each leg.

*Pavana* means "wind", and *Mukta* means "liberation." This asana evokes the position of the fetus, which is free to breathe the air from the outside. We take both knees with our hands; with an inspiration we take the legs toward the thorax, and with a full breath we raise the head to the knees. We exhale to undo the pose. With this asana, we stretch the entire spine. It is indicated to relax the nervous system.

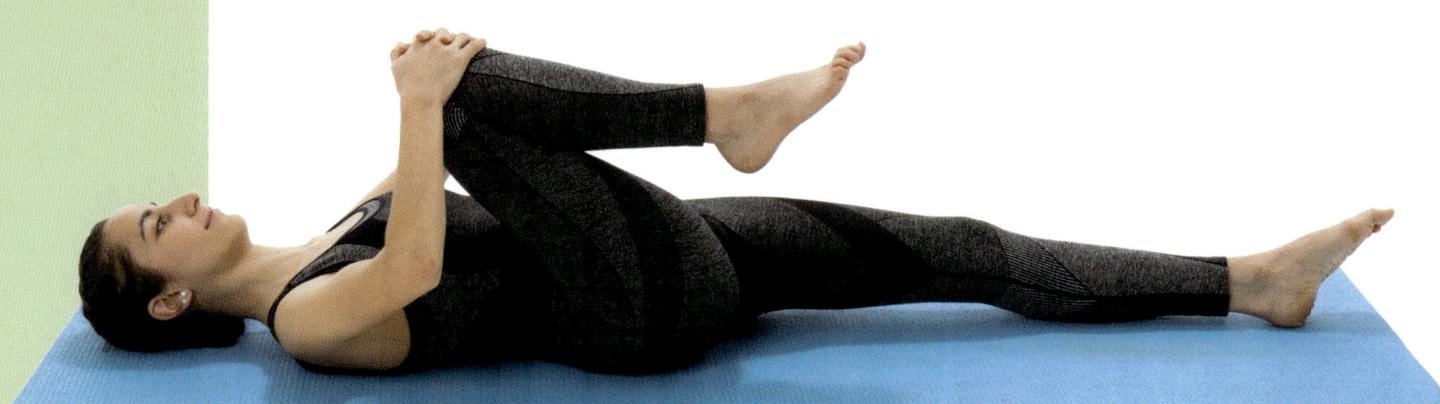

Apanasana is a moving asana that allows us to regenerate prana while also helping us as a *vinyasa* (warm-up movement). This activates the Muladhara Chakra.

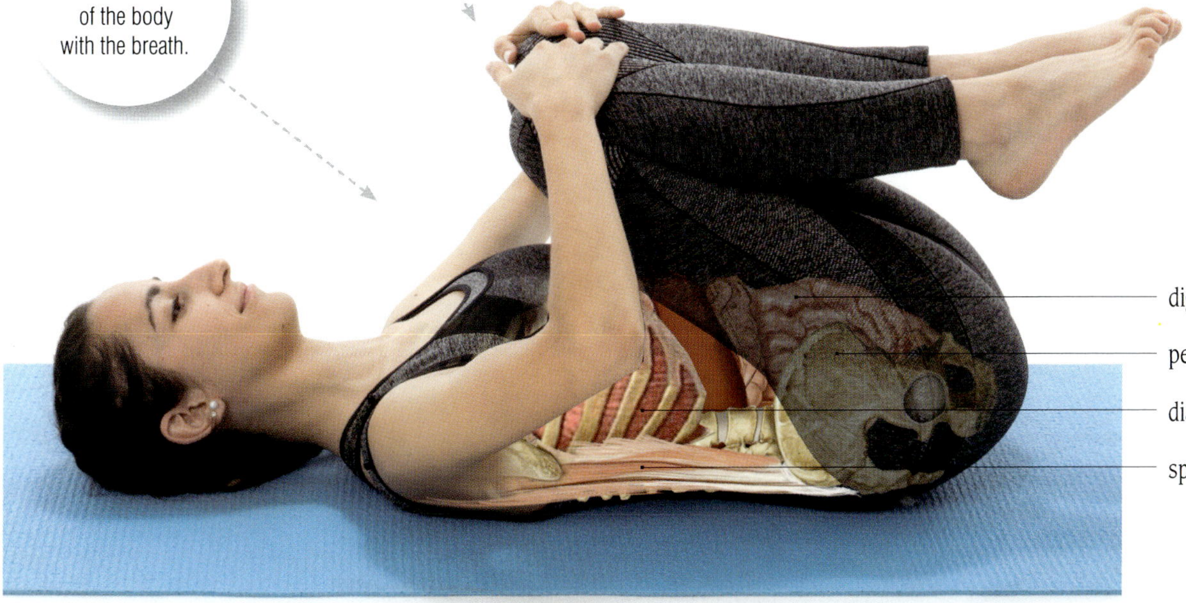

Stimulation of the exhalation process by pressing the legs toward the torso, while the abdominal organs are massaged.
It connects the movement of the body with the breath.
digestive system
pelvis
diaphragm
spine

Elongation and mobility of the lumbar area.
digestive system
pelvis
diaphragm
spine

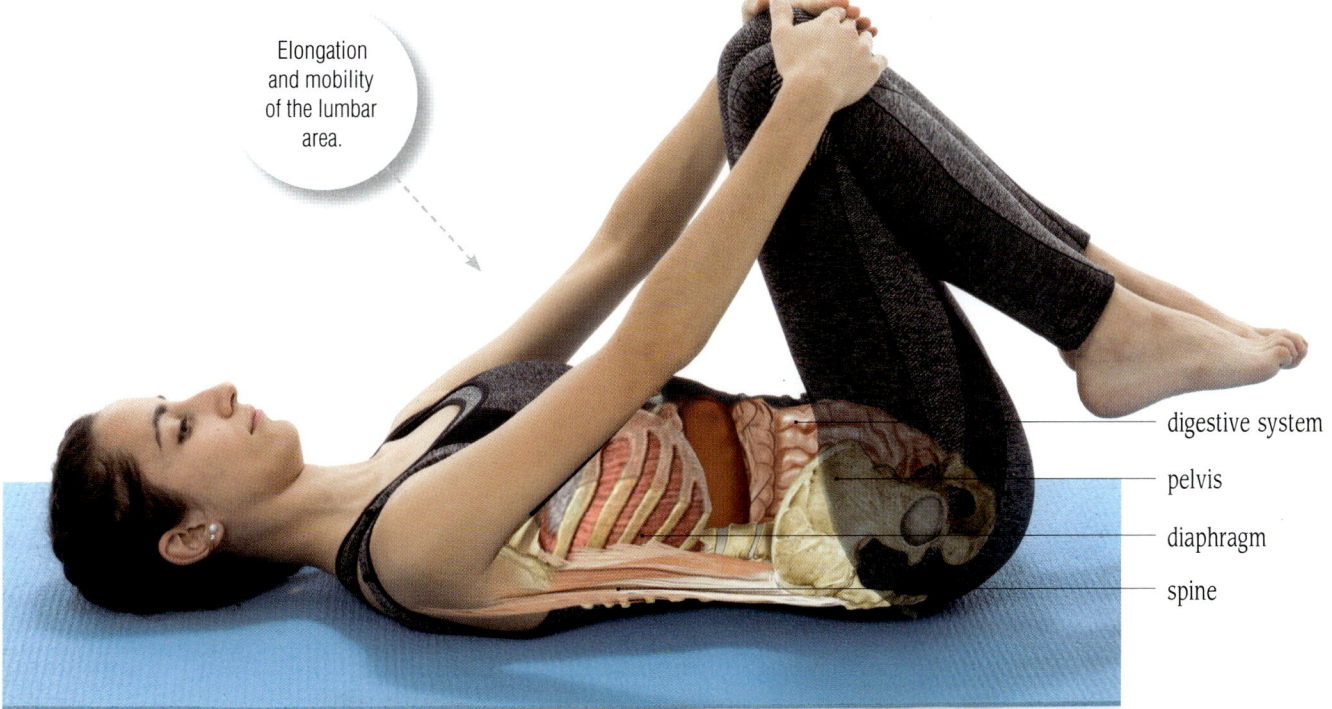

Asanas

BASIC ASANAS

# Marjariasana

Also known as *Cakravakasana*, the cat pose, or *Vyaghrasana*, the tiger pose. The movement that is done in this pose reminds us of two felines, and that is where the names come from.

## BENEFITS

- Provides greater mobility and flexibility to the spine.
- Strengthens the muscles of the back, making the neck and back tensions disappear.
- Tones the abdominal muscles.
- Decongestions spinal nerves which has a beneficial effect on the nervous system.
- Beneficial for pregnant women and for those with heart problems and asthma attacks.

## WARNINGS

- Weakness or problems in the wrists: possibility of supporting the fists on the ground.
- Neck injuries: perform the pose by maintaining neutral alignment of the neck.

### CLASSIFICATION
Basic pose. *Vinyasa* (dynamic articulatory pose of the spine).

### TECHNIQUE
We kneel on the floor, placing the legs separated under the joints of the hips. We support the hands on the floor, separated from each other and in line with the shoulders. The arms and the thighs should be perpendicular on the floor.

**Position 1.** While exhaling we bend the entire back, starting with the head, then the neck, the dorsal region, and then the lumbar. The back is raised to its maximum extension, forming an arc.

**Position 2.** While exhaling we arc the entire back, from the coccyx, and pass this movement onto the entire spine until, reaching the head, we raise the head without tucking the neck. Arms and legs remain still. We continue the exercise by slowly alternating the positions.

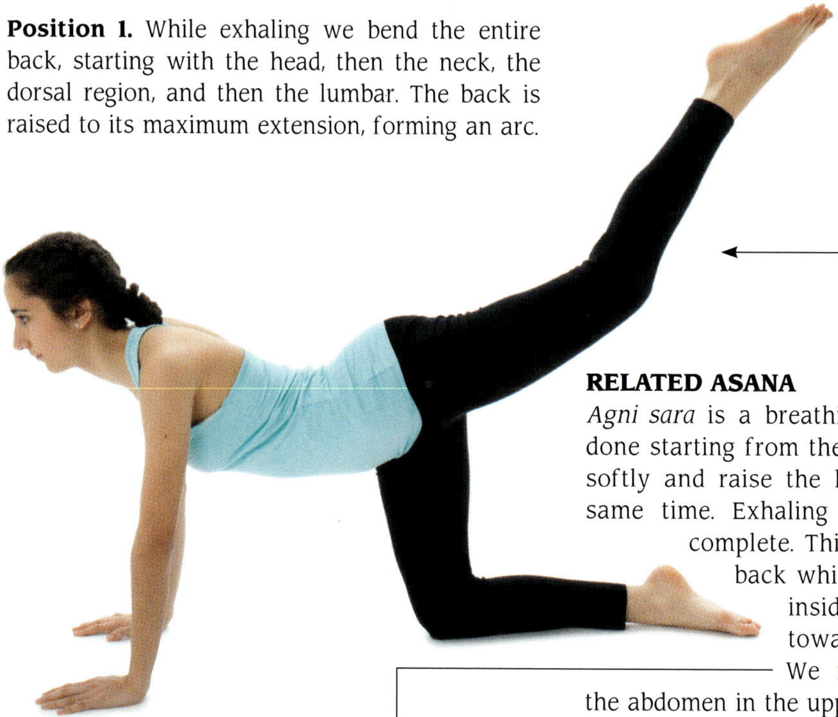

### RELATED ASANA
*Agni sara* is a breathing exercise that can be done starting from the Marjariasana. We inhale softly and raise the head and left leg at the same time. Exhaling must be energetic and complete. This is done by arching the back while keeping the leg on the inside and moving the knee toward the nose.

We first exhale by pressing the abdomen in the upper part of the pubis, then the middle area of the abdomen, the upper area, and, finally, we exhale all the air from the chest. We inhale again, this time following the inverse order: we take in air into the chest, starting from the upper abdomen and middle part, while lifting the head and leg.

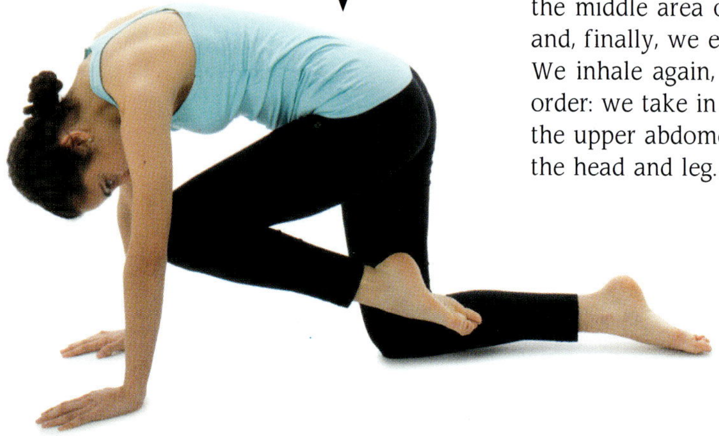

BASIC ASANAS: Marjariasana 57

Practicing Marjarasana strengthens the coordination of movements and stimulates the moving of energy through the entire spine. It primarily activates the chakras of Manipura and Anahata.

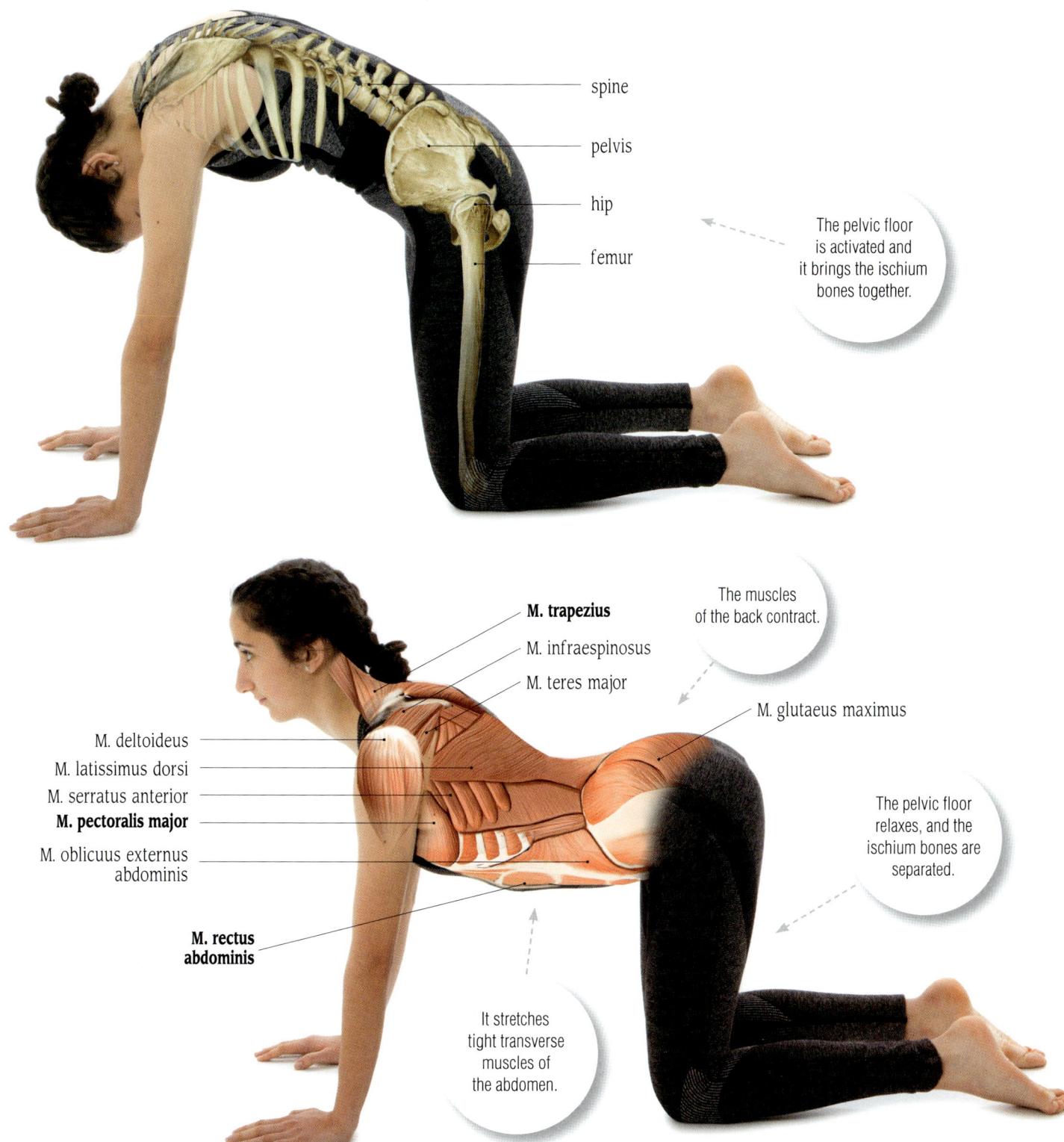

# Basic Asanas

# Adho Mukha Svanasana

*Adho Mukha* means "with the head down," and *svana* means "dog." This asana evokes the position of a dog when it is stretching.

**BENEFITS**
- Stimulates the body and reduces fatigue.
- Increases blood flow to the head.
- Strengthens the muscles of the arms, legs, and back.

**WARNINGS**
- Hypertension.
- Inflammation of knees, shoulders, or wrists.

**CLASSIFICATION**
Symmetrical pose, semi-inverted.

**TECHNIQUE**
We start from the same position as Marjariasana. We place the knees a little behind the hip joint and the hands at the level of the shoulders, with the fingers extended. We start from the tips of the feet and, while pressing with the strength of the hands on the ground, we lift the knees and move the pelvis backward and up. We move the weight of the body toward the soles of the feet and stretch the legs by pressing the heels toward the floor. The arm is rotated externally. The body should form a triangle.

**COUNTERPOSE**
Bhujangasana.

**ADAPTATIONS**
In the event of tension in the hamstrings or limited flexibility, we can hold this position with bent knees.

Partner pushes softly into position.

BASIC ASANAS: Adho Mukha Svanasana 59

In Adho Mukha the energy flows from the base of the spine to the head, and activates the Manipura Chakra.

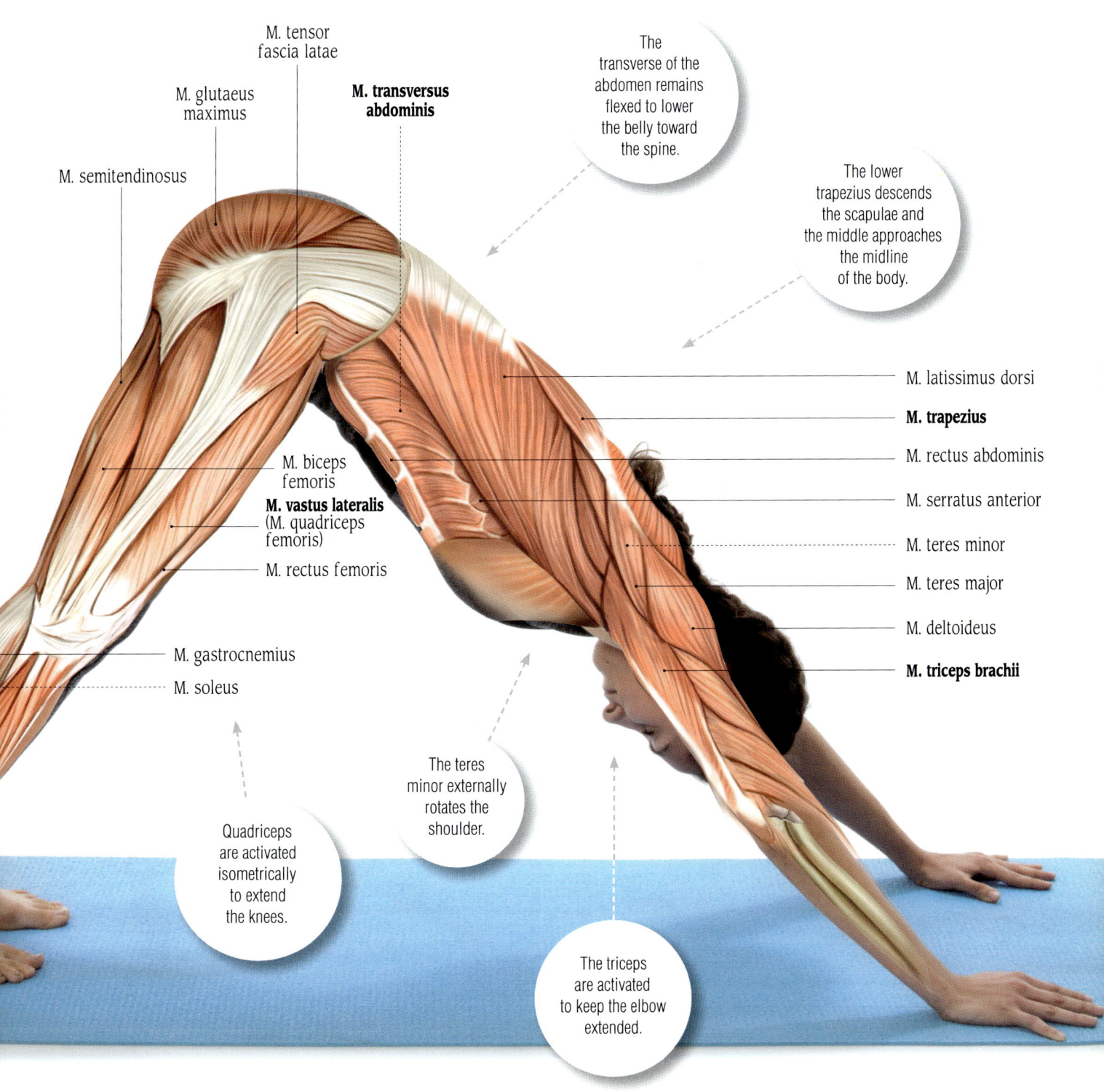

BASIC ASANAS

# Virabhadrasana I and II

*Virabhadra* is a hero that, according to the mythical legend, was created from a lock of hair from the god Siva (poem *Kumara Sambhava*). There are three warrior poses, dedicated to *Virabhadra*.

**BENEFITS**
- Strengthens the knees and hip joints, and the muscles of the feet and legs.
- Develops balance.
- Relieves shoulder and back stiffness.
- Increases respiratory capacity.

**WARNINGS**
- Back injuries, or coronary problems: preferable to practice pose II.

**CLASSIFICATION**
Virabhadrasana I: basic pose for balance, asymmetric with extension. Virabhadrasana II: basic pose for strength, asymmetric.

**TECHNIQUE**
**Virabhadrasana I:** Starting from Tadasana, we take a step forward, and the lower leg moves forward and bends at the knee until the thigh is parallel to the ground. We rotate the rear foot 45º out. The bent knee should not pass the vertical position of the ankle, while it remains in line with the 2nd and 3rd toe of the foot. We raise and stretch the arms above the head, with the palms of the hands together. We look up. We release the pose and repeat it with the other side.

**Virabhadrasana II:** Starting from Tadasana, we open the legs laterally, and rotate the foot, leg, and right hip 90º while the left foot rotates 45º. We bend the right knee without passing the ankle. We stretch the arms to the side with the tips of the fingers at the height of the shoulders. We rotate the head to the right side, looking toward the tips of the fingers. To complete the opposite side, we return to the position with the legs open, with the feet parallel, and proceed in the same way for the left side.

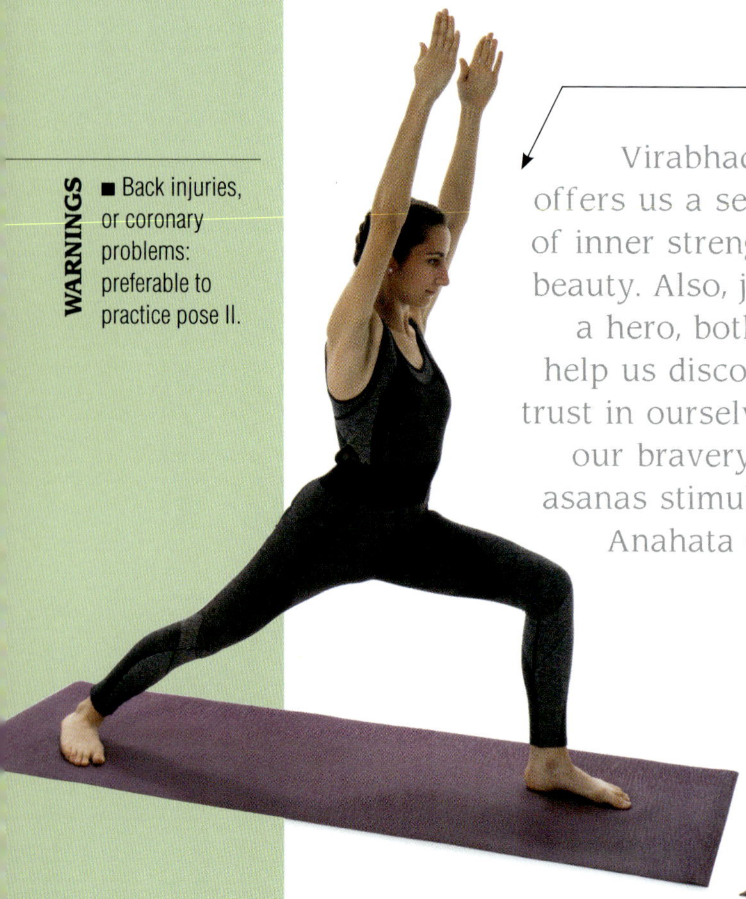

**ADAPTATIONS**
**Variations of Virabhadrasana I.** If there is too much tension in the shoulders and the neck, you can practice the asana with the arms parallel while looking forward.

A more simple variation would be to place the hands on the hips.

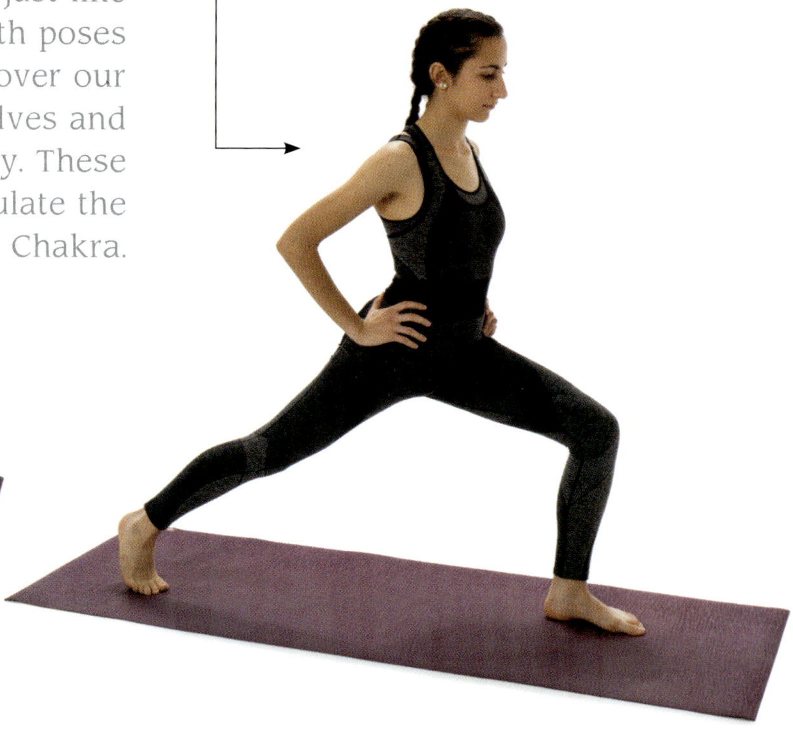

*Virabhadrasana offers us a sensation of inner strength and beauty. Also, just like a hero, both poses help us discover our trust in ourselves and our bravery. These asanas stimulate the Anahata Chakra.*

BASIC ASANAS: Virabhadrasana I and II

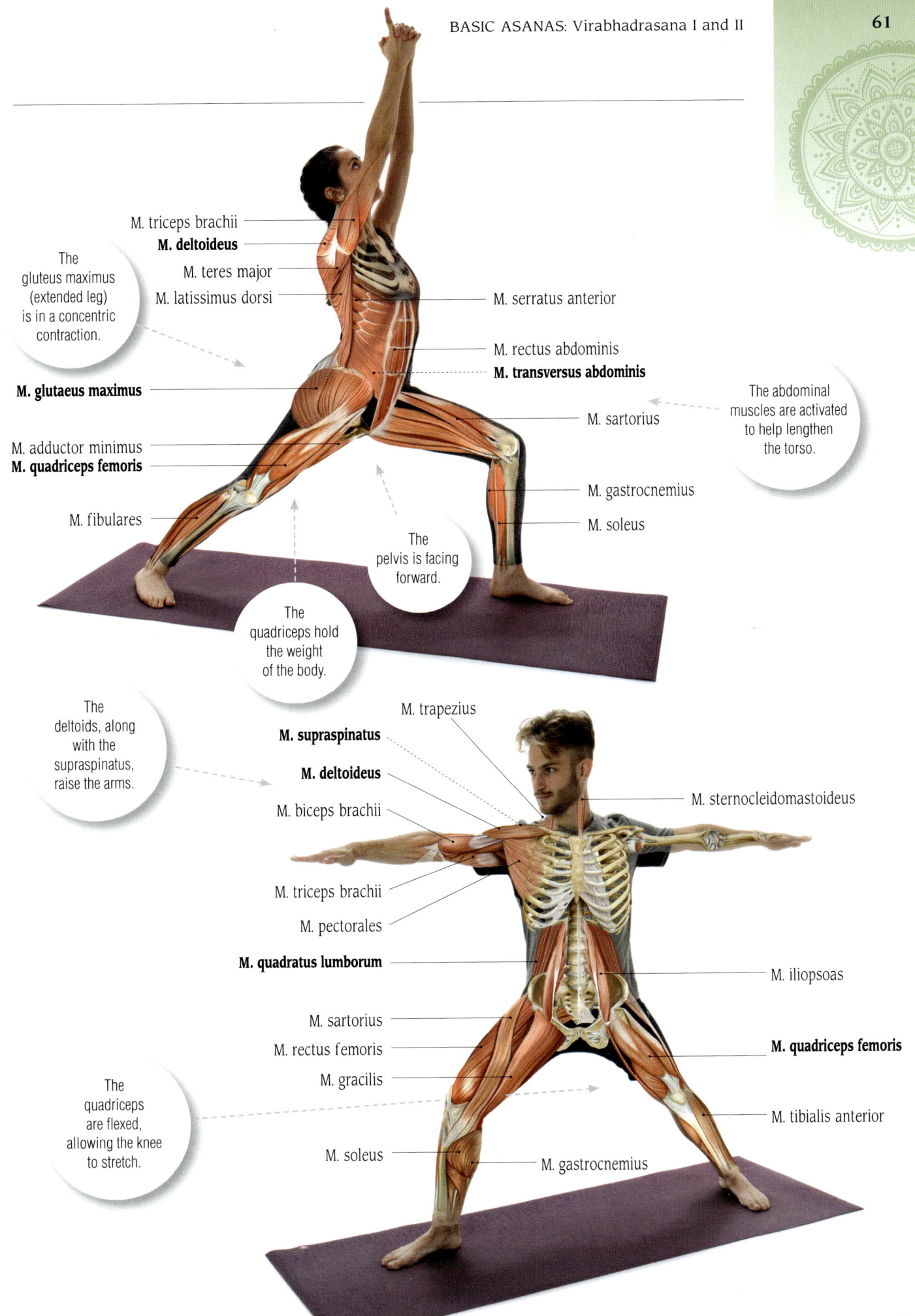

BASIC ASANAS

# Virabhadrasana III

This pose, like the two previous ones, is also dedicated to the hero *Virabhadra*.

**BENEFITS**
- Tones the abdominal muscles.
- Strengthens the feet, ankles, and legs.
- Provides agility and energy, and promotes physical and mental balance.
- Develops concentration.

**WARNINGS**
- Joint problems or osteoarthritis of the feet, legs, hips, and shoulders; practice with caution.

**CLASSIFICATION**
Basic pose for balance, asymmetric with extension.

**TECHNIQUE**
We start in the position with the legs of Virabhadrasana I, we lean the trunk forward little by little and raise the leg behind, moving the entire body forward. We stretch the leg that remains standing on the floor. We also stretch the arms forward along with the palms of the hands.

The body and elevated leg should remain parallel to the ground. The elevated leg rotates on the inside with the groin facing down. All the weight of the body rests on the standing foot. We hold the pose and breathe calmly and release it to proceed to the other side.

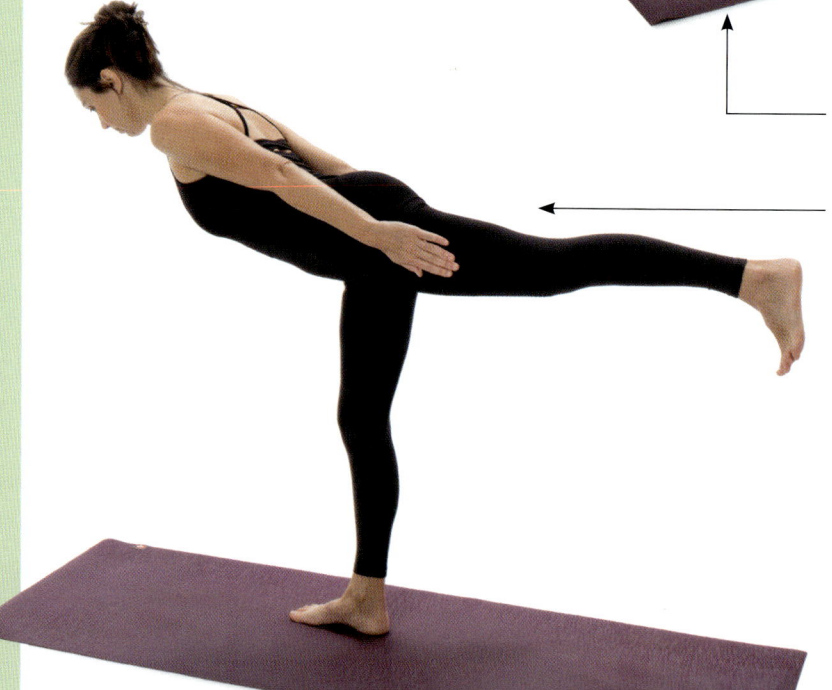

**ADAPTATIONS**
Variation with the arms extended parallel together.

With osteoarthritis or problems in the shoulders, it is preferable to use the variation with the arms on the side of the body. If we lack balance, we will support the arms on a wall or on the back of a chair and, little by little, we will advance in the pose.

BASIC ASANAS: Virabhadrasana III

Virabhadrasana III develops balance and inner harmony while providing strength and certainty. It revitalizes the Manipura Chakra.

The triceps straighten the elbows and the anterior and middle deltoids raise the arm. The erector muscles of the spine straighten the back and the lumbar spine stabilizes the torso and pelvis.

The gluteus maximus and hamstrings are active to support the raised leg.

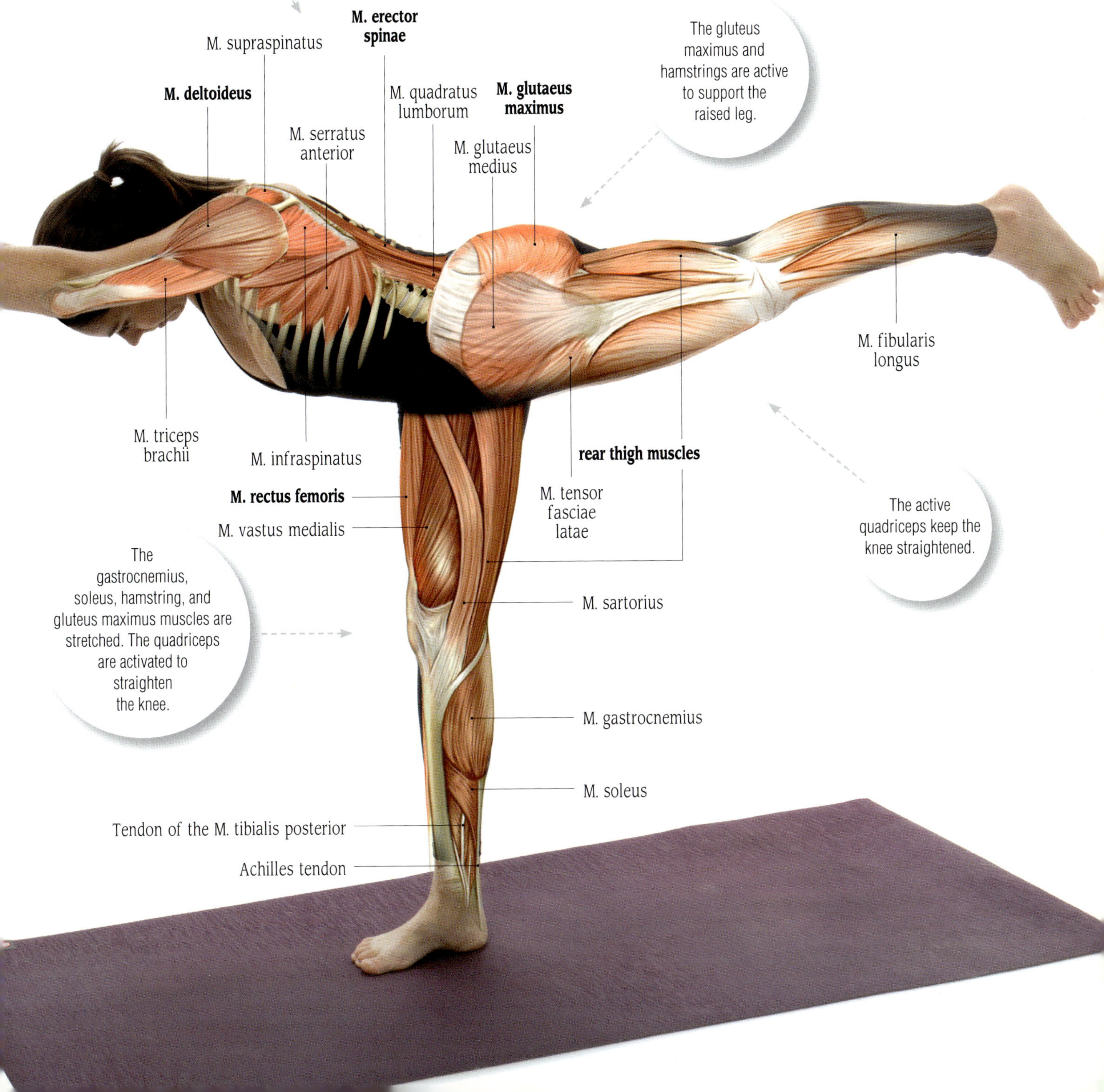

The gastrocnemius, soleus, hamstring, and gluteus maximus muscles are stretched. The quadriceps are activated to straighten the knee.

The active quadriceps keep the knee straightened.

- M. supraspinatus
- M. erector spinae
- M. deltoideus
- M. quadratus lumborum
- M. glutaeus maximus
- M. serratus anterior
- M. glutaeus medius
- M. triceps brachii
- M. infraspinatus
- M. fibularis longus
- M. rectus femoris
- rear thigh muscles
- M. vastus medialis
- M. tensor fasciae latae
- M. sartorius
- M. gastrocnemius
- M. soleus
- Tendon of the M. tibialis posterior
- Achilles tendon

BASIC ASANAS

# Malasana

*Mala* means "wreath." This is the wreath pose, since your arms make a crown that seems to hang on your neck. This asana creates an offering to your inner self; it is also a good way to prepare for meditation.

**BENEFITS**
- Tones the abdominal muscles, stimulates digestion, and relieves constipation.
- Relieves back pain.
- Encourages stretching of the lower back, pelvis, and pelvic floor. Since the feet are separated, it is very appropriate for pregnant women.
- Calms the nervous system.

**WARNINGS**
- Problems of hips, knees and shoulders.

**CLASSIFICATION**
Basic squatting pose, symmetrical.

**TECHNIQUE**
We start from the squatting position, the feet are together and flat on the floor. We raise the buttocks, maintaining our balance. Separate your legs and move your core forward, until the armpits pass your knees. Take the back part of your ankles in your hands, while your head lowers until you support your forehead on the floor. Hold this position for a few minutes. To release this pose, place your hands on the floor, under your shoulders, and exhale while you lift your head little by little.

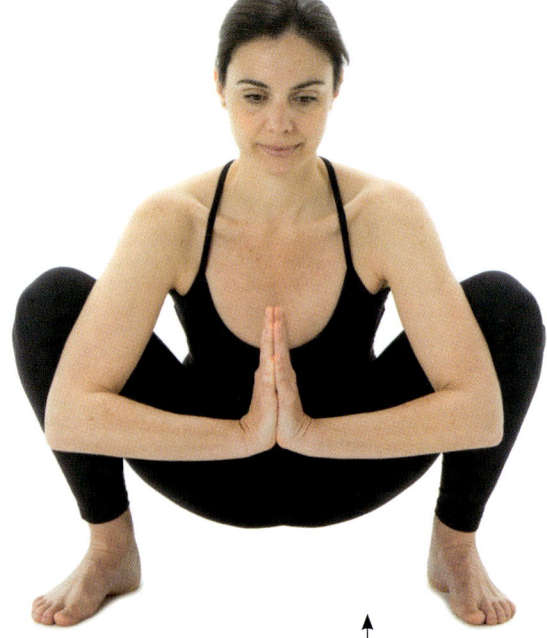

**RELATED ASANA**
Upavesasana is an asana related to Malasana. To perform this, squat with your feet separated and your elbows resting on the inside part of your knees, your hands are together in *namasté*. Lightly press outward with your elbows that are on your knees, in this way you will open your hip. This is a very appropriate pose for pregnant women.

If you have a tight Achilles tendon, you can place a support under your heel.

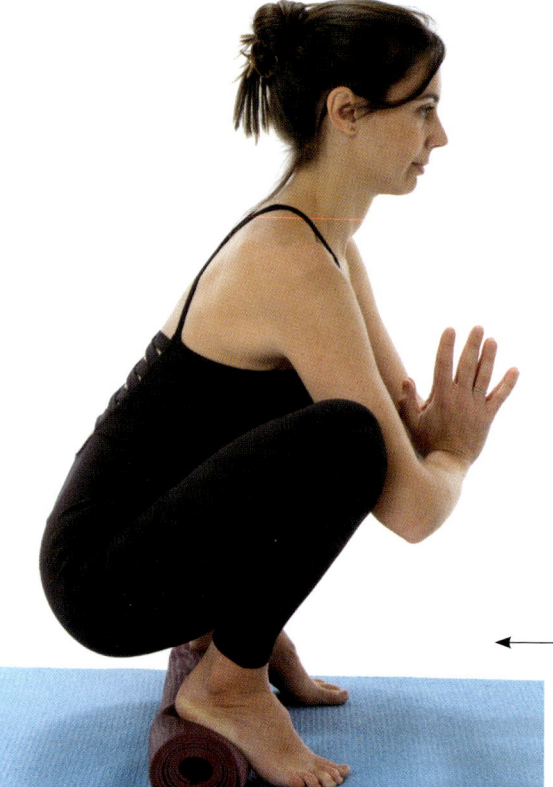

BASIC ASANAS: Malasana

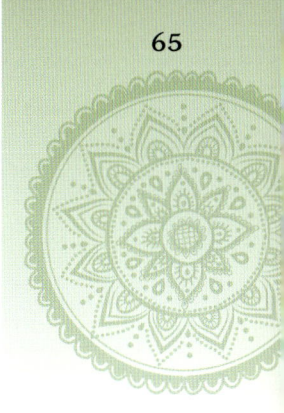

Malasana affects and stimulates the opening of the Muladhara Chakra and invigorates the Svadisthana Chakra. It offers us inner stability, balance, and safety.

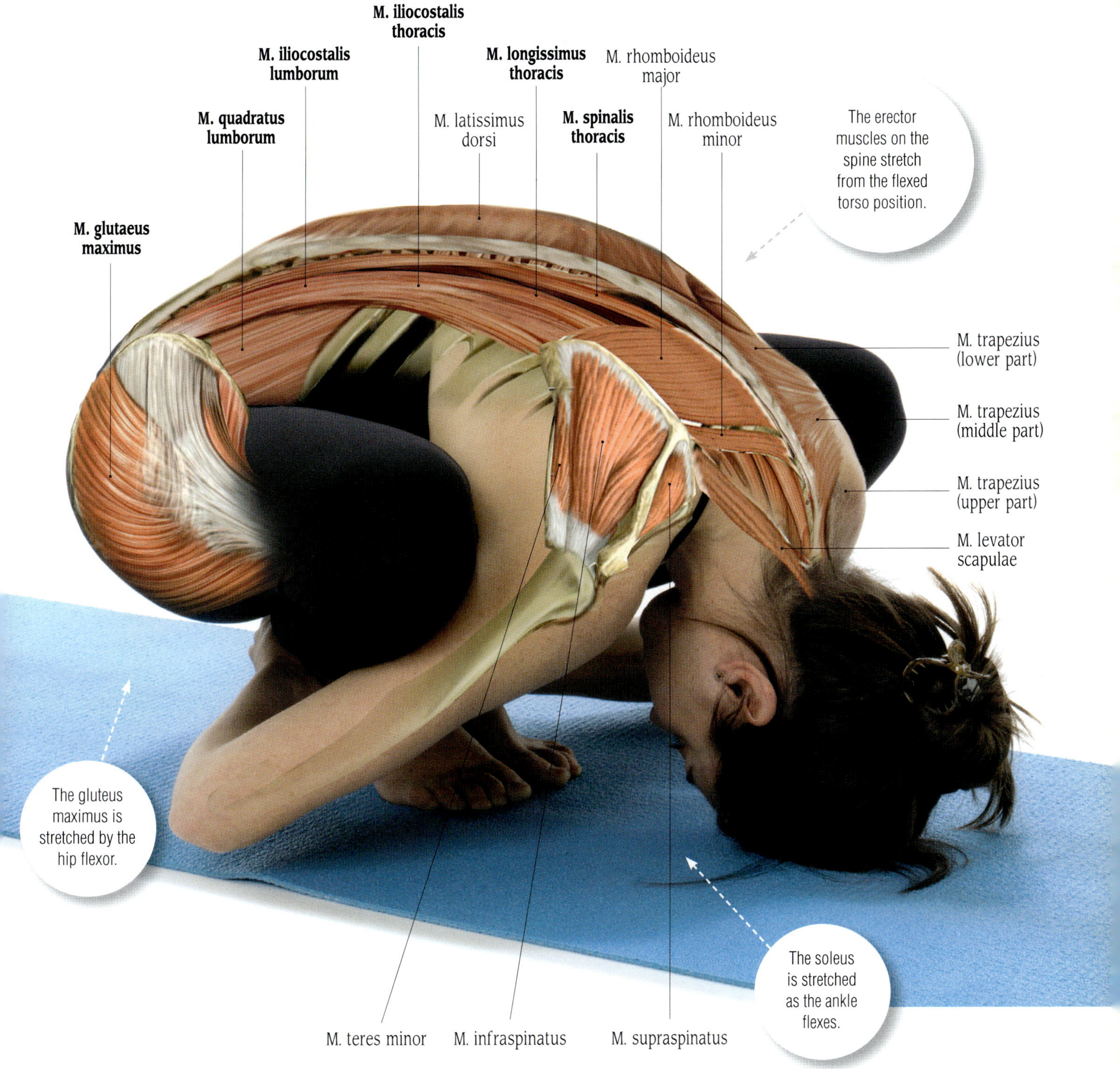

- **M. glutaeus maximus**
- **M. quadratus lumborum**
- **M. iliocostalis lumborum**
- **M. iliocostalis thoracis**
- M. latissimus dorsi
- **M. longissimus thoracis**
- **M. spinalis thoracis**
- M. rhomboideus major
- M. rhomboideus minor
- M. trapezius (lower part)
- M. trapezius (middle part)
- M. trapezius (upper part)
- M. levator scapulae
- M. teres minor
- M. infraspinatus
- M. supraspinatus

The erector muscles on the spine stretch from the flexed torso position.

The gluteus maximus is stretched by the hip flexor.

The soleus is stretched as the ankle flexes.

BASIC ASANAS

# Utkatasana

*Utkata* means "power," "ferocity," and "valor." It is also called the seat pose, since it looks like you are sitting while holding the pose. It is a pose that offers us strength and stability.

**BENEFITS**
- Strengthens the muscles of the legs and ankles.
- Corrects inadequate posture of the legs and small deformations.
- Tones the abdominal muscles and expands the thorax, which increases the lung capacity.
- Develops stability, balance, and strength.
- Stimulates blood circulation.

**WARNINGS**
- Weakness in the knees, although the constant and gentle practice of this asana can strengthen them.
- Sciatic nerve and problems in the lower back; practice it with caution leaning on a wall.

### CLASSIFICATION
Pose of strength, symmetric on the foot.

### TECHNIQUE
We start from Tadasana. While inhaling, we raise the arms above the head along with the palms of the hands. We can complete a Ksepana mudra. We observe that the shoulders move down and the thorax expands. While exhaling, the knees bend and the trunk lowers while keeping the pelvis down. In order for the feet and knees to remain parallel, press the heels against the floor, keeping your weight on them. The spine stretches and with every breath we see the thorax expand. The shoulders should face down and back, the body should be leaning forward.

To finish this pose, with a breath, we slowly stretch the legs, lower the arms, and return to the Tadasana pose. For a few seconds we observe sensations that this asana offers.

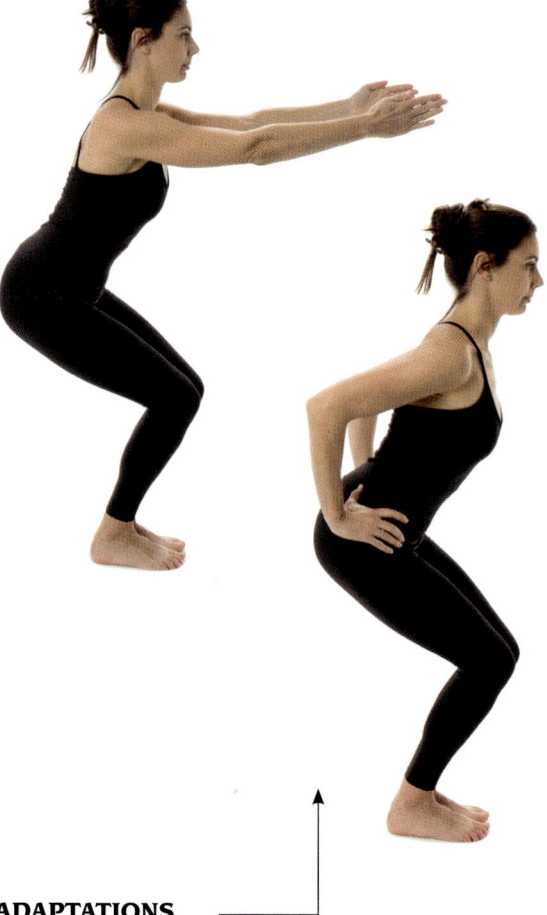

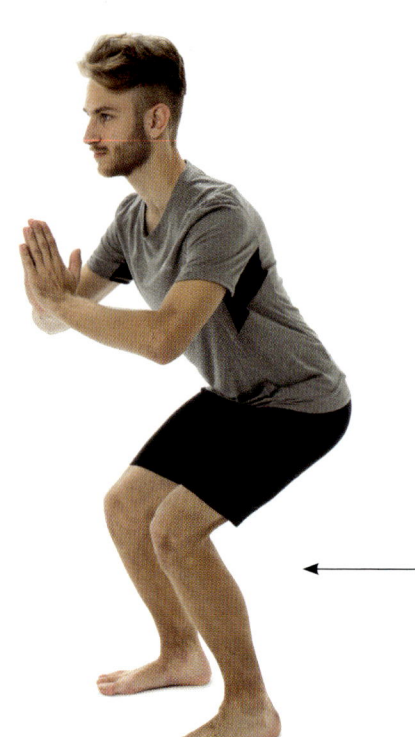

### ADAPTATIONS
This asana can be practiced with variations. For people with little stability or balance, it is recommended to use a wall for support. Also, if there is limited balance, or weakness in the shoulders and neck, the arms can be stretched forward. For the previous case, to intensify the opening of the thorax, the arms may be supported on the waist. This last variation will be used if there is any discomfort in the back and arms.

### VARIATION
One variation would be the Urvasana pose. Starting from Samasthiti, with the legs separated, we lower the trunk in the same way as Utkatasana. This variation is recommended to strengthen the legs for women.

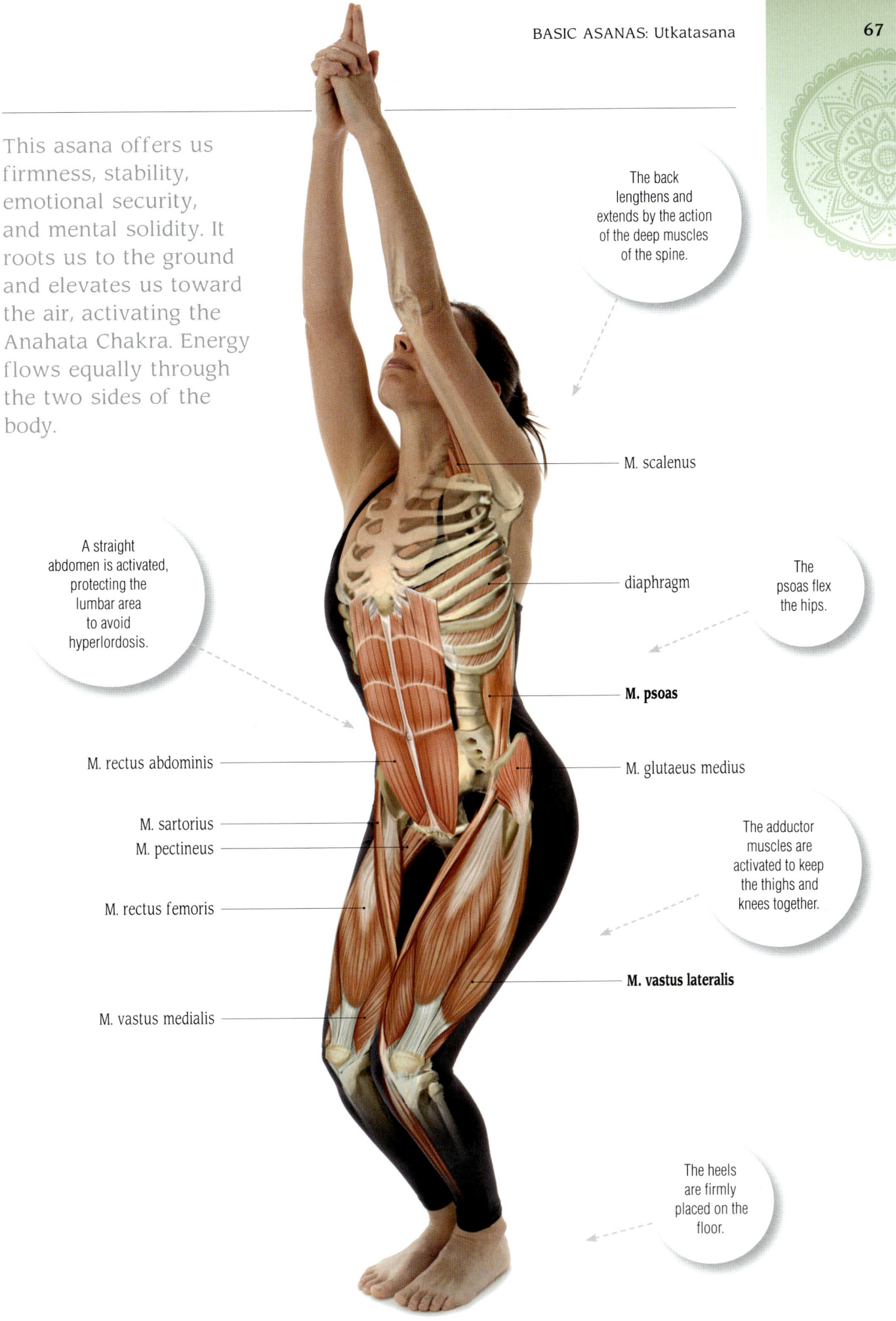

BASIC ASANAS: Utkatasana

This asana offers us firmness, stability, emotional security, and mental solidity. It roots us to the ground and elevates us toward the air, activating the Anahata Chakra. Energy flows equally through the two sides of the body.

The back lengthens and extends by the action of the deep muscles of the spine.

M. scalenus

diaphragm

The psoas flex the hips.

A straight abdomen is activated, protecting the lumbar area to avoid hyperlordosis.

**M. psoas**

M. rectus abdominis

M. glutaeus medius

M. sartorius

M. pectineus

The adductor muscles are activated to keep the thighs and knees together.

M. rectus femoris

**M. vastus lateralis**

M. vastus medialis

The heels are firmly placed on the floor.

ASANAS OF STRENGTH

# Navasana

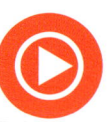

*Nava* means "ship," or "boat." This is known as ship pose, since by doing it, the body imitates the shape of a boat with oars. It is an asana that gives us energy, balance, and vigor.

**BENEFITS**
- Strengthens the muscles of the back, abdomen, neck, groin, and quadriceps.
- Stimulates the digestive system (intestines, gallbladder, spleen, liver), benefiting digestion. Invigorates the kidneys.
- Improves blood flow and invigorates the heart.
- Promotes balance and reduces pressure

**WARNINGS**
- Inflammation or hernias in the groin or abdomen.
- Pregnancy.
- Problems in the lumbar region.

**CLASSIFICATION**
Pose of strength, symmetric, a flexed trunk, and balancing.

**TECHNIQUE**
We start sitting on the ground with the legs crossed. We move the weight of the body toward the coccyx in a way that is distributed between the ischium bones. We hold for a moment with the hands on the knees and, while raising the thorax, stretch the legs. The legs and the body should form a 90º angle. The arms stretch on each side, parallel to the ground, with the palms of the hands facing the knees. The pose is held with the sternum raised and the back straight. We become aware of the asana.

We release the pose by bending the legs and placing the feet back on the ground.

**COUNTER POSE**
Pranatasana.

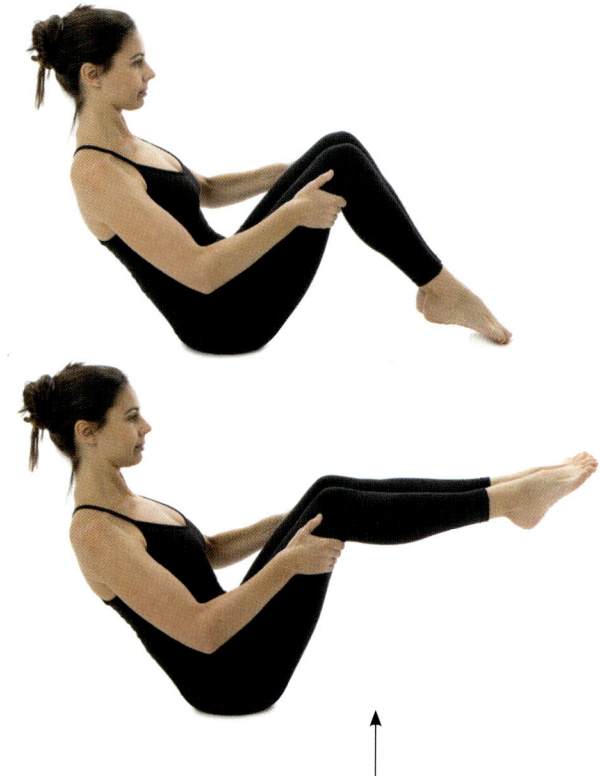

**ADAPTATIONS**
To progress to this pose, we start by lightly supporting the tips of the toes on the ground while we raise the back. For the second movement, we start with the feed on the ground and raise the legs so that the calves are parallel to the ground.

If we observe any lack of balance, we can alternatively support our hands on the ground.

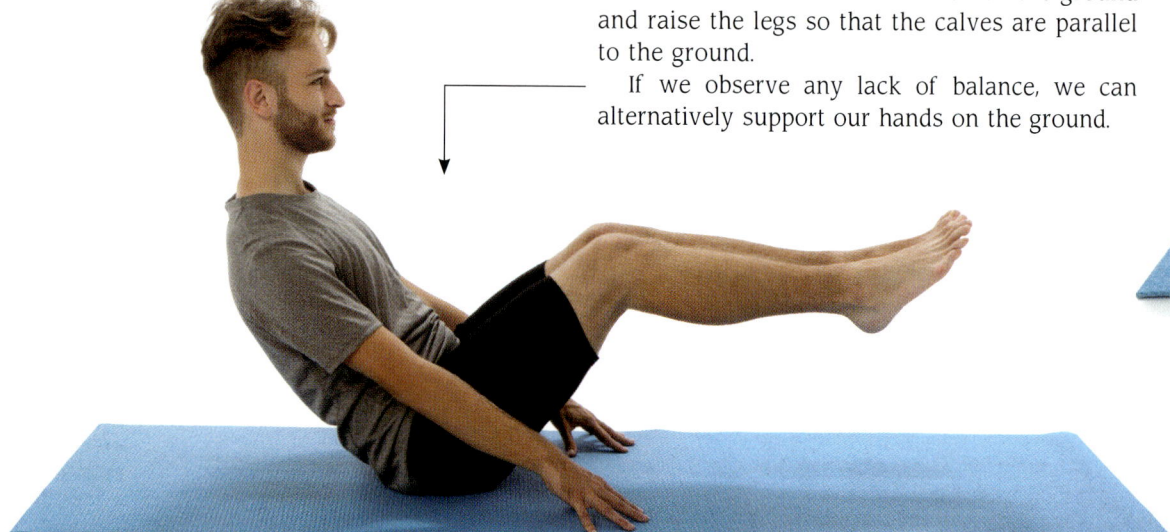

ASANAS OF STRENGTH: Navasana

Navasana reinvigorates, offers physical balance, mental concentration and physical and emotional strength. It stimulates the Muladhara Chakra, which causes the movement of energy in an ascending direction.

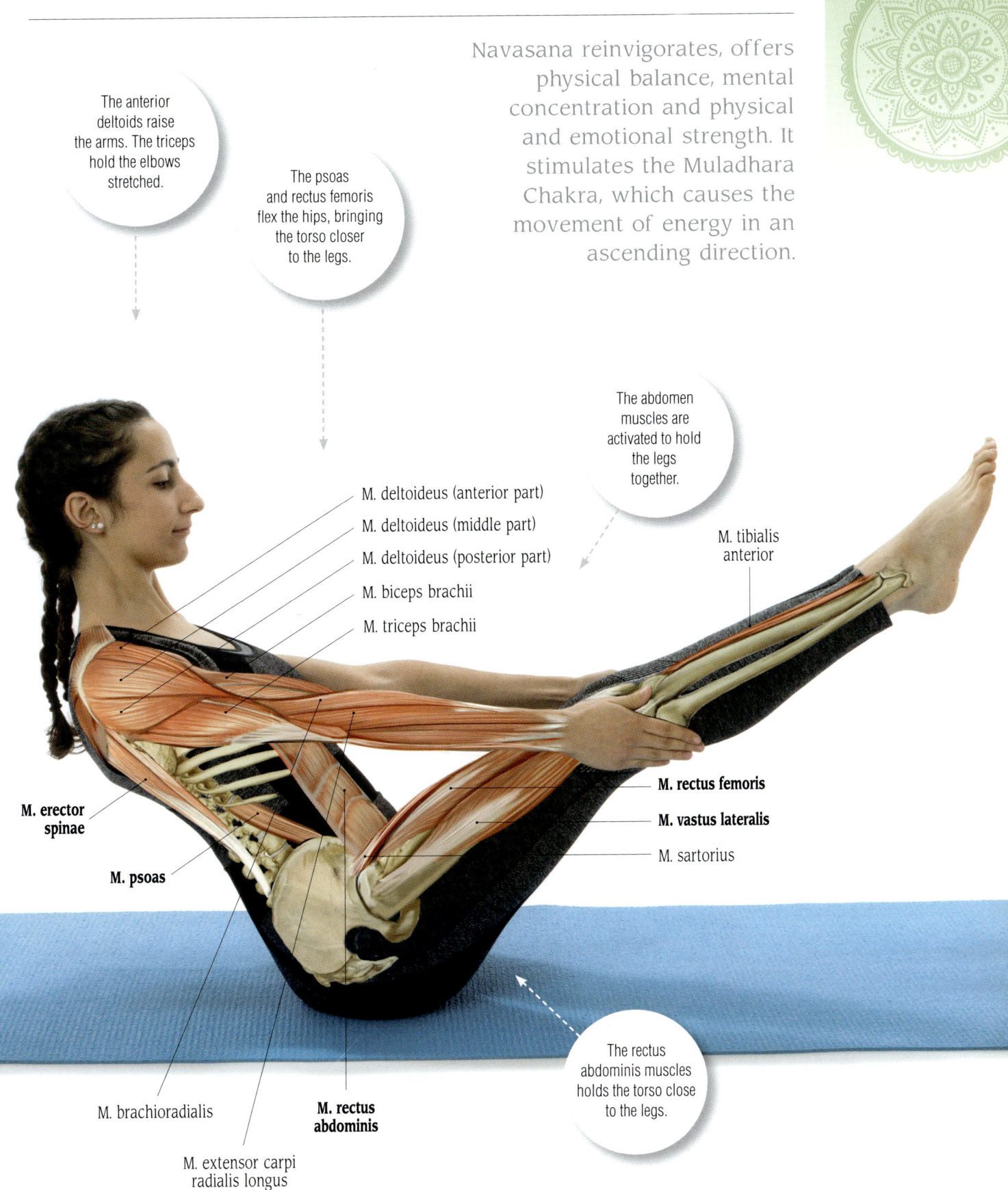

- The anterior deltoids raise the arms. The triceps hold the elbows stretched.
- The psoas and rectus femoris flex the hips, bringing the torso closer to the legs.
- The abdomen muscles are activated to hold the legs together.
- The rectus abdominis muscles holds the torso close to the legs.

Labels:
- M. deltoideus (anterior part)
- M. deltoideus (middle part)
- M. deltoideus (posterior part)
- M. biceps brachii
- M. triceps brachii
- M. tibialis anterior
- M. erector spinae
- M. psoas
- M. rectus femoris
- M. vastus lateralis
- M. sartorius
- M. brachioradialis
- M. rectus abdominis
- M. extensor carpi radialis longus

ASANAS OF STRENGTH

# Vasishtasana

*Vasishta* refers to one of the seven great sages, author of various Vedic hymns; this asana is dedicated to him. The name *Vashista* means "his most excellent," or "the best one."

**BENEFITS**

- Strengthens wrists, arms, shoulders, and legs.
- Strengthens the muscles responsible for keeping the body erect.
- Develops and perfects balance, and creates awareness of the lateral plane.
- Stimulates blood circulation and breathing.

**WARNINGS**

- Inflammations in the joints of the arms and shoulders.
- Ailments in the back.
- General weakness.

**CLASSIFICATION**
Asana of strength, asymmetrical, lateral balance.

**TECHNIQUE**
We place the palms of the hands on the ground and the feet are stretched. We rotate the body laterally so that the palms of the right hand and the outside part of the right foot are supported; the left foot rests on the right. We raise the left arm vertically, until it is in line with the right arm; the spine and the legs also remain in a single plane and aligned together. Keep this pose for a few breaths and release from the pose. We repeat the pose on the other side.

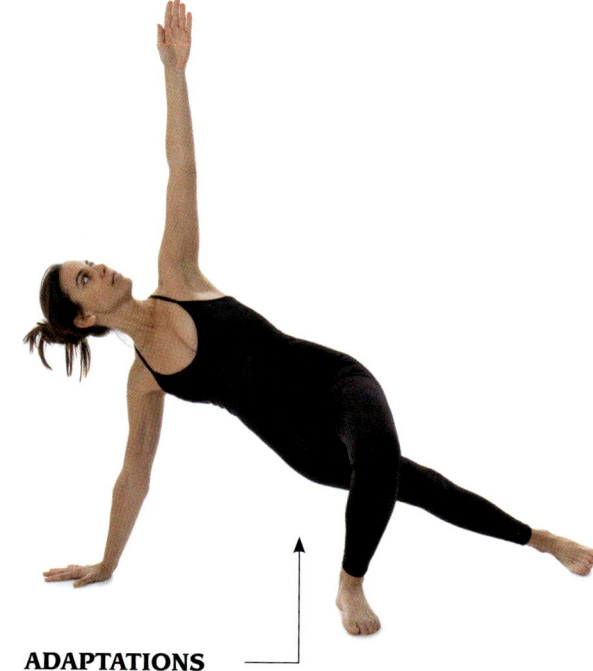

**ADAPTATIONS**
If we lack balance, we can use the other leg for support, moving it forward and placing the sole of the foot on the ground. We can also use a wall for support.

**VARIATION**
We hold the pose with the arm supported on the body.
Another more advanced variation is to bend the leg up and hold the knee with the hand. We rotate the head and look up.

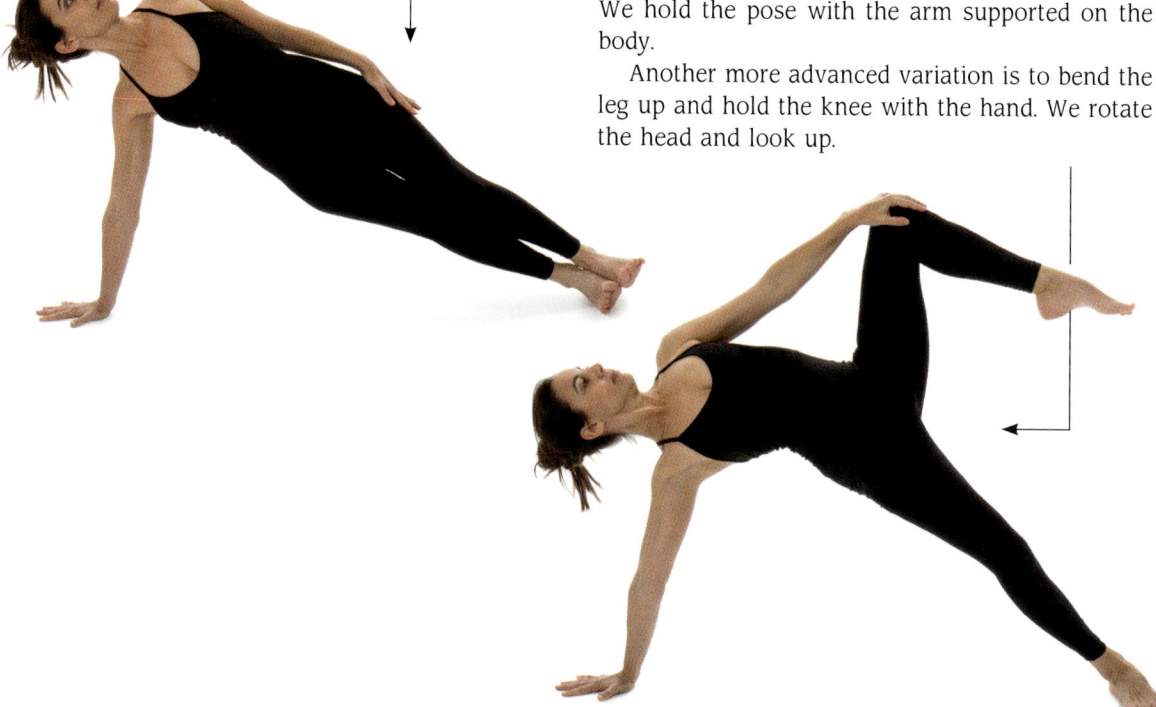

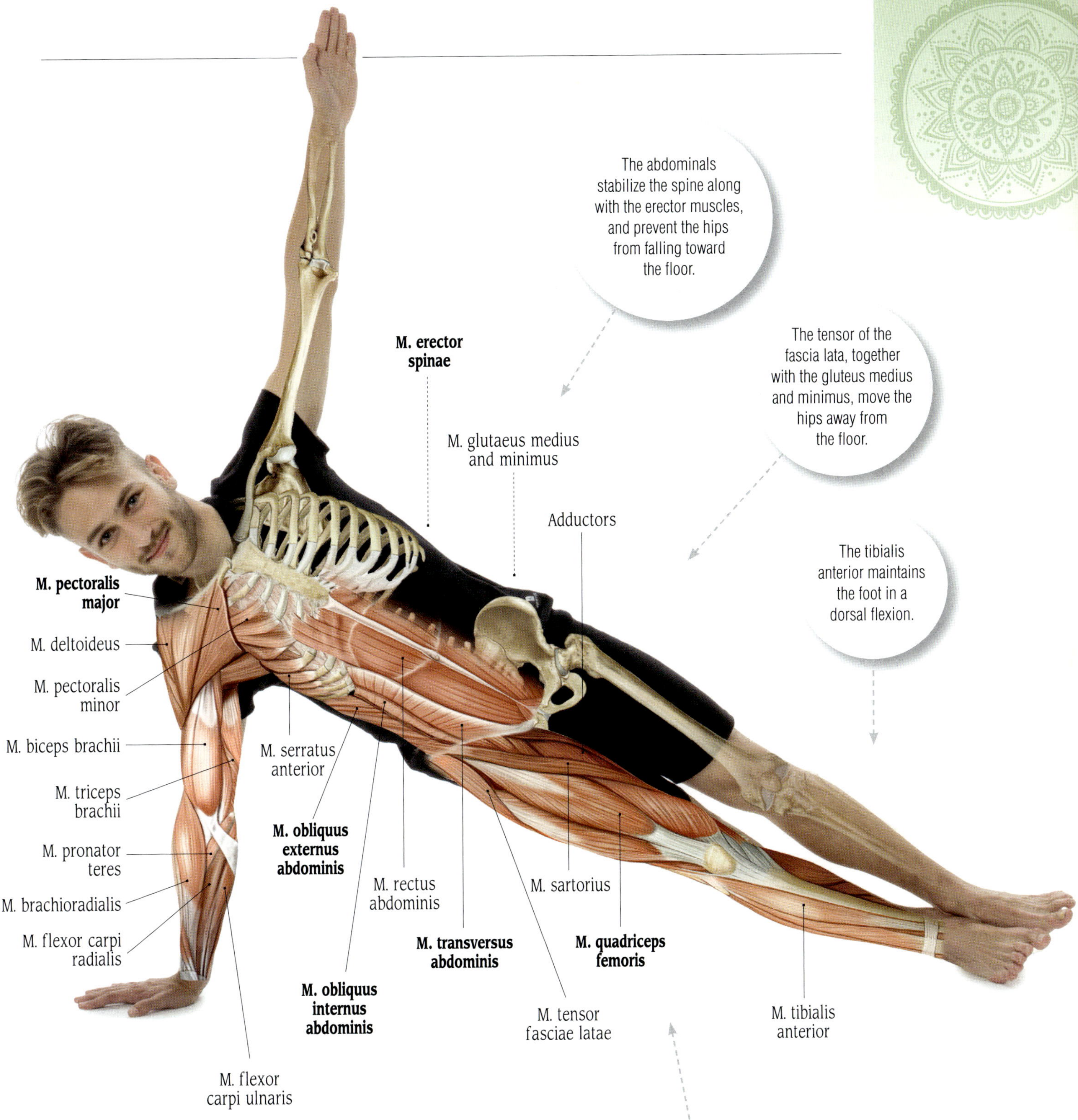

ASANAS OF STRENGTH: Vasishtasana 71

The abdominals stabilize the spine along with the erector muscles, and prevent the hips from falling toward the floor.

The tensor of the fascia lata, together with the gluteus medius and minimus, move the hips away from the floor.

The tibialis anterior maintains the foot in a dorsal flexion.

**M. erector spinae**

M. glutaeus medius and minimus

Adductors

**M. pectoralis major**

M. deltoideus

M. pectoralis minor

M. biceps brachii

M. triceps brachii

M. pronator teres

M. brachioradialis

M. flexor carpi radialis

M. serratus anterior

**M. obliquus externus abdominis**

M. rectus abdominis

**M. obliquus internus abdominis**

**M. transversus abdominis**

M. tensor fasciae latae

M. sartorius

**M. quadriceps femoris**

M. tibialis anterior

M. flexor carpi ulnaris

The quadriceps are activated to straighten the knees, while the adductors hold the legs together.

Vasishtasana strengthens mental and emotional balance, contributing to our inner strength. It also offers us a sensation of control of the mind over the body. We work the Manipura Chakra with this pose.

Asanas

ASANAS OF STRENGTH

# Chaturanga Dandasana

*Chatu* means "four," *anga* is "member" or "extremity" and *danda* means "staff" or "cane." It is the cane pose on four members.

**BENEFITS**
- Strengthens the muscles of the back and abdomen.
- Strengthens arms, wrists, and shoulders.
- Develops the chest muscles.
- Tones the abdominal muscles.
- Increases physical endurance.

**WARNINGS**
- General weakness, or in recovery processes of a disease.
- Injuries to wrists, arms, or shoulders.

**CLASSIFICATION**
Pose of strength, symmetric.

**TECHNIQUE**
We start in an Advasana, with the palms of the hands on the ground and in line with the shoulders. We keep the feet on the ground and stretch the arms to make the shape of a table. We bend the arms little by little until the body is parallel with the floor. The elbows should remain close to the body. If we want to accentuate this pose, we move the body forward slowly until the feet are supported on the tips of the toes. We remain in this position for a few seconds with the body stiff like a rod. We release the pose. We can repeat it a few times.

**RELATED ASANAS**
Chatuspadasana, or a four-footed pose, is a related asana. It would be the place to start the Chaturanga Dandasana pose. In this asana, the pelvis should not remain hanging below or above. The palms of the hands press against the floor strongly.

**VARIATION**
Perform the pose with the knees supported on the ground with the elbows flexed.

Chaturanga Dandasana is an asana that increases our energy and gives us inner strength. Develops our self-esteem. It stimulates the Manipura Chakra and the Anahata Chakra.

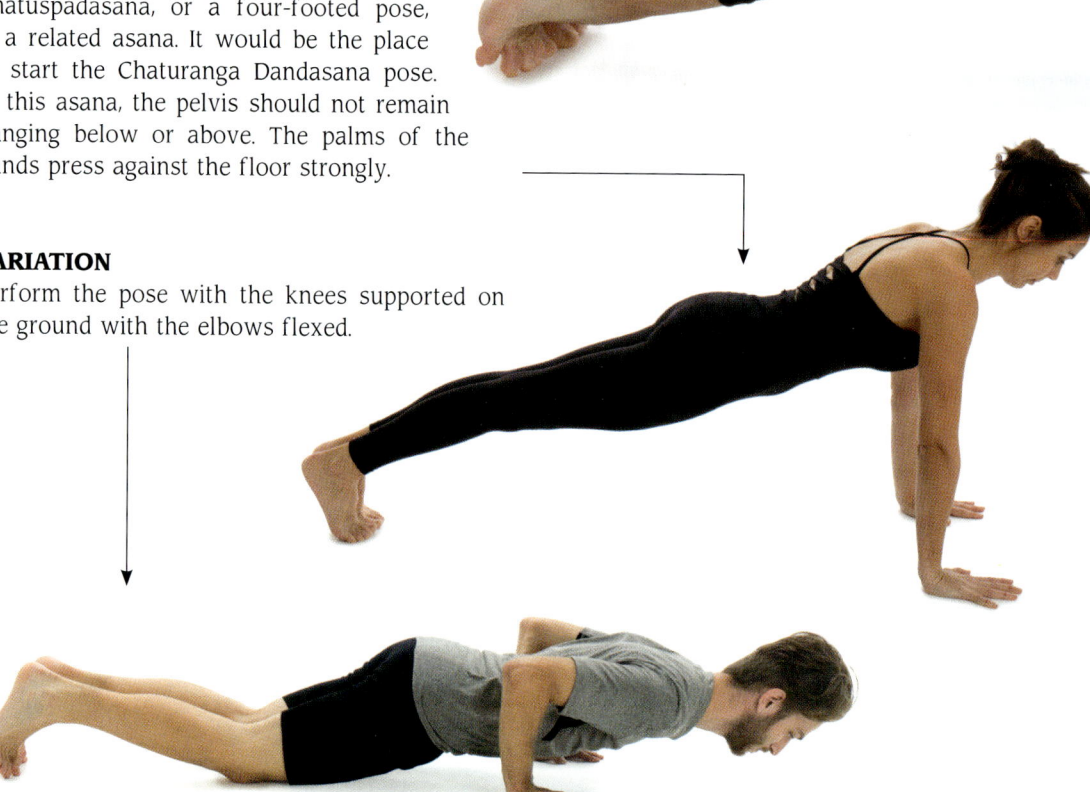

KRAFT ERFORDERNDE ASANAS: Chaturanga Dandasana 73

The serratus anterior holds the scapulae close to the rib cage.

- M. extensor carpi radialis longus
- M. brachioradialis
- M. erector spinae
- **M. serratus anterior**
- M. supraspinatus
- **M. triceps brachii**
- M. infraspinatus
- M. glutaeus maximus
- M. quadratus lumborum
- M. deltoideus (posterior part)
- M. deltoideus (middle part)
- M. deltoideus (anterior part)
- **M. pectoralis major**
- M. vastus lateralis
- M. rectus femoris
- **M. transversus abdominis**
- M. rectus abdominis
- M. brachialis
- M. extensor digitorum
- M. biceps brachii

The quadriceps keep the knees straight.

The effort is done by the erector muscles of the trunk, while the lumbar square and the abdominals stabilize the spine.

The pectoralis major and minor are activated, supporting the weight of the body, while the triceps and the biceps work together to stabilize the elbow.

Asanas

ASANAS OF BALANCE

# Vrikasana

*Vrika* means "tree;" it is the pose of the tree. This asana firmly roots us to the earth, at the same time that it elevates us to heaven; it evokes a tree, whose roots penetrate the ground while its branches grow upwards.

**BENEFITS**

- Strengthens and tones the feet and the muscles of the legs.
- Develops balance and concentration.
- Increases physical endurance.

**WARNINGS**

- Lack of balance; practice near the wall or with the backrest of a chair.
- Articular problems in the feet or legs; practice it with caution.
- Osteoarthritis of the shoulders; it is preferable not to raise the arms.

**CLASSIFICATION**
Basic pose for balance, asymmetric, standing.

**TECHNIQUE**
We start from Tadasana, and become aware of the weight our feet on the ground. Little by little, we move the weight to the left foot, bend the knee of the right leg, turn the leg out through the hip joint and place the foot in the lotus position or, if there is not enough flexibility, in the inner part of the left thigh, near the groin. The toes point toward the ground. We hold our gaze fixed at a point at eye level in order to maintain balance. We put our hands together and, while inhaling, we raise our arms above our heads. We maintain the position for as long as it is comfortable and then we undo it in the opposite direction. We repeat with the opposite side.

**VARIATIONS**
In the softer variation, we place the foot on the inner part of the thigh, with the fingers pointing toward the floor.

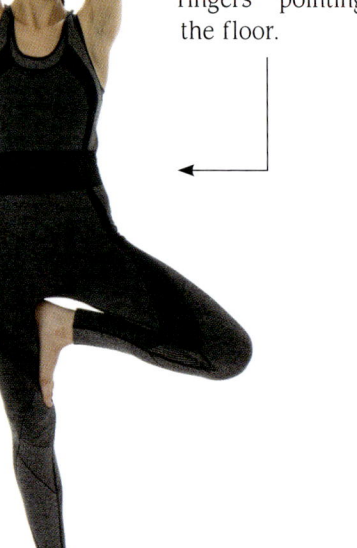

This other variation has the hands in *namaste*, in front of the chest, which gives us greater stability. If it is difficult for us to maintain balance, we can place our feet close to the ground with our fingers supported, or we can move the pose closer to a solid support, such as a wall or a chair.

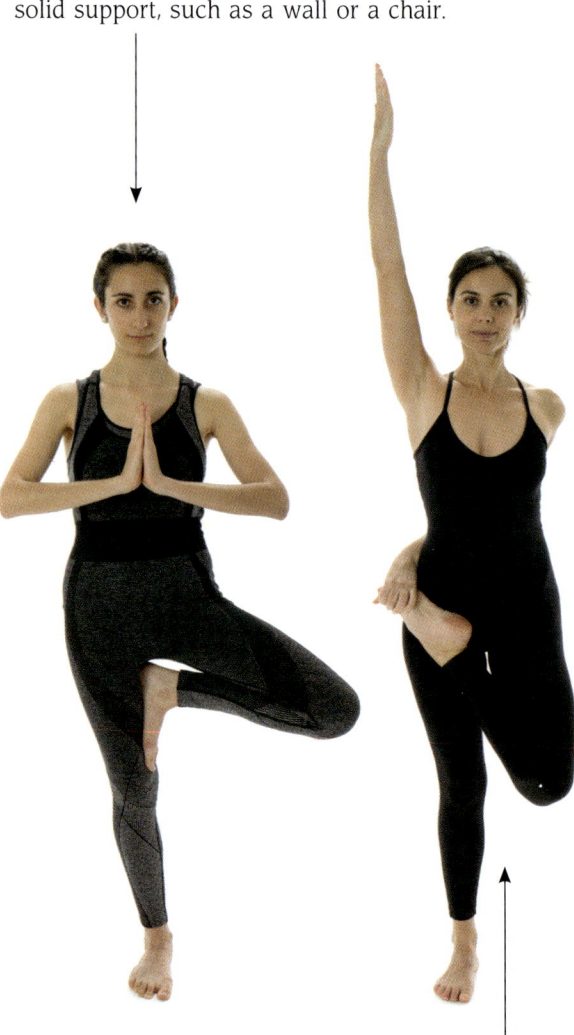

A more advanced position asks us to place the foot above the opposite hip, in lotus. We put our arms behind our backs and we reach for the foot with our hands. The other arm remains stretched up. Do not practice it if you have a meniscal problem.

ASANAS OF BALANCE: Vrikasana

Vrikasana develops inner balance and serenity. Practicing this helps us become calm at a mental level. We activate the Muladhara Chakra and energy flows between the three lower chakras (Muladhara, Svanisthana, and Manipura).

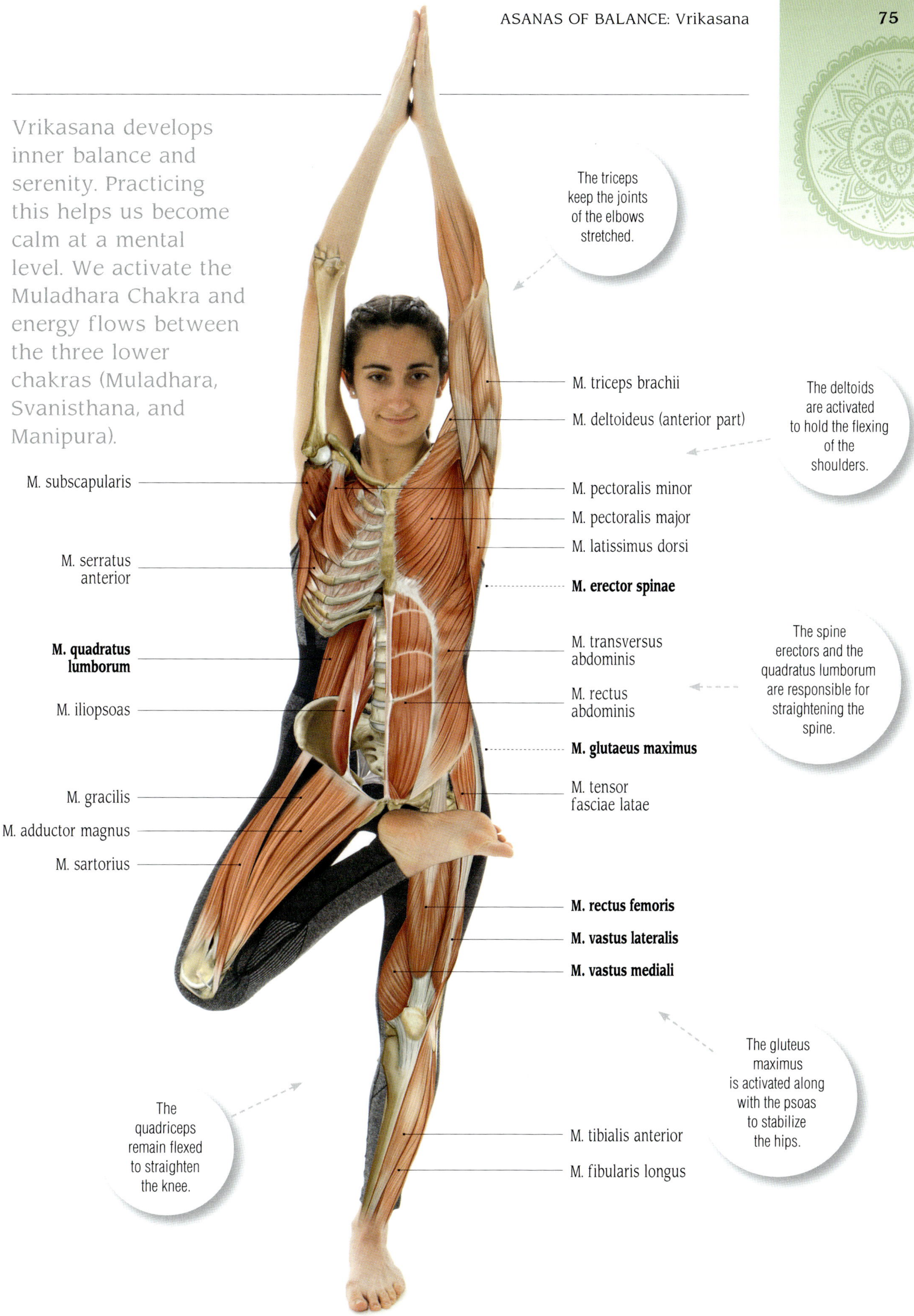

- M. subscapularis
- M. serratus anterior
- **M. quadratus lumborum**
- M. iliopsoas
- M. gracilis
- M. adductor magnus
- M. sartorius

- The triceps keep the joints of the elbows stretched.
- M. triceps brachii
- M. deltoideus (anterior part)
- The deltoids are activated to hold the flexing of the shoulders.
- M. pectoralis minor
- M. pectoralis major
- M. latissimus dorsi
- **M. erector spinae**
- M. transversus abdominis
- M. rectus abdominis
- **M. glutaeus maximus**
- M. tensor fasciae latae
- The spine erectors and the quadratus lumborum are responsible for straightening the spine.
- **M. rectus femoris**
- **M. vastus lateralis**
- **M. vastus mediali**
- M. tibialis anterior
- M. fibularis longus
- The gluteus maximus is activated along with the psoas to stabilize the hips.
- The quadriceps remain flexed to straighten the knee.

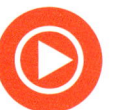

ASANAS OF BALANCE

# Garudasana

Garuda means "eagle," or "king of the birds." *Garuda* also represents the vehicles of the golden body of the god Visnu. This asana offers us balance while at the same time wisdom and a sharp and clear vision just like an eagle or a falcon seated on a rock.

**BENEFITS**
- Eliminates stiffness of the shoulders, arms, and wrists, increasing their mobility.
- Strengthens the muscles of the legs.
- Tones the abdominal area.

**WARNINGS**
- Weakness of knees, shoulders, and arms.
- Vertigo or balance problems.
- Cardiovascular problems; practice with prudence.
- Pregnancy.

**CLASSIFICATION**
Basic pose for balance, asymmetric, standing.

**TECHNIQUE**
We start from Tadasana. We bend the right knee, while aware of the support of the soles of the feet on the ground. We move our weight to the left leg and lift the right. We roll the right leg onto the left in such a way that the lower part of the leg is supported on the right thigh. The foot moves back and curls up in the rear area so that the toe touches the inner part of the opposite ankle. We hug the front of the body, the right arm on top of the left, so they are twisted together. We put the hands together. To release this pose, we can open the arms and stretch them back to stimulate the back. We repeat with the opposite side.

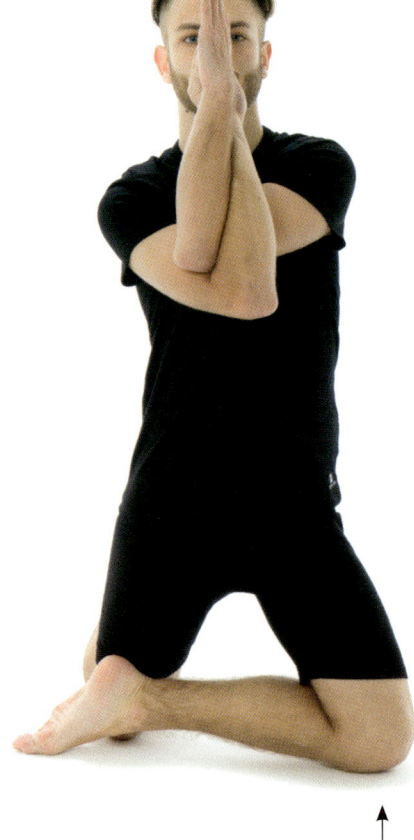

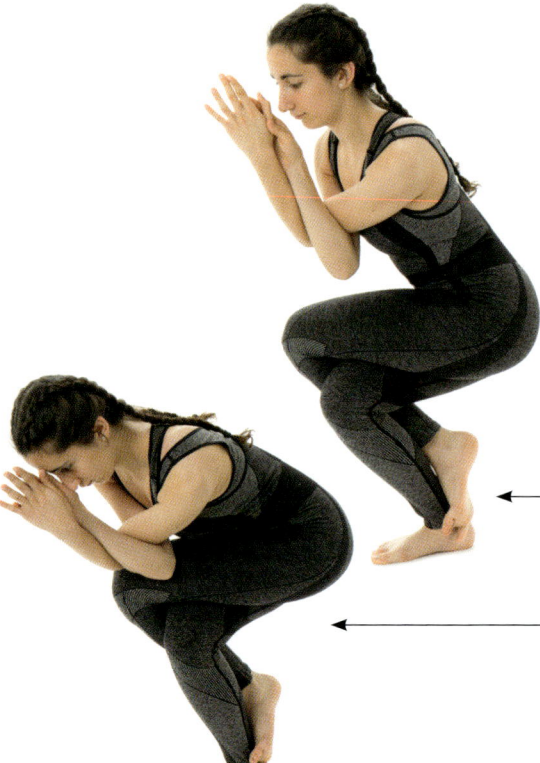

**VARIATION**
This variation for the legs opens the lateral hip. This offers more stability with a connection to the ground.

In this more advanced posture, we flex the hip and joints in the knees, the trunk remains straight. We practice this pose with care.

With the other variation, we go deeper into the asana. While keeping the spine straight, we bring the elbows close to the knees. The thumb is in the Ajna Chakra. We remain in this pose for a while. It is not appropriate for those who have cardiovascular problems.

ASANAS OF BALANCE: Garudasana 77

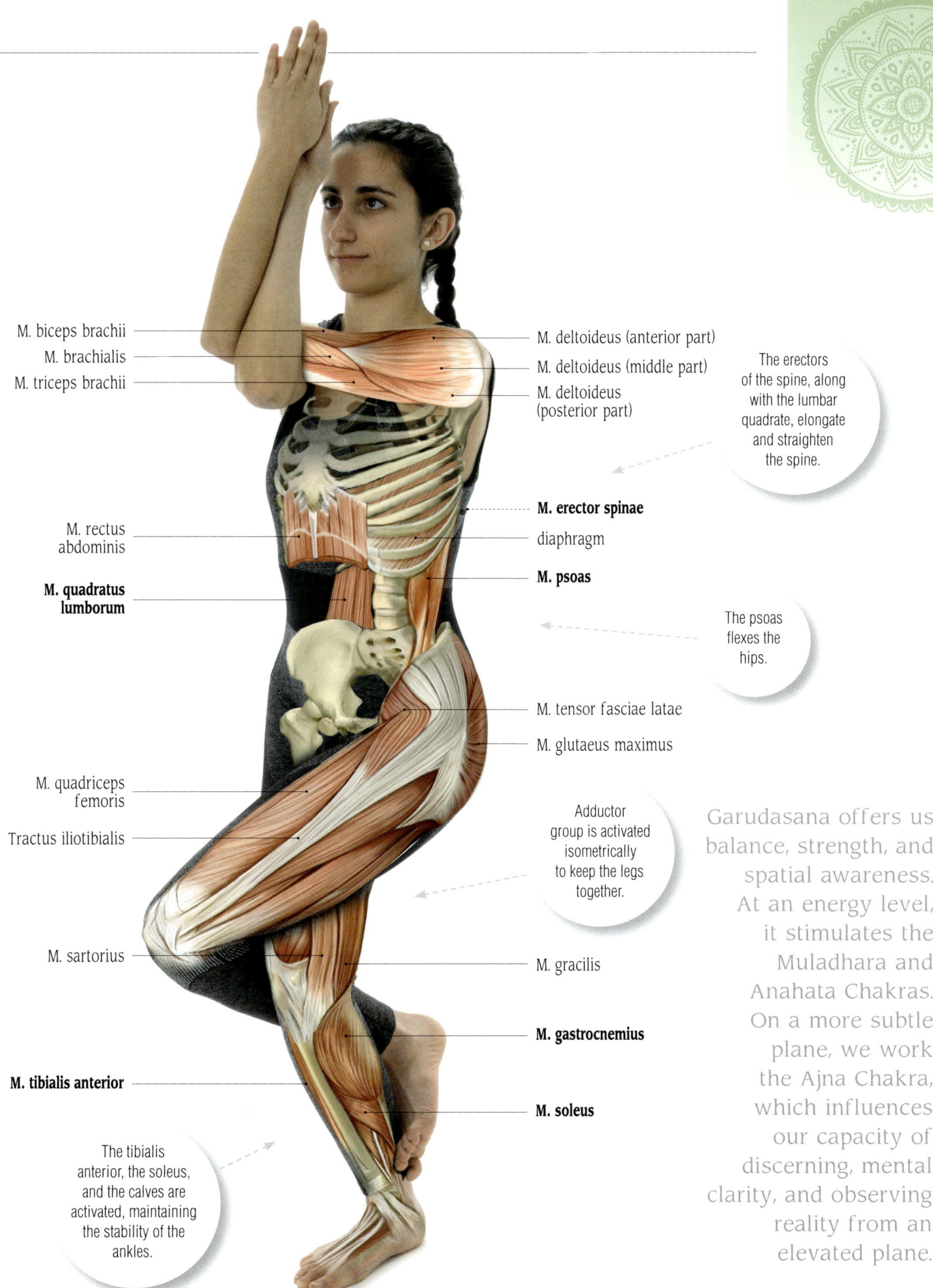

M. biceps brachii
M. brachialis
M. triceps brachii

M. deltoideus (anterior part)
M. deltoideus (middle part)
M. deltoideus (posterior part)

The erectors of the spine, along with the lumbar quadrate, elongate and straighten the spine.

M. erector spinae
diaphragm
M. psoas

M. rectus abdominis
**M. quadratus lumborum**

The psoas flexes the hips.

M. tensor fasciae latae
M. glutaeus maximus

M. quadriceps femoris
Tractus iliotibialis

Adductor group is activated isometrically to keep the legs together.

M. sartorius
M. gracilis

**M. gastrocnemius**

**M. tibialis anterior**
**M. soleus**

The tibialis anterior, the soleus, and the calves are activated, maintaining the stability of the ankles.

Garudasana offers us balance, strength, and spatial awareness. At an energy level, it stimulates the Muladhara and Anahata Chakras. On a more subtle plane, we work the Ajna Chakra, which influences our capacity of discerning, mental clarity, and observing reality from an elevated plane.

## ASANAS OF LATERAL FLEXING AND TRIKONAS

# Parighasana

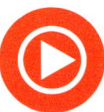

*Parigha* refers to the hinge that is used to close a door. In this pose, the body adopts a position appearing to be a bolt that closes a door. It symbolizes the quality of opening or closing a door.

**BENEFITS**
- Tones muscles and abdominal muscles.
- Provides flexibility to the spine and pelvis.
- Stretches and strengthens the leg muscles.
- Invigorates the spinal nerves.

**WARNINGS**
- Problems in the knees: place a folded blanket on the floor.
- Lower back injuries.

**CLASSIFICATION**
Lateral flexing pose, asymmetric, kneeling.

**TECHNIQUE**
We place the knees on the floor. We stretch the right leg to the side, leaving the foot supported and facing forward. The left leg remains perpendicular to the ground. We breathe in and open the arms laterally; the right arm searches for the right leg, while the left arm rotates and elevates above the head, accompanied by the lateral flexing of the trunk. We should not bend the trunk forward; the legs, the trunk, the arms, and the head should be on the same plane. We hold this pose a few seconds and then release. We proceed to do the same on the other side.

**VARIATION**
Variation with lateral flexing in which we support the hand on the floor, and we stretch the arm following the natural curvature of the torso.

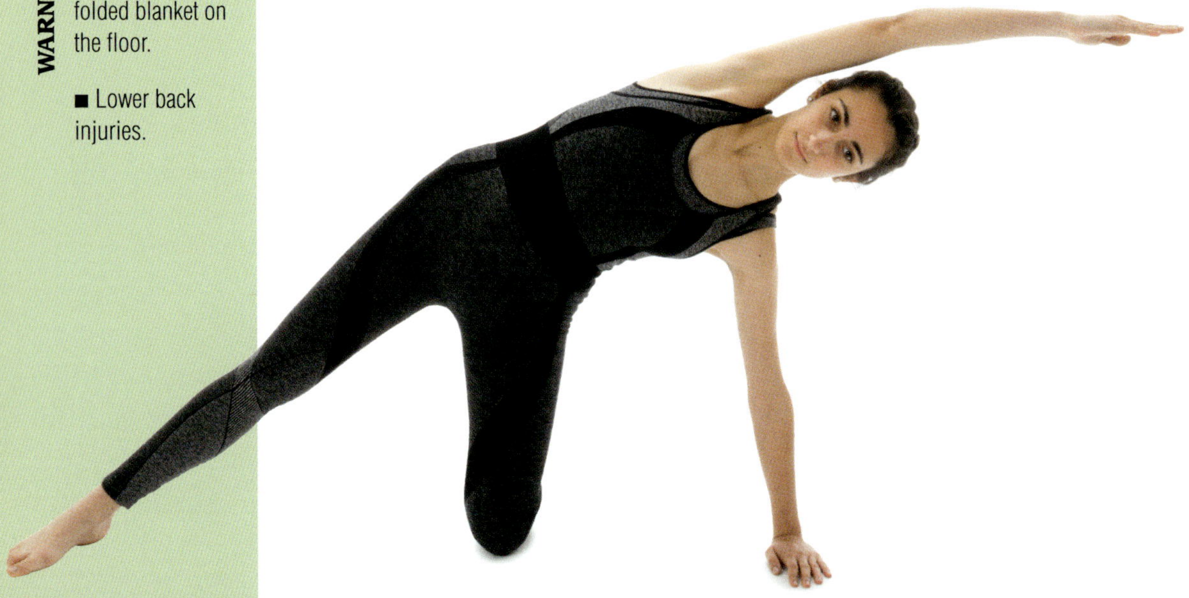

**RELATED ASANA**
Nitambasana. Asana of lateral flexing with the feet together. To perform this pose, we stretch the arms up as high as possible, we twist the pelvis backward and flex the spine laterally to make a slight arc. We can practice this while on the floor, with one arm supporting one side of the body.

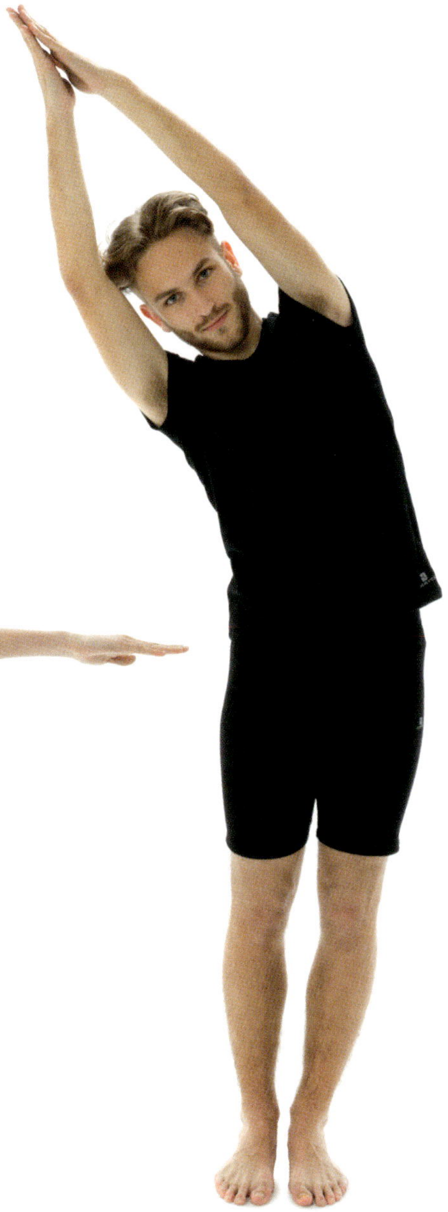

## ASANAS OF LATERAL FLEXING AND TRIKONAS: Parighasana

Parighasana symbolizes change. This pose offers us an adaptation and flexibility facing the changes of life. It balances the energetic activity of the two sides of the body. There is an energy exchange between the Manipura Chakra and the Anahata Chakra.

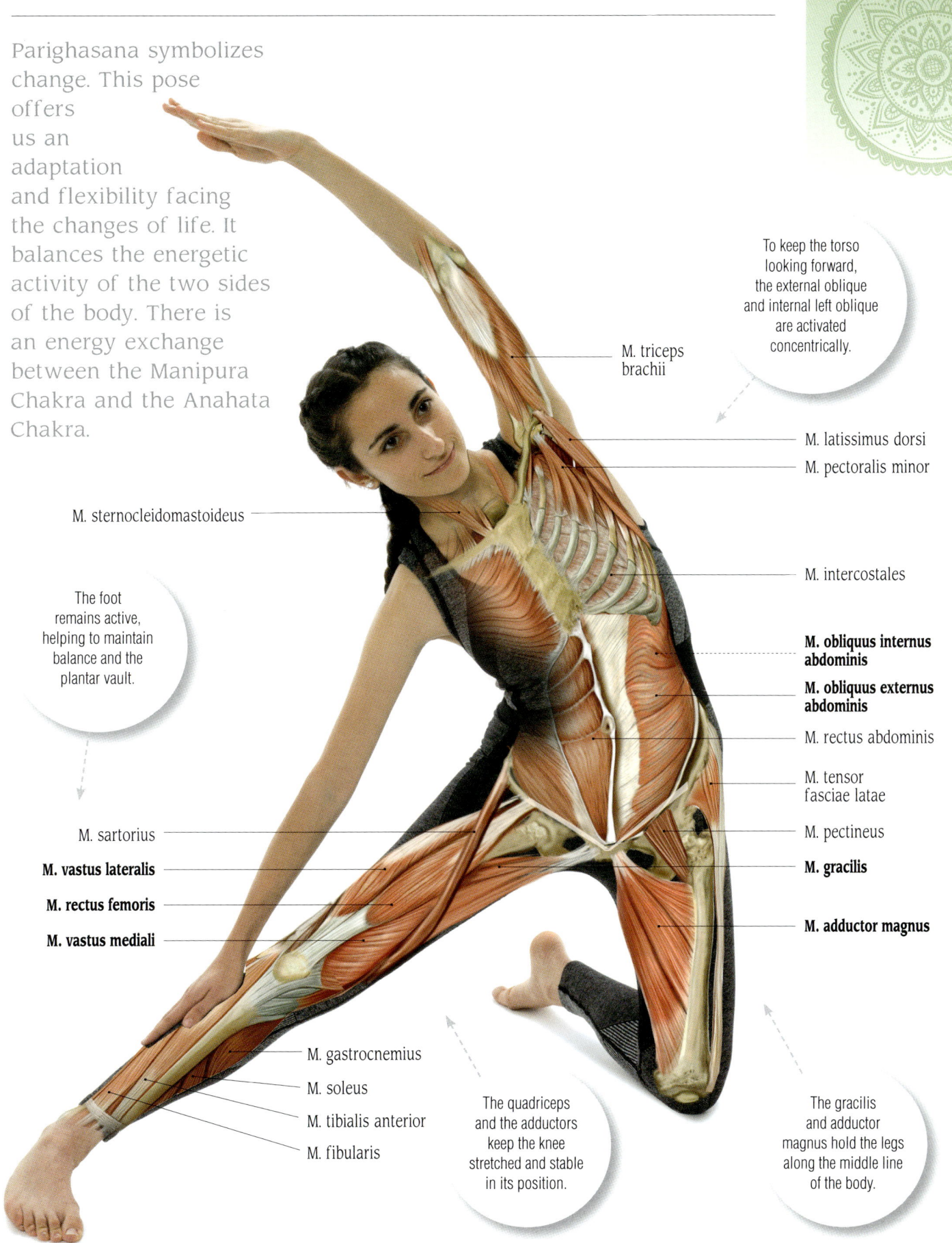

To keep the torso looking forward, the external oblique and internal left oblique are activated concentrically.

- M. triceps brachii
- M. latissimus dorsi
- M. pectoralis minor
- M. sternocleidomastoideus
- M. intercostales
- **M. obliquus internus abdominis**
- **M. obliquus externus abdominis**
- M. rectus abdominis
- M. tensor fasciae latae
- M. pectineus
- **M. gracilis**
- **M. adductor magnus**

The foot remains active, helping to maintain balance and the plantar vault.

- M. sartorius
- **M. vastus lateralis**
- **M. rectus femoris**
- **M. vastus mediali**
- M. gastrocnemius
- M. soleus
- M. tibialis anterior
- M. fibularis

The quadriceps and the adductors keep the knee stretched and stable in its position.

The gracilis and adductor magnus hold the legs along the middle line of the body.

ASANAS OF LATERAL FLEXING AND TRIKONAS

# Utthita Trikonasana

*Utthita* means "extended," and *trikona* is "triangle." This is the extended triangle pose, which invokes harmony along the three planes of the human being: physical, mental, and spiritual.

## BENEFITS

- Strengthens the muscles of the abdomen, legs, and pelvis.
- Increases the stretch of the back of the legs.
- Mobilizes the hip joints.
- Makes the spine flexible (it is appropriate for scoliosis).
- Develops balance.

## WARNINGS

- Severe problems in the lumbar region, displaced vertebrae, or neck problems.
- Inflammation of the abdomen, inguinal hernia.

## CLASSIFICATION

Lateral flexing pose, asymmetric, standing.

## TECHNIQUE

We start from Tadasana. We separate the legs laterally. With a breath we raise the arms to the height of the shoulders, with the palms of the hands facing the ground. We rotate the right foot a little to the inside and the left foot 90º to the right. With an exhale, we bend the trunk and bring the left hand to the right ankle. If we have plenty of flexibility, we can support the hand on the ground. The left arm remains up, with the palm of the hand facing ahead. We rotate the head and look toward the left hand. In the final position, the legs, the trunk, the arms, and the head are in the same plane. We hold this pose a few seconds and release it per the following: first, we tense the muscles of the legs, the thighs and the hips, and then we raise the body little by little. We can also release from this pose by bending the stretched knee. We repeat the pose on the other side.

## ADAPTATIONS

If we have limited flexibility, we can use a support to start this asana. If we experience dizziness or injuries to the cervicals, it would be helpful to look forward.

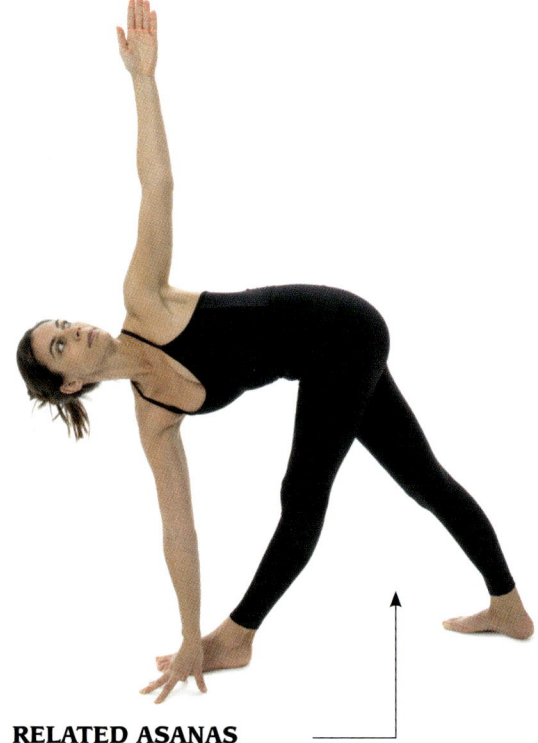

## RELATED ASANAS

*Parivritta Trikonasana* means "triangle looking ahead" and it is a twisting asana related to Utthita. This pose follows a feeling contrary to Utthita. We start the same way, with the legs separated, rotating the feet, with the arms crossed, but this time we rotate the body to move the right hand to the left ankle (or the ground). We stretch the left arm up and align it with the right. We rotate the head slowly and look at the hand. This pose requires strength and flexibility.

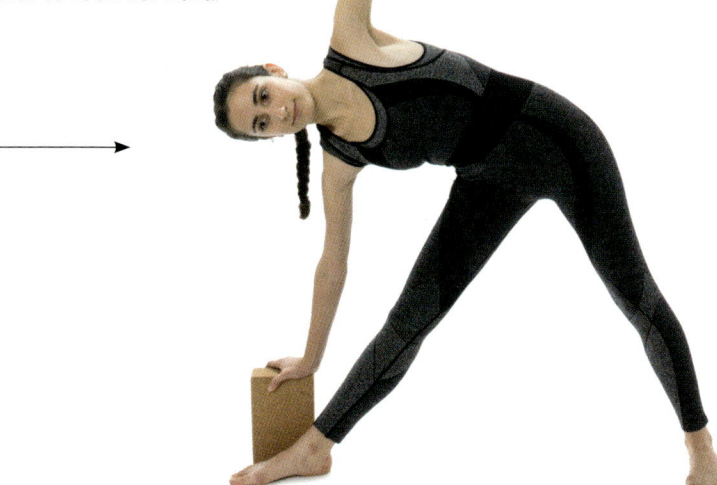

# ASANAS OF LATERAL FLEXING AND TRIKONAS: Utthita Trikonasana

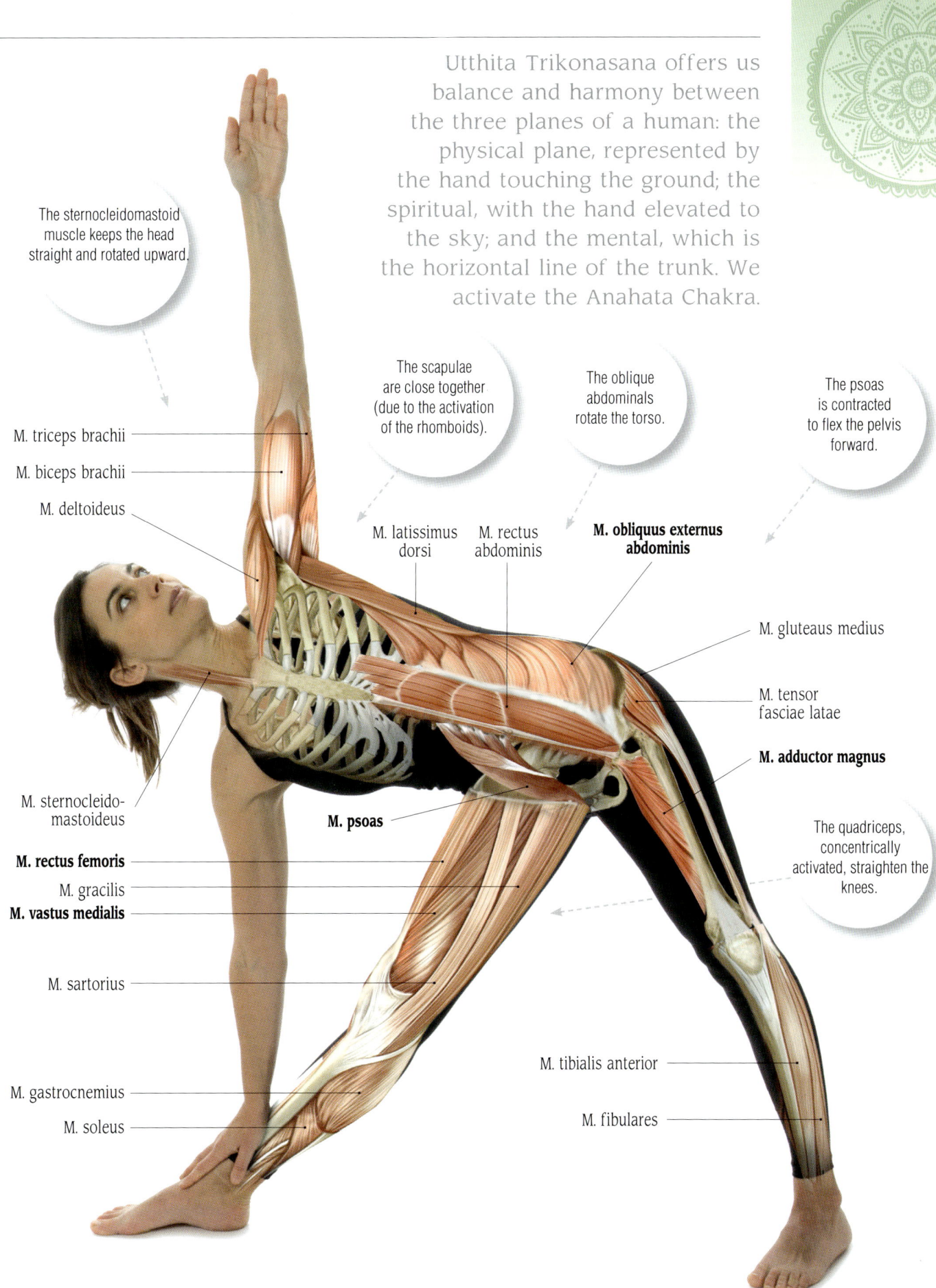

Utthita Trikonasana offers us balance and harmony between the three planes of a human: the physical plane, represented by the hand touching the ground; the spiritual, with the hand elevated to the sky; and the mental, which is the horizontal line of the trunk. We activate the Anahata Chakra.

The sternocleidomastoid muscle keeps the head straight and rotated upward.

The scapulae are close together (due to the activation of the rhomboids).

The oblique abdominals rotate the torso.

The psoas is contracted to flex the pelvis forward.

The quadriceps, concentrically activated, straighten the knees.

- M. triceps brachii
- M. biceps brachii
- M. deltoideus
- M. latissimus dorsi
- M. rectus abdominis
- **M. obliquus externus abdominis**
- M. gluteus medius
- M. tensor fasciae latae
- **M. adductor magnus**
- M. sternocleido-mastoideus
- **M. psoas**
- **M. rectus femoris**
- M. gracilis
- **M. vastus medialis**
- M. sartorius
- M. tibialis anterior
- M. gastrocnemius
- M. fibulares
- M. soleus

Asanas

ASANAS OF LATERAL FLEXING AND TRIKONAS

# Utthita Parsva Konasana

*Parsva* means "side" and *kona* means "angle." Its name refers to the extended pose in a lateral angle.

**BENEFITS**

- Stretches the side with intensity.
- Strengthens and stretches the muscles of the feet, legs, thighs, hips, and trunk.
- Provides strength and endurance.
- Stimulates the organs of the abdominal cavity.

**WARNINGS**

- Back injuries: use an adaptation.
- Headache.

**CLASSIFICATION**
Lateral flexing pose, asymmetric, standing.

**TECHNIQUE**
We start from Tadasana. We open the legs, rotate the right foot out 90º and the left foot inward 45º. We extend the arms in a cross. We bend the right knee making a right angle that is aligned with the ankle. We lean the trunk until we place the right hand on the ground, next to the right foot, and we stretch the left arm parallel with the trunk. The palm of the left hand should stay low. We slowly rotate the head and look up. To release the pose, we can place both hands on the ground and rise up little by little. We repeat with the opposite side.

**ADAPTATION**
If we cannot place the hand on the ground, or have some pain in the back, we need to use a cork block, placing it on the inside of the right foot. The arm may stretch up or be parallel with the body.

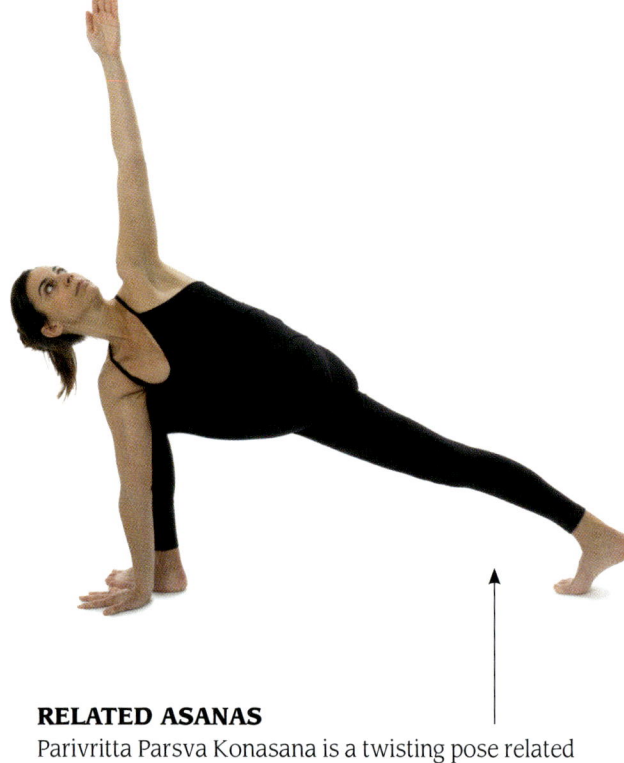

**RELATED ASANAS**
Parivritta Parsva Konasana is a twisting pose related to the previous pose. It is a pose of a twisting lateral angle. It is structured like the previous one, but we rotate the trunk to bring the left arm above the right knee with the palm of the left hand supported on the ground next to the right foot. It is a much more intense pose than Utthita.

This variation of Parivritta Parsva Konasana is a twisting asana, asymmetric, kneeling. We place the hands in *namasté*.

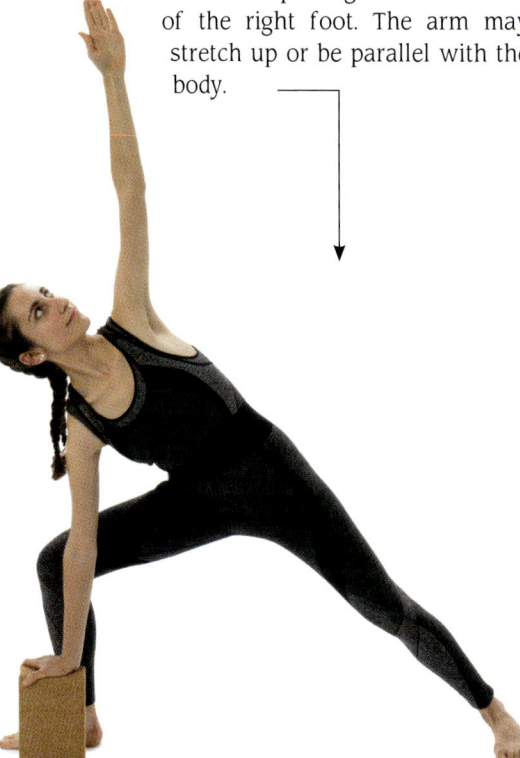

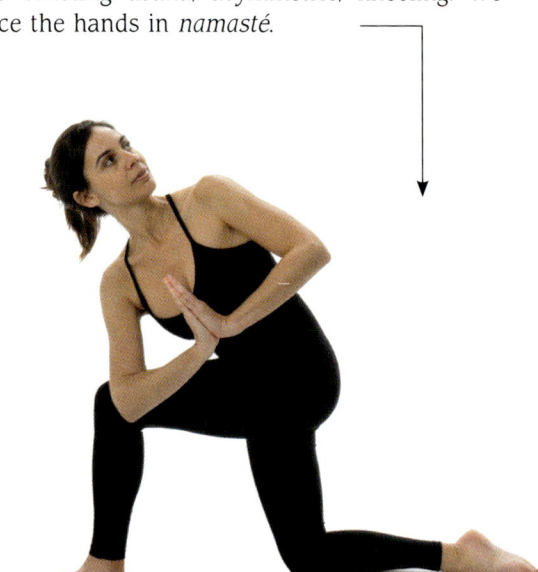

## ASANAS OF LATERAL FLEXING AND TRIKONAS: Utthita Parsva Konasana

Utthita Parsva Konasana allows for the channels of Ida and Pingala to open, which benefits the flow of energy through the central channel of Sushumna. At the mental level, it offers us stability and a connection to our masculine and feminine side, creating a balance between the opposite energies (Sun/Moon, Earth/sky).

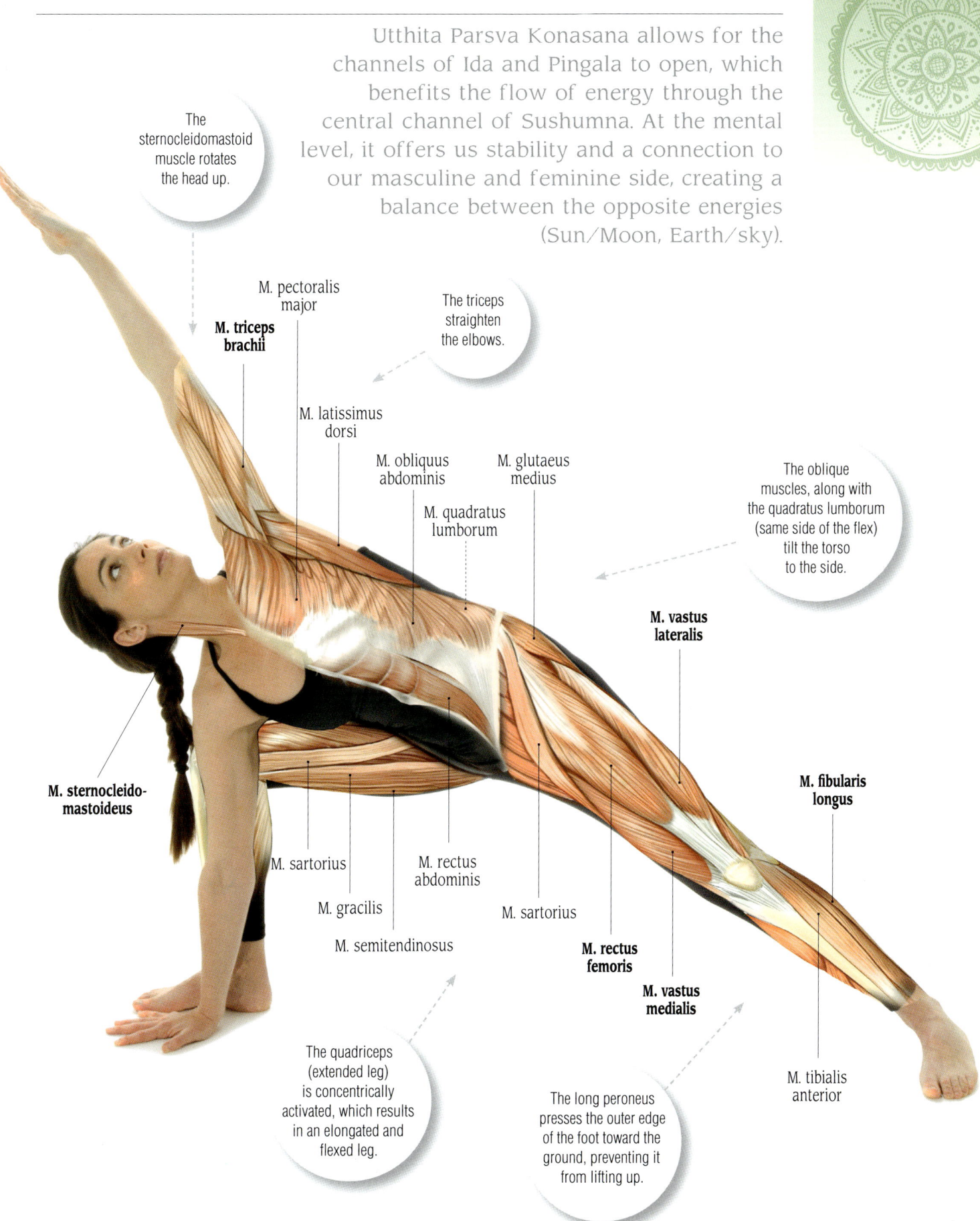

- The sternocleidomastoid muscle rotates the head up.
- The triceps straighten the elbows.
- The oblique muscles, along with the quadratus lumborum (same side of the flex) tilt the torso to the side.
- The quadriceps (extended leg) is concentrically activated, which results in an elongated and flexed leg.
- The long peroneus presses the outer edge of the foot toward the ground, preventing it from lifting up.

Labels: M. triceps brachii, M. pectoralis major, M. latissimus dorsi, M. obliquus abdominis, M. glutaeus medius, M. quadratus lumborum, M. vastus lateralis, M. sternocleidomastoideus, M. sartorius, M. gracilis, M. semitendinosus, M. rectus abdominis, M. sartorius, M. rectus femoris, M. vastus medialis, M. fibularis longus, M. tibialis anterior

Asanas

ASANAS OF EXTENSION VARIATION

# Setu-Bandhasana

*Setu* means "bridge" and *bandha* means "close" and also "formation." The pose simulates the building of a bridge.

**BENEFITS**
- Strengthens muscles at the base of the pelvis, the lumbar area, and the legs.
- Keeps the spine flexible.
- Prepares for practicing pranayama and bandhas.

**WARNINGS**
- Hypertension.
- Cataracts or eye problems.
- Migraines and headaches, inflammations of the head.
- Cervical injuries.

**CLASSIFICATION**
Inverted symmetrical pose, extended chest.

**TECHNIQUE**
We start from Savasana, placing the arms on the floor next to the body with the palms of the hands facing down. We bend the knees to place the feet on the ground, parallel together, close to the buttocks, and in line with the hips. With a breath, we flex the muscles at the base of the pelvis, raising the coccyx, and the sacrum bone, and we lift the entire lumbar spine and chest off of the ground, from bottom to top, vertebra by vertebra. We place the hands on the back, at the level of the pelvis. We move the sternum close to the chin. The weight of the body is distributed between the feet and the shoulders. We hold this pose with intermittent breathing. To release it, while exhaling, we slowly return the back to the floor, vertebra by vertebra.

**COUNTER POSE**
Apanasana.

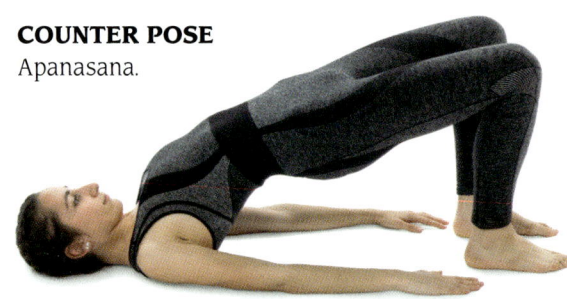

**VARIATION**
For the variation Dwi Pada Pitham, the arms are stretched along the side of the body, with the palms of the hands facing the floor. It is important to keep the base of the big toe well grounded. Raise the sternum toward the chin and elevate the gluteals away from the ground. We can practice this pose dynamically by inhaling while we raise the pelvis and the spine vertebra by vertebra and exhaling as we lower the spine inversely.

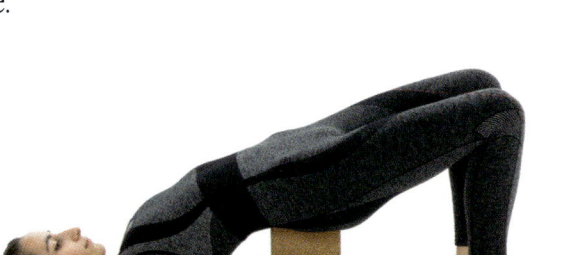

**ADAPTATIONS**
We place a cork block under us in order to hold the pose without over-exerting the back.

**RELATED ASANAS**
Urdhva Dhanurasana. In this pose, the body is curved upward like an arc. We start from the initial position of the previous poses. We place the palms of the hands under the shoulders and the feet on the ground, as close to the buttocks as possible. When exhaling, we start to raise the trunk while resting the head on the floor for a moment. With the following exhale, we press the hands and feet against the floor and raise the trunk while arching the back. The weight of the body falls on the palms of the hands and the feet. It is an intense pose that should not be done if you have back problems or hernias or while pregnant.

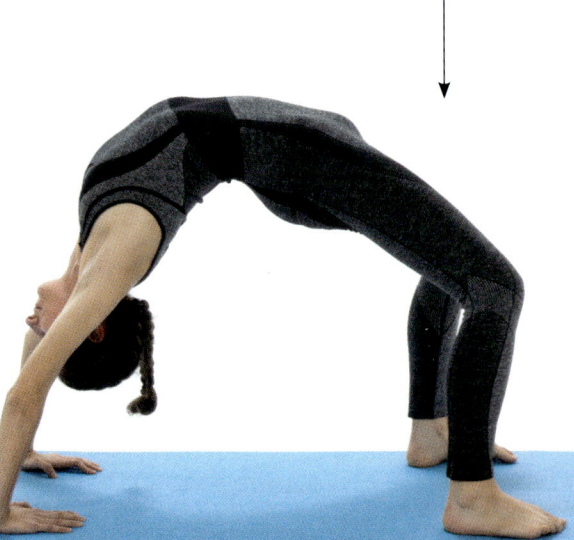

ASANAS OF EXTENSION: Setu-Bandhasana

In Setu-Bandhasana, energy flows from the Muladhara Chakra toward Vishuddha, stimulating the Anahata Chakra and the Manipura to Muladhara Chakra. This asana liberates emotions and provides us mental strength, energy, and a sensation of balance and inner peace.

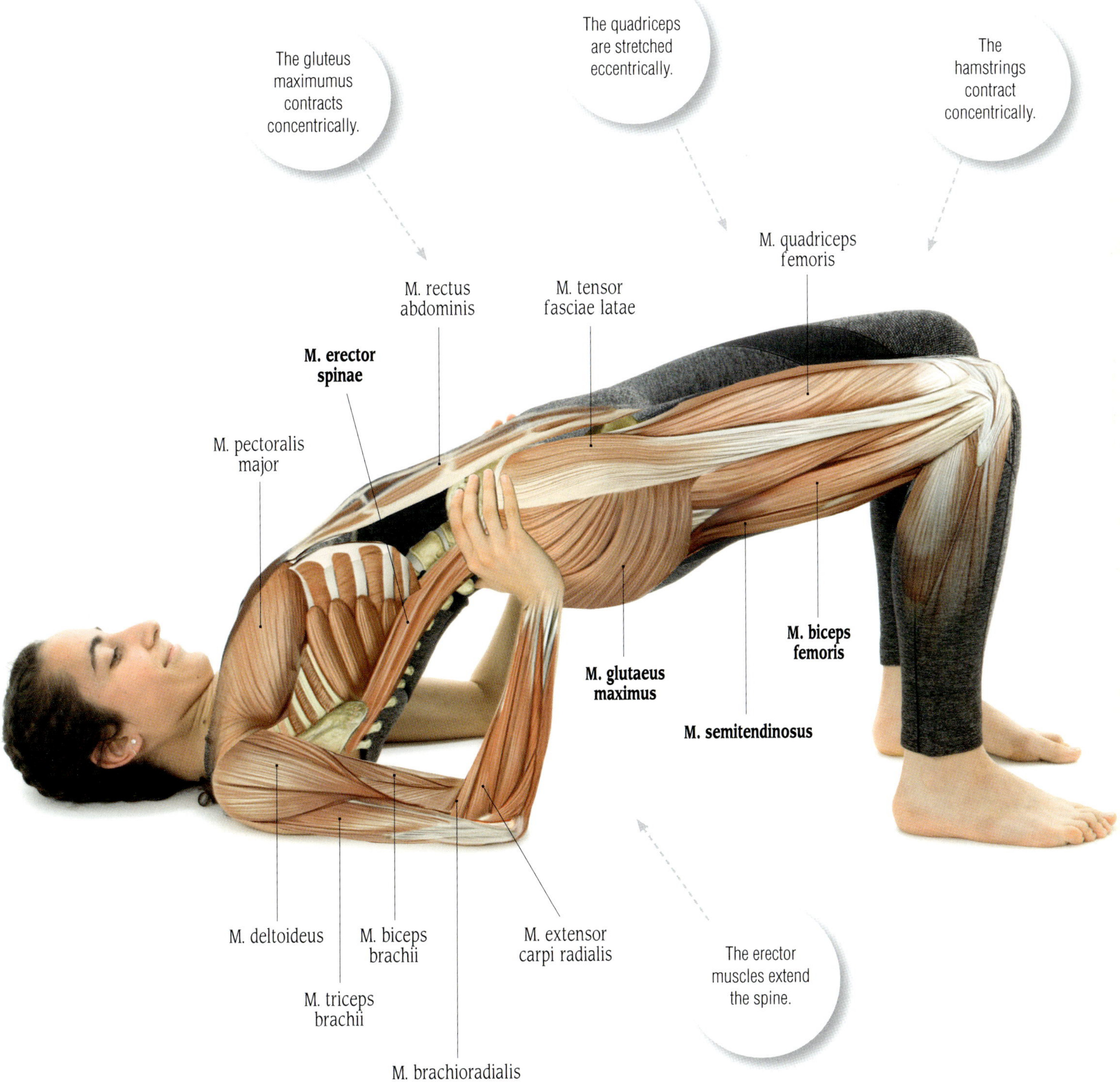

- The gluteus maximumus contracts concentrically.
- The quadriceps are stretched eccentrically.
- The hamstrings contract concentrically.
- The erector muscles extend the spine.

Labels:
- M. rectus abdominis
- M. tensor fasciae latae
- M. quadriceps femoris
- **M. erector spinae**
- M. pectoralis major
- **M. biceps femoris**
- **M. glutaeus maximus**
- **M. semitendinosus**
- M. deltoideus
- M. biceps brachii
- M. extensor carpi radialis
- M. triceps brachii
- M. brachioradialis

Asanas

ASANAS OF EXTENSION

# Purvottanasana

*Purva* means "east," *ut* means "intense," and *tana* is "stretch." This pose stretches the entire rear part of the body, lengthening it. It is also known as the Sun pose, since it is practiced facing the east, with the rising sun.

**BENEFITS**
- Strengthens wrists and ankles.
- Strengthens the back muscles.
- Expands the chest and develops breathing.
- Stimulates circulation.

**WARNINGS**
- Articular problems in arms or wrists.
- General weakness.
- Neck injuries: do not drop your head back.

**CLASSIFICATION**
Symmetric pose, extended chest.

**TECHNIQUE**
Starting from Dandasana, we lightly flex the knees and place the soles of the feet on the ground. While exhaling, we press the palms of the hands on the floor and flex the pelvis muscles; in this way, we elevate the trunk and the pelvis. The soles of the feet should keep maximum contact with the ground. The whole rear part of the body is flat like a table, with the arms stretched perpendicularly to the ground. We can align the head with the trunk. We hold the pose. To release it, while exhaling, we bend the elbows and knees and return to sitting on the floor.

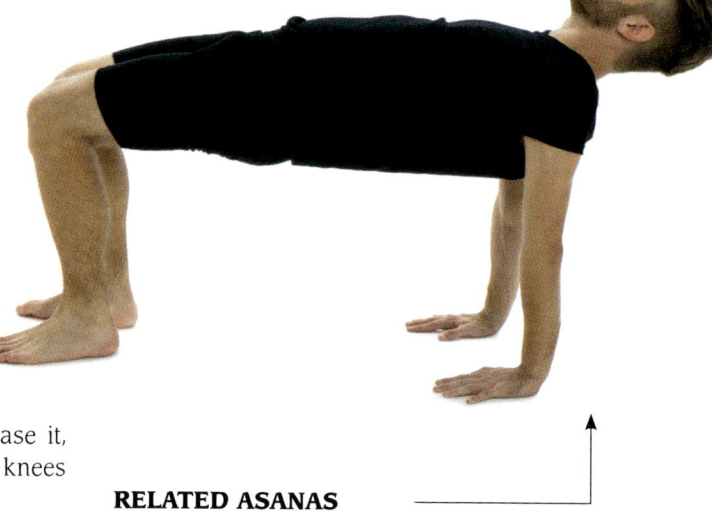

**RELATED ASANAS**
Chatus Pada Pitham is the table pose on four *(chatus)* feet *(pada)*. It is important to keep the thighs parallel at the level of the hips, the arms stretched, and the soles of the feet in contact with the floor. The head can be in line with the body.

In this variation, the fists are closed, and the thumb is outstretched. This is recommended if wrist problems are present or if arms are short.

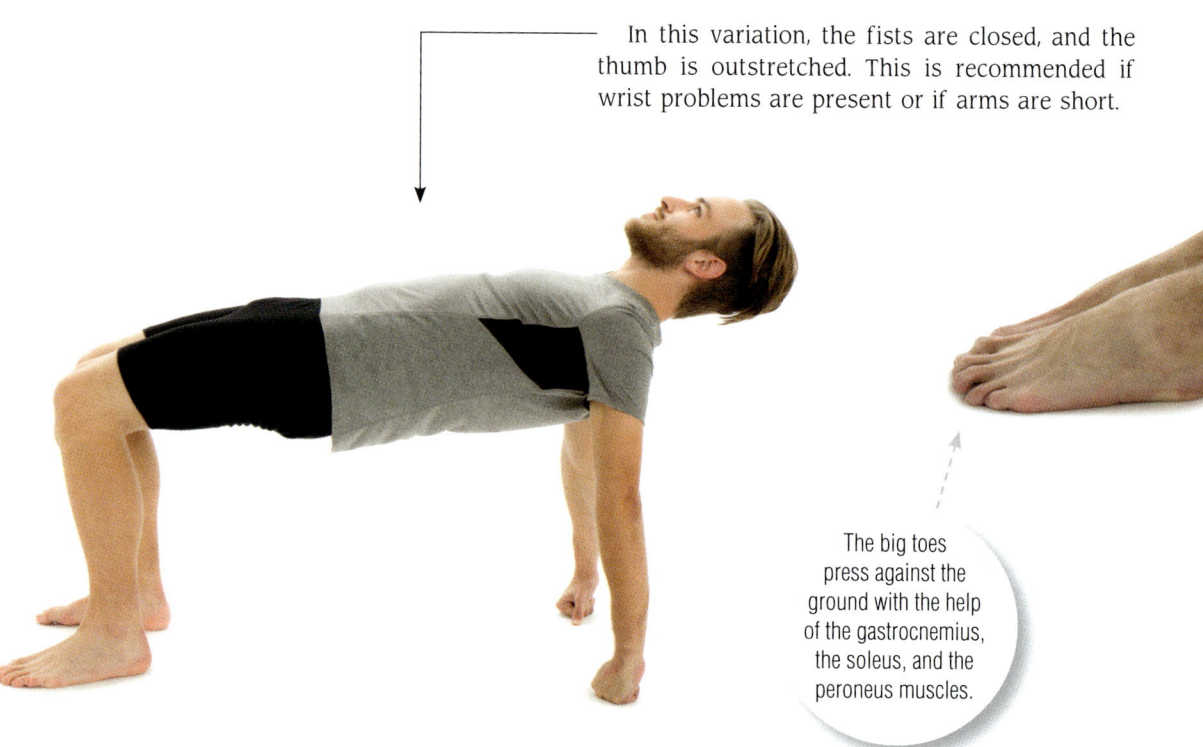

The big toes press against the ground with the help of the gastrocnemius, the soleus, and the peroneus muscles.

ASANAS OF EXTENSION: Purvottanasana

Purvottanasana influences the Anahata Chakra. It offers us energy and emotional balance. It has a sedative effect on the nervous system.

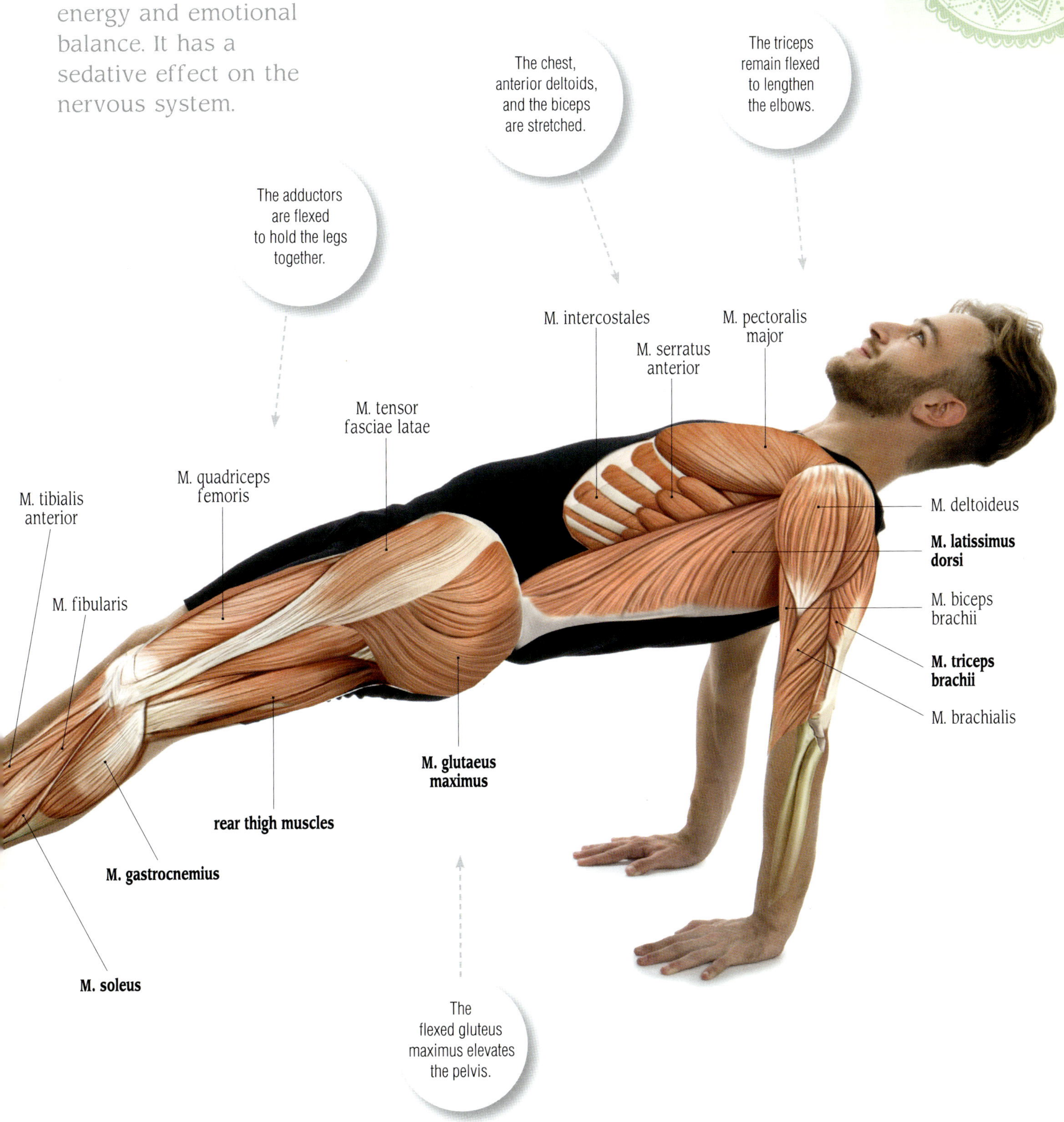

The adductors are flexed to hold the legs together.

The chest, anterior deltoids, and the biceps are stretched.

The triceps remain flexed to lengthen the elbows.

M. intercostales
M. serratus anterior
M. pectoralis major
M. tensor fasciae latae
M. quadriceps femoris
M. deltoideus
**M. latissimus dorsi**
M. tibialis anterior
M. biceps brachii
M. fibularis
**M. triceps brachii**
M. brachialis
**M. glutaeus maximus**
**rear thigh muscles**
**M. gastrocnemius**
**M. soleus**

The flexed gluteus maximus elevates the pelvis.

ASANAS OF EXTENSION

# Bhujangasana

Bhujanga means "snake." It is known as the "cobra pose," since the shape of the body appears like a snake that is raised from the ground. This pose symbolizes the strength of the practitioner.

**BENEFITS**
- Tones and relaxes the spine, and strengthens the muscles of the back and the legs.
- Expands the thorax.
- Stimulates digestion and kidney function.
- Invigorates the nervous system.

**WARNINGS**
- Problems in the lumbar spine (hernias, sciatica): perform it with caution.
- Hernias or inflammations in the abdominal area.
- Angina of the chest.

**CLASSIFICATION**
Thoracic extension in a prone position.

**TECHNIQUE**
We start in the Advasana pose, placing the legs together and stretching the feet. We place the hands under the shoulders. While inhaling, we first raise the head and then the thorax, focusing on raising one vertebra at a time. Initially, we only use the strength of the back, and little by little, we advance by pressing the palms of the hands against the floor and pushing with the arms. The buttocks and thighs are contracted. The shoulders should remain back and down, in a way that creates broadness in the thorax. The pubis stays in contact with the ground, and the spine extension should be spread equally, making sure not to create any pronounced lumbar lordosis. The head is in an anatomic position, and it isn't too far backward or shrugging. We look toward the horizon. We hold the pose by supporting the weight of the body with the arms. While exhaling, we slowly release the pose.

**COUNTER POSE**
Pranatasana.

**VARIATION**
The sphinx is a softer variation, since the elbows, forearms, and palms rest on the floor. We look toward the horizon.

**RELATED ASANAS**
Urdhva Mukha Svanasana is similar the dog pose. To practice it, we start in Advasana, with the feet separated and the palms of the hands place on both sides of the waist. While inhaling, we raise the head, the trunk, the pelvis, and the knees. The buttocks should be flexed in a way that all the weight of the body rests on the palms of the hands and the toes. It is an advanced pose.

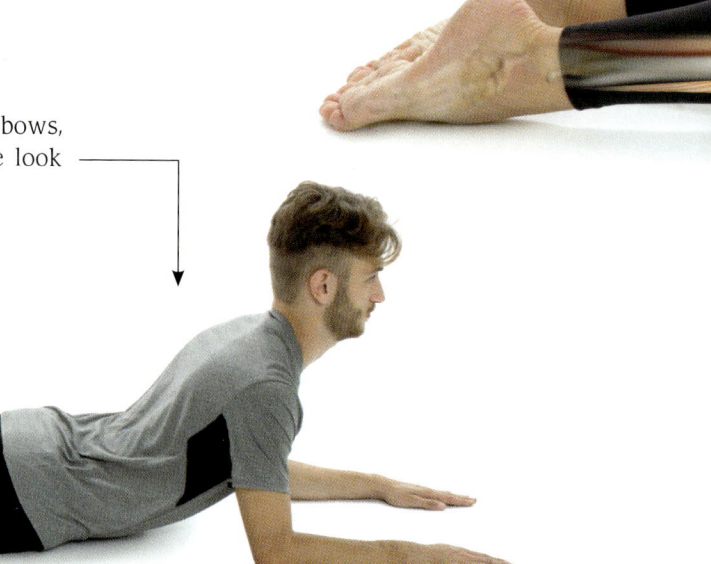

ASANAS OF EXTENSION: Bhujangasana

Bhujangasana helps to harmonize the three planes of a human being (physical, mental, and spiritual), offering confidence in ourselves, an open mind, vitality, and strength. Energy is first focused in the Manipura Chakra and ascends up to the Vishuddha Chakra.

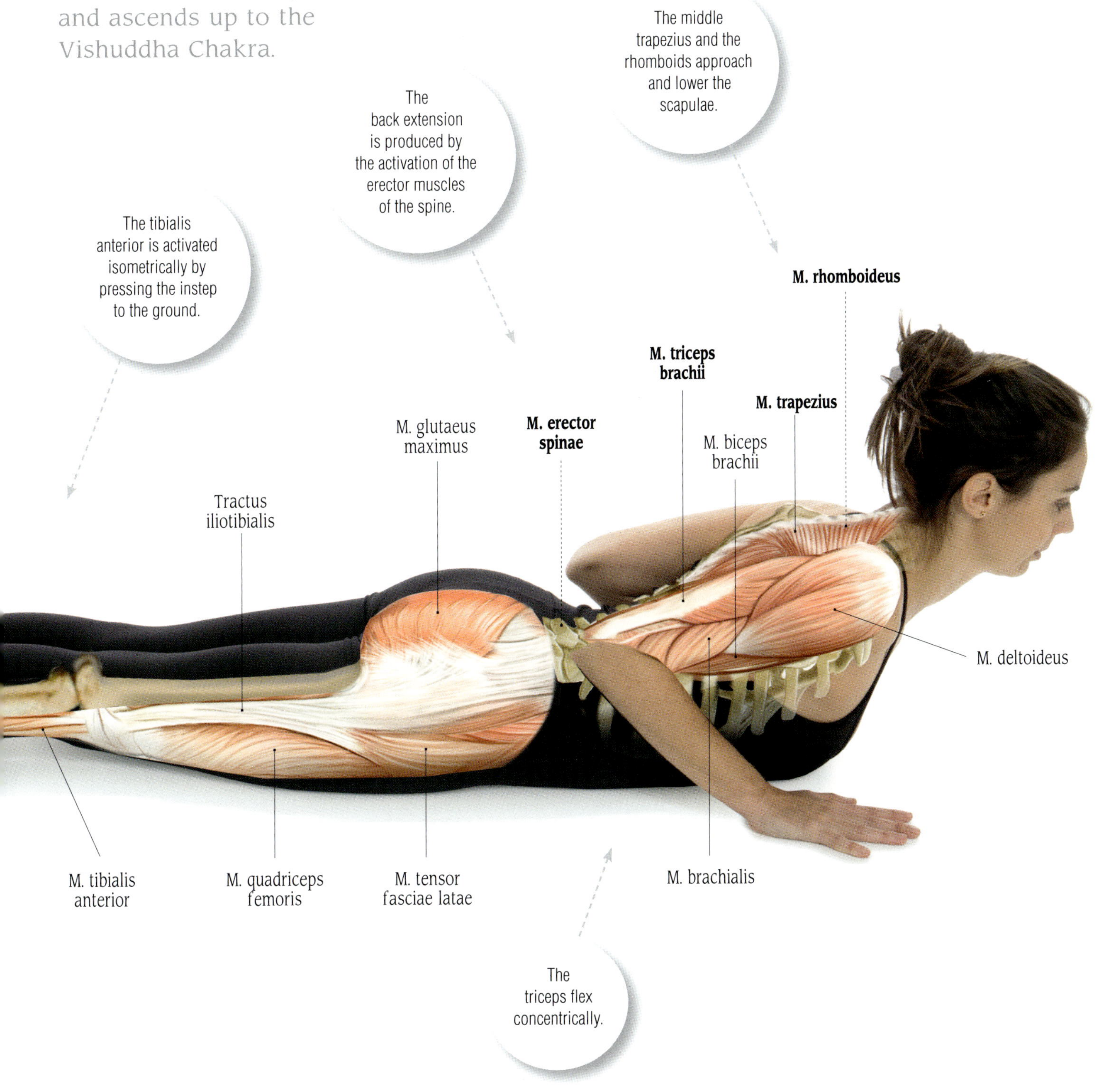

The middle trapezius and the rhomboids approach and lower the scapulae.

The back extension is produced by the activation of the erector muscles of the spine.

The tibialis anterior is activated isometrically by pressing the instep to the ground.

The triceps flex concentrically.

- **M. rhomboideus**
- **M. triceps brachii**
- **M. trapezius**
- M. glutaeus maximus
- **M. erector spinae**
- M. biceps brachii
- Tractus iliotibialis
- M. deltoideus
- M. tibialis anterior
- M. quadriceps femoris
- M. tensor fasciae latae
- M. brachialis

## ASANAS OF EXTENSION

# Matsyasana

*Matsya* means "fish." It is an asana dedicated to the incarnation of the god Vishnu in the shape of a fish. It evokes the continuity and substance of life.

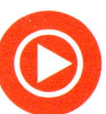

**BENEFITS**
- Strengthens the muscles of the neck, shoulders, and back.
- Expands the thorax, improves pulmonary ventilation.
- Thoroughly stretches the abdominal muscles.

**WARNINGS**
- Cervical problems.
- Injuries or problems in the joints of the knees, shoulders, and hips: use variations.
- Hypertension or hyperthyroidism: practice with caution, placing a cushion under the head.
- Ulcers, hernias, dizziness.

**CLASSIFICATION**
Extended thorax pose, symmetric, a face-up position.

**TECHNIQUE**
We start the pose seated in Padmasana (if it is difficult to do this pose from the lotus, we will do it with the legs extended). We lay on the floor and support ourselves with the forearms on the floor, arching the back and raising the thorax and the neck, placing the upper part of the head on the floor. Each hand searches for the opposite foot. With each breath, we try to expand the thorax region more and more. To release this pose, we support our body with the elbows, lower the head to the floor carefully, and rest on our back. We return to the initial pose and release the lotus.

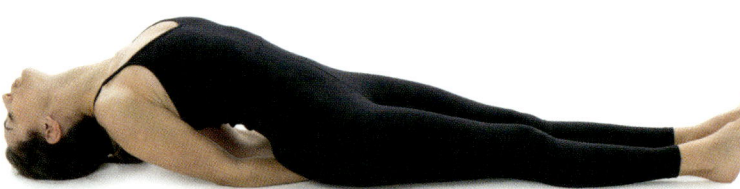

**VARIATION**
With stretched legs, we hold the weight of the body on the elbows and buttocks.

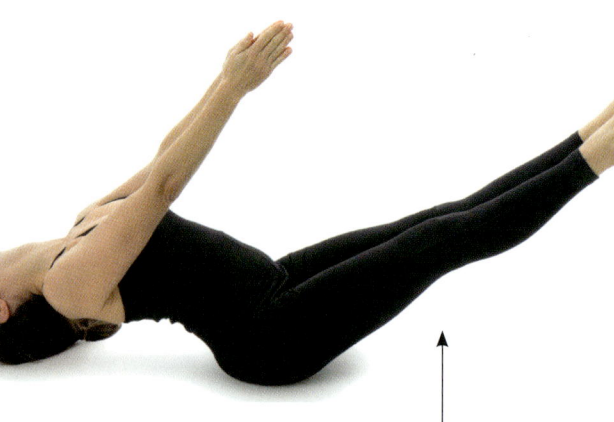

**RELATED ASANAS**
Uttana Padasana. This is an advanced pose that is done with the arms and legs elevated upward. We start in Matsyasana, holding the spine arched, extending the legs and the arms with the palms of the hands together, forming a 45° angle with the ground.

**ADAPTATIONS**
We use a doubled-up blanket or a cork block. Indicated for people with back problems. We let the arms fall relaxed at the sides, with the palms of the hands facing up. The legs can remain bent on the sides with the soles of the feet together (Baddha Konasana), or stretched.

ASANAS OF EXTENSION: Matsyasana

Matsyasana gives us a sensation of rest and calmness while at the same time, it opens us up to the universe. It stimulates the Anahata Chakra and activates the Vishuddha Chakra.

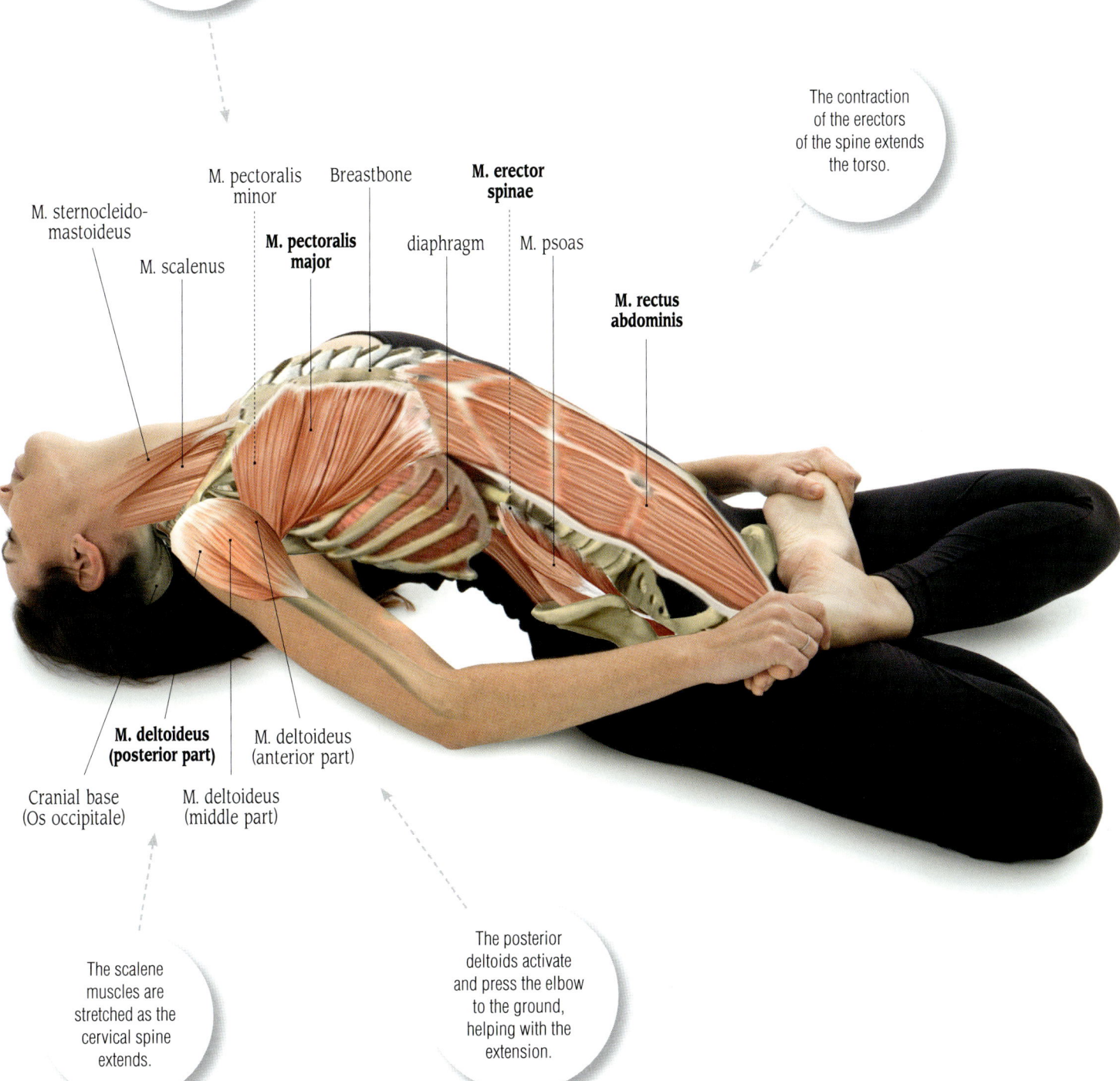

The chest stretches as the torso and arms extend.

The contraction of the erectors of the spine extends the torso.

The scalene muscles are stretched as the cervical spine extends.

The posterior deltoids activate and press the elbow to the ground, helping with the extension.

- M. sternocleido-mastoideus
- M. scalenus
- M. pectoralis minor
- **M. pectoralis major**
- Breastbone
- **M. erector spinae**
- diaphragm
- M. psoas
- **M. rectus abdominis**
- **M. deltoideus (posterior part)**
- M. deltoideus (anterior part)
- Cranial base (Os occipitale)
- M. deltoideus (middle part)

CLOSED OR FORWARD-FLEXING ASANAS

# Parsvottanasana

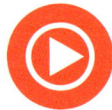

*Parsva* means "lateral," *ut* means "intense," and *tan*, "extend." It is an asana in which we practice an intense stretch throughout the entire lateral and posterior parts of the body. The hands are in a position of an inverted *namasté*, helping to open the thorax and the shoulders.

**BENEFITS**
- Intense stretching of the posterior muscles of the back, buttocks, and the back of the legs.
- Strengthens the muscles of the legs, feet, and those responsible for standing erect.

**WARNINGS**
- Injuries or back problems (e.g., sciatica, herniated discs).
- Blood pressure problems.

**CLASSIFICATION**
Semi-inverted pose, symmetric, flexed from the waist to the feet.

**TECHNIQUE**
We start in the Tadasana pose, separating the legs laterally to approximately one meter in distance. We rotate the trunk and the right foot about 90º, while the left foot rotates 75º. We place the palms of the hands next to the back, between the scapula, and open the elbows outward (the inverse Namaskara mudra). We breathe in and grow upward, contracting the muscles at the base of the pelvis. While exhaling, we lean with a straight spine toward the stretched leg. We hold the pose. To release it, we fold the knees a little and elevate the trunk with a flat back.

**ADAPTATIONS**
In case it is not possible to put the palms together behind the back, we put the hands on each opposite elbow.

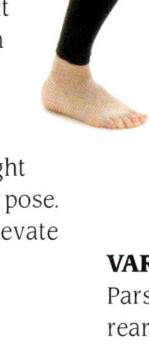

**VARIATION**
Parshva Uttanasana. We place the lightly flexed rear leg and the out stretched arms on the floor.

**ADAPTATION**
If we feel pain or weakness in the back, and we lack flexibility in the muscles of the legs, we can support ourselves on the cork block or a seat.

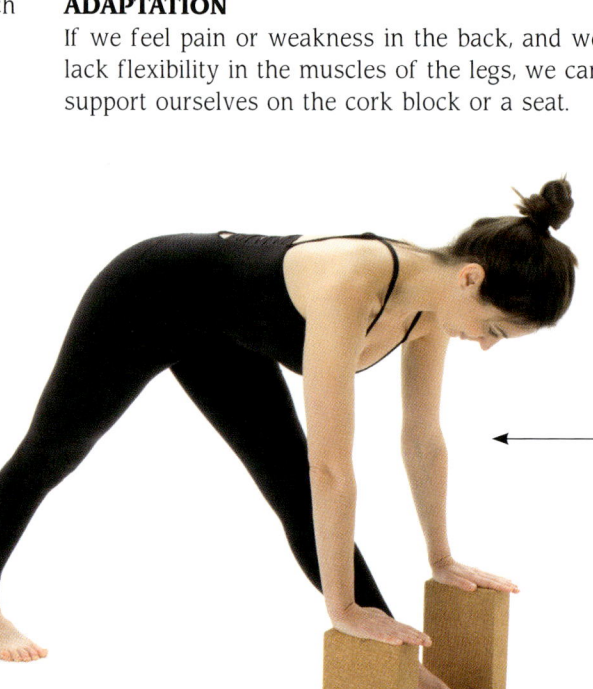

## CLOSED OR FORWARD-FLEXING ASANAS: Parsvottanasana

Parsvottanasana provides balance and resistance, creating confidence in the practitioner in the face of uncertainty. It also strengthens inner introspection. Energy circulates through Svadhistana in the direction of the Ajna Chakra.

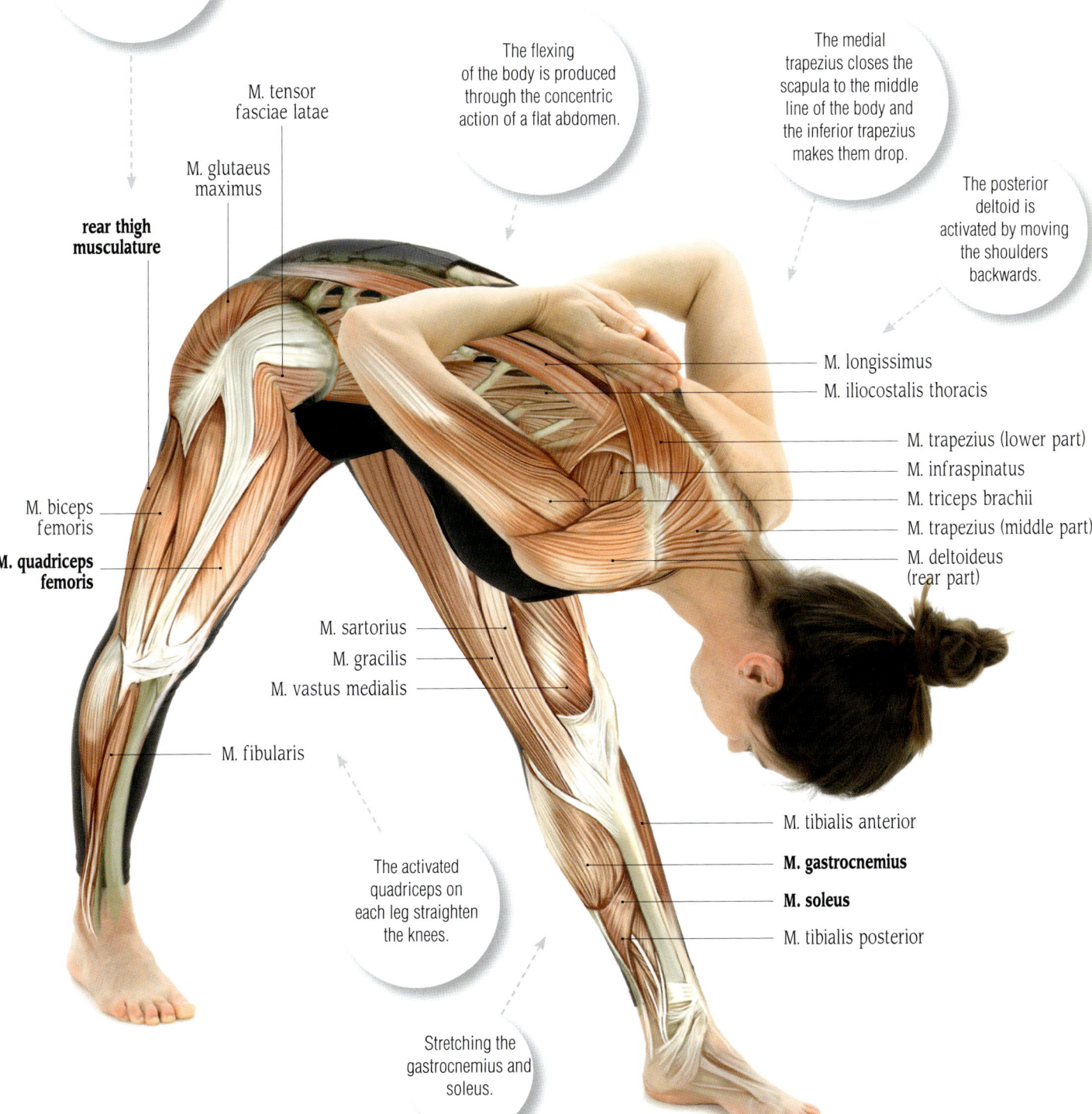

The flexing of the torso causes an intense stretch to the hamstring muscles.

The flexing of the body is produced through the concentric action of a flat abdomen.

The medial trapezius closes the scapula to the middle line of the body and the inferior trapezius makes them drop.

The posterior deltoid is activated by moving the shoulders backwards.

- M. tensor fasciae latae
- M. glutaeus maximus
- **rear thigh musculature**
- M. biceps femoris
- **M. quadriceps femoris**
- M. sartorius
- M. gracilis
- M. vastus medialis
- M. fibularis
- M. longissimus
- M. iliocostalis thoracis
- M. trapezius (lower part)
- M. infraspinatus
- M. triceps brachii
- M. trapezius (middle part)
- M. deltoideus (rear part)
- M. tibialis anterior
- **M. gastrocnemius**
- **M. soleus**
- M. tibialis posterior

The activated quadriceps on each leg straighten the knees.

Stretching the gastrocnemius and soleus.

CLOSED OR FORWARD-FLEXING ASANAS

# Paschimottanasana

*Paschima* means "west," which is the back part of the body, *ut* is "intense," and *tan* is "stretch." This asana intensely stretches the rear part of the body. It is known as the tweezer pose.

### BENEFITS

- Stretches and tones the muscles of the back and legs.
- Stimulates the abdominal organs, providing great benefits in the digestive process.
- Reduces the heart rate by relaxing the nervous system.

### WARNINGS

- Severe or degenerative diseases of the spine (e.g., arthritis, lumbago, herniated disc, sciatica).
- Inflammations in the abdominal region.
- Advanced pregnancy.

### CLASSIFICATION
Closing pose, flexed forward, symmetrical, seated.

### TECHNIQUE
We start in a seated pose with the legs bent. We try to make the buttocks stick out so that we sit on the ischium bones. We stretch the back. We take the toes with the thumb, index, and middle finger on each hand. We raise the thorax and bring the shoulders down and back. Little by little, we slide the legs back so that, the abdomen and thighs touch. We advance in this pose until we can feel the abdomen separate from the thighs, and we hold this position when it happens. Finally, we can loosen from this pose by letting the head and trunk fall onto the legs. To release, bend the legs again and we straighten our body slowly.

### ADAPTATIONS
In the case of a rigid back or tight hamstring muscles, we can sit on a mat or a cushion to relax and allow the pelvis to rotate forward and the trunk lower with gravity. We can use a rope that helps to stretch and lengthen the back.

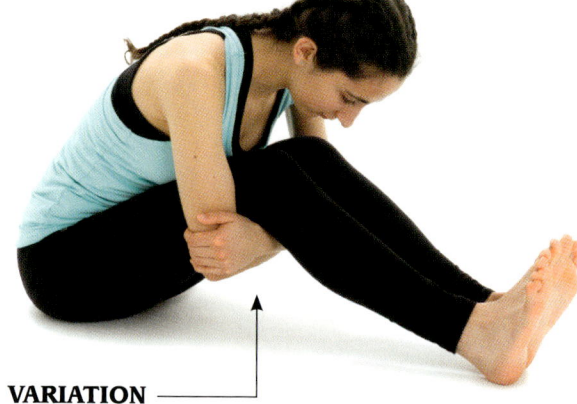

### VARIATION
We can hug the legs with the arms without separating the abdomen from the thighs, and thus advance this pose.

### RELATED ASANAS
Janu Sirsasana. While seated in Dandasana, we place the right heel next to the perineum, supporting the sole on the left thigh. With a breath, we raise the arms and the hands stretch for the left foot. With every exhale, we advance the pose. When finished, we proceed to do the same on the other side.

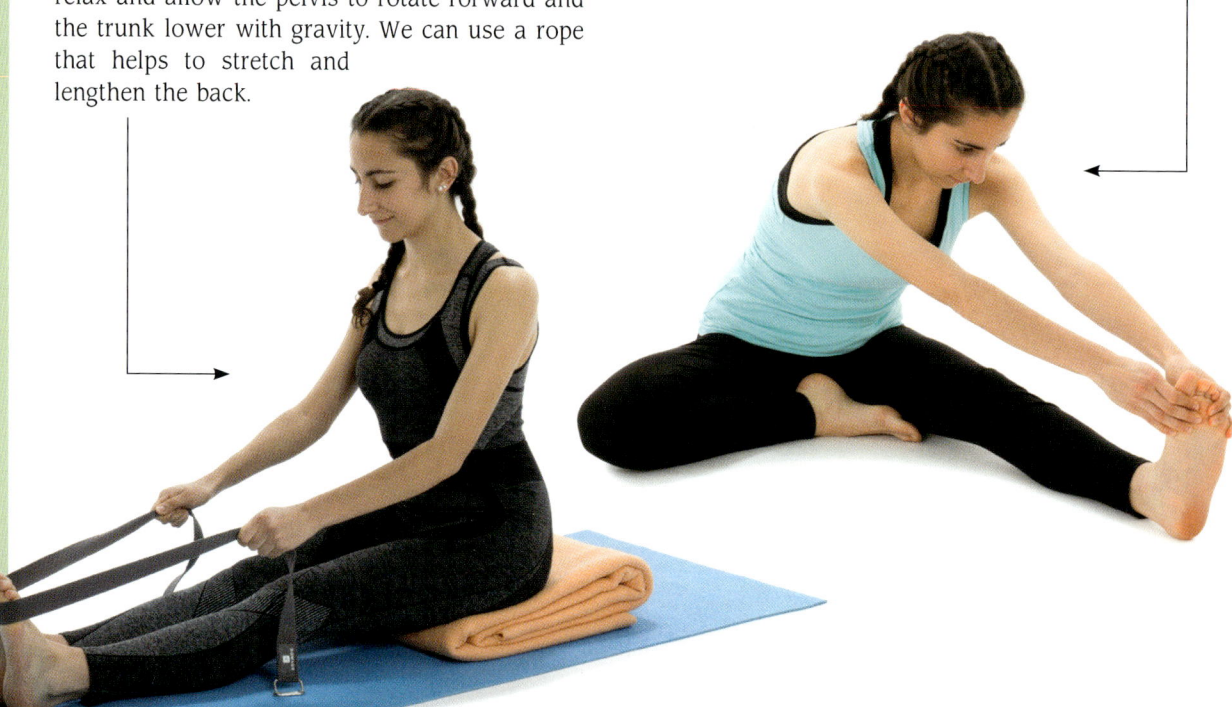

CLOSED OR FORWARD-FLEXING ASANAS: Paschimottanasana

Paschimottanasana stimulates the Svadhistana and Manipura Chakras and the pranic flow in the Sushumna nadi, harmonizing energy in the body. It provides internalized states of mental tranquility.

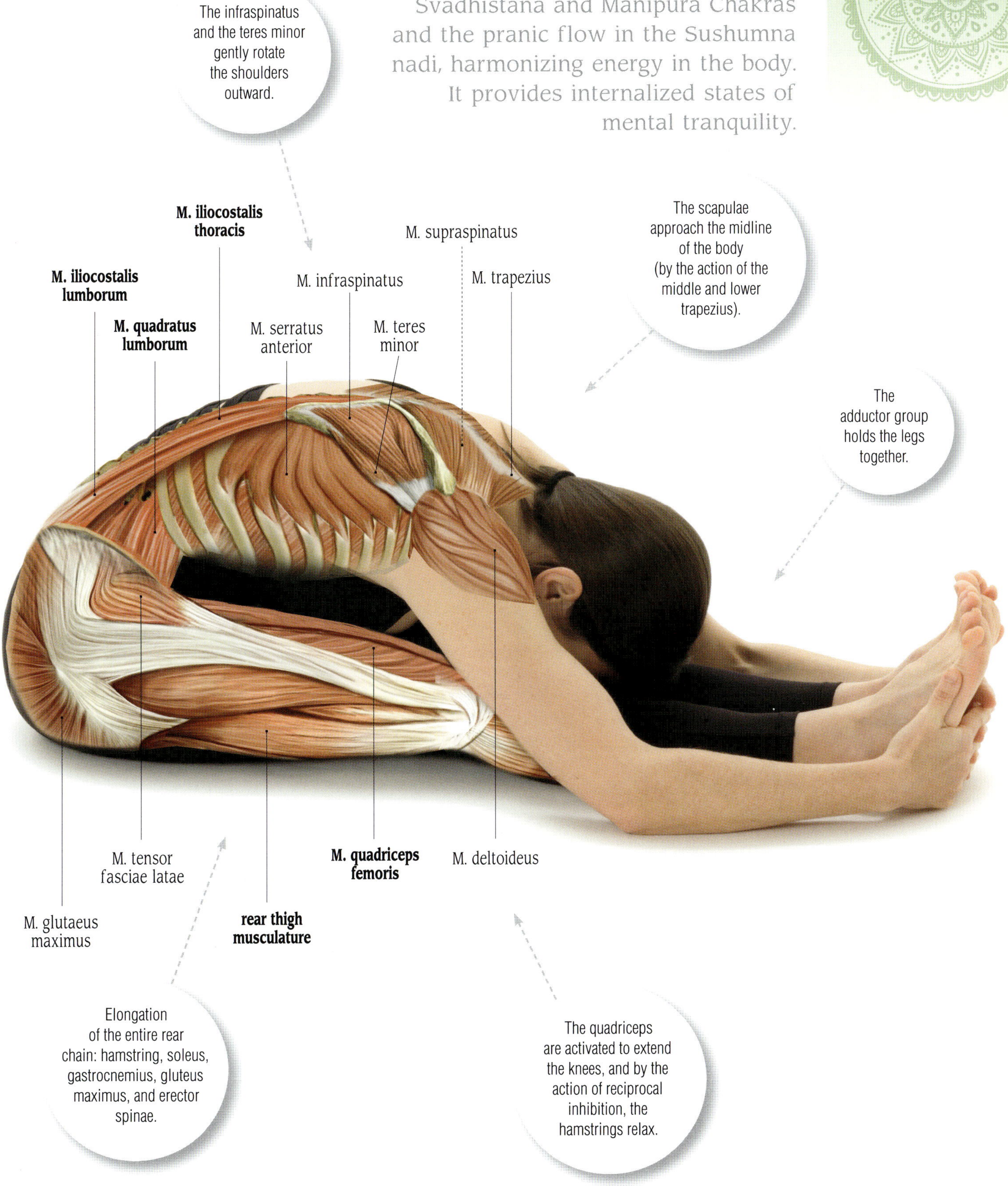

The infraspinatus and the teres minor gently rotate the shoulders outward.

The scapulae approach the midline of the body (by the action of the middle and lower trapezius).

The adductor group holds the legs together.

The quadriceps are activated to extend the knees, and by the action of reciprocal inhibition, the hamstrings relax.

Elongation of the entire rear chain: hamstring, soleus, gastrocnemius, gluteus maximus, and erector spinae.

- M. iliocostalis lumborum
- M. quadratus lumborum
- M. iliocostalis thoracis
- M. serratus anterior
- M. infraspinatus
- M. teres minor
- M. supraspinatus
- M. trapezius
- M. tensor fasciae latae
- M. quadriceps femoris
- M. deltoideus
- rear thigh musculature
- M. glutaeus maximus

## Asanas

CLOSED OR FORWARD-FLEXING ASANAS

# Balasana

It is also called Pranatasana. Balasana is known as the child's pose, since the body retreats on itself into a fetal position.

**BENEFITS**
- Stretches and relaxes the back.
- Stimulates the digestive function.
- Invigorates the blood circulation of the organs of the head.
- Relaxes the nervous system.

**WARNINGS**
- Inflammation in the abdominal region.
- High blood pressure, headaches, or colds: put your head higher.
- Pregnancy: practice with your legs separated.

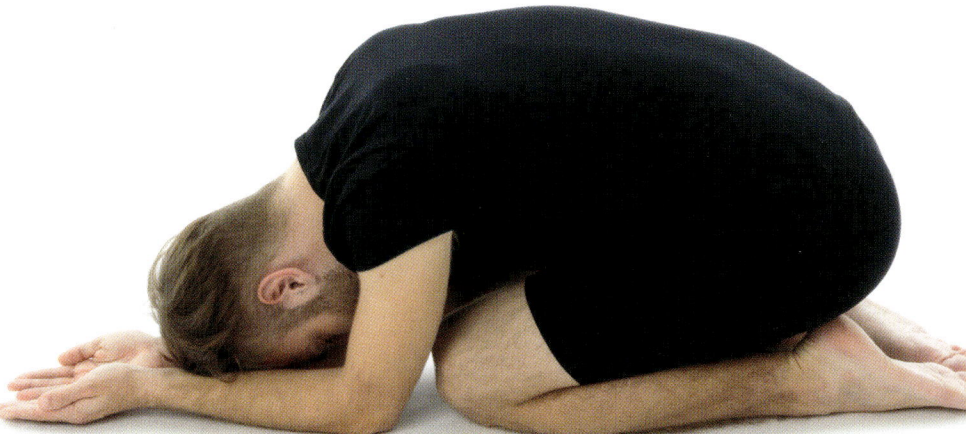

### CLASSIFICATION
Closed pose, symmetric, seated on the heels.

### TECHNIQUE
We start sitting on the heels with the legs together. We place the hands on the ground and let the abdomen fall to the thighs, then we rest the forehead on the ground. We place the arms on both sides of the trunk, with the palms facing up. We relax the arms and the entire back, close the eyes, and observe our breathing. To release the pose, we place the hands on the ground, next to the knees, and with the strength in our arms, we rise slowly, little by little.

### ADAPTATIONS
We place the forearms as close to one another as possible, and we support the head on them with the palms of the hands facing up.

If it is not possible to put the head on the ground, we use a cork block or two fists, and we rest the head on them.

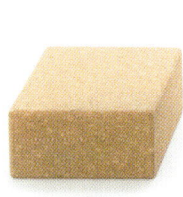
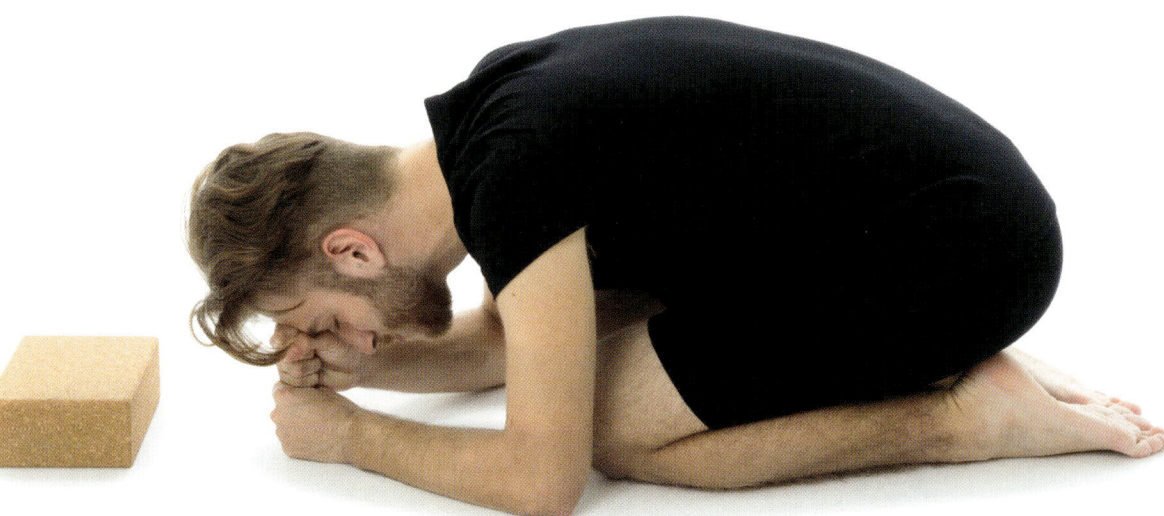

## CLOSED OR FORWARD-FLEXING ASANAS: Balasana

In Balasana, the Vishuddha Chakra is activated, which offers energy to the upper chakras and creates a calming effect on the mind. It is also a posture of introspection and a withdrawal of the senses, since it offers a state of inner peace.

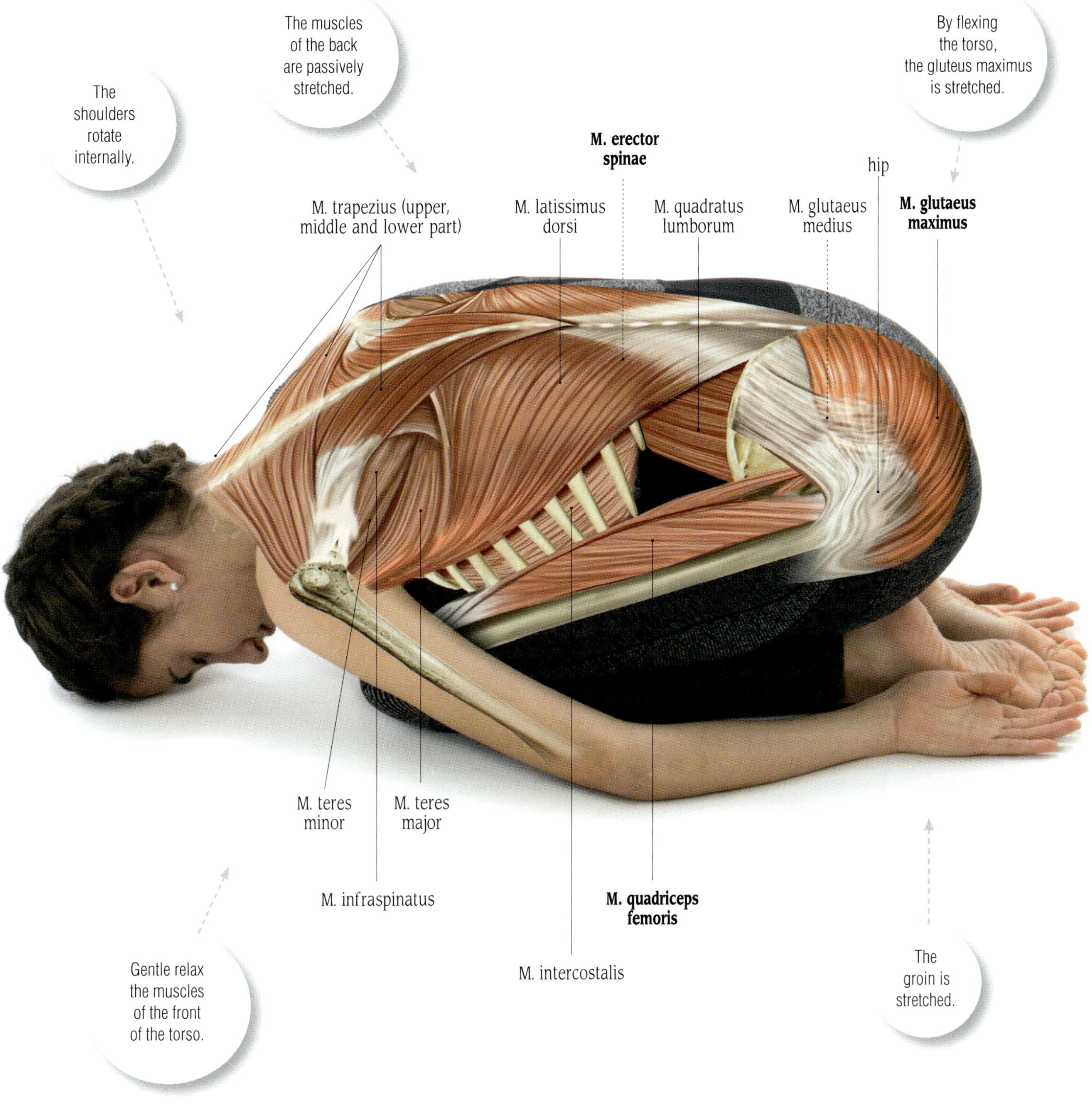

- The shoulders rotate internally.
- The muscles of the back are passively stretched.
- By flexing the torso, the gluteus maximus is stretched.
- Gentle relax the muscles of the front of the torso.
- The groin is stretched.

Labels:
- M. trapezius (upper, middle and lower part)
- M. latissimus dorsi
- **M. erector spinae**
- M. quadratus lumborum
- M. glutaeus medius
- hip
- **M. glutaeus maximus**
- M. teres minor
- M. teres major
- M. infraspinatus
- **M. quadriceps femoris**
- M. intercostalis

CLOSED OR FORWARD-FLEXING ASANAS

# Kurmasana

*Kurma* means "turtle." This asana is dedicated to Kurma, the incarnation of Vishnu in the form of a turtle. The pose allows us to protect our interior.

**BENEFITS**
- Stretches and tones the muscles of the back.
- Increases flexibility in the spine.
- Stimulates the abdominal organs.
- Calms the nervous system.

**WARNINGS**
- Ailments in the abdominal organs.
- Lesions in the spine (e.g., sciatica, herniated disc).
- Problems in the shoulder joints: use the variations.
- Advanced pregnancy.

**CLASSIFICATION**
Closed pose, symmetric, seated.

**TECHNIQUE**
Starting in Dandasana, we separate the legs and fold the knees while moving the feet toward the trunk. With a hand on each knee, we stretch the spine while raising the thorax. We lean the trunk forward and place each hand and arm under the corresponding knee. If we have sufficient flexibility in the shoulders, spine, and hips, we can stretch the arms to the ground with the palms facing down. We progressively lean the trunk further forward, supporting the forehead, the chin, and, lastly, the chest on the ground. After this, we stretch the legs. With every breath, we intensify the pose.

**ADAPTATIONS**
It may serve to prepare the pose. With the legs separated and the knees bent, we move the arms under each leg and take hold of the foot by the heel with the corresponding hand.

We can adapt the pose with or without a cork block. We put the soles of the feet together and let the trunk fall forward. We move the hands and forearm under the legs, and the hands reach for each foot or grab the block. We remain relaxed in the pose.

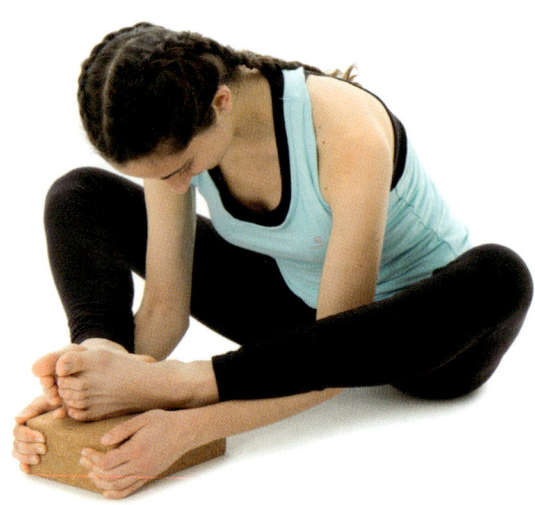

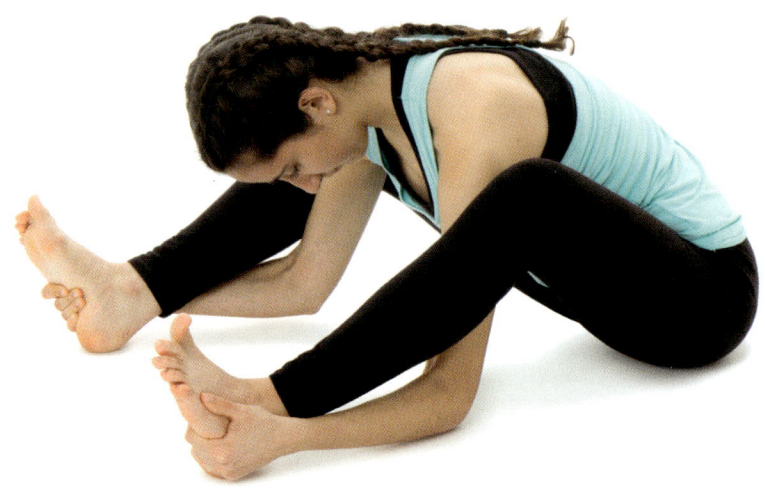

CLOSED OR FORWARD-FLEXING ASANAS: Kurmasana

Kurmasana allows us to withdraw our senses from the outside world, freeing us from external worries and pleasures. In this way, we find our inner space. This asana stimulates the Svadhisthana, Manipura, and Anahata Chakras.

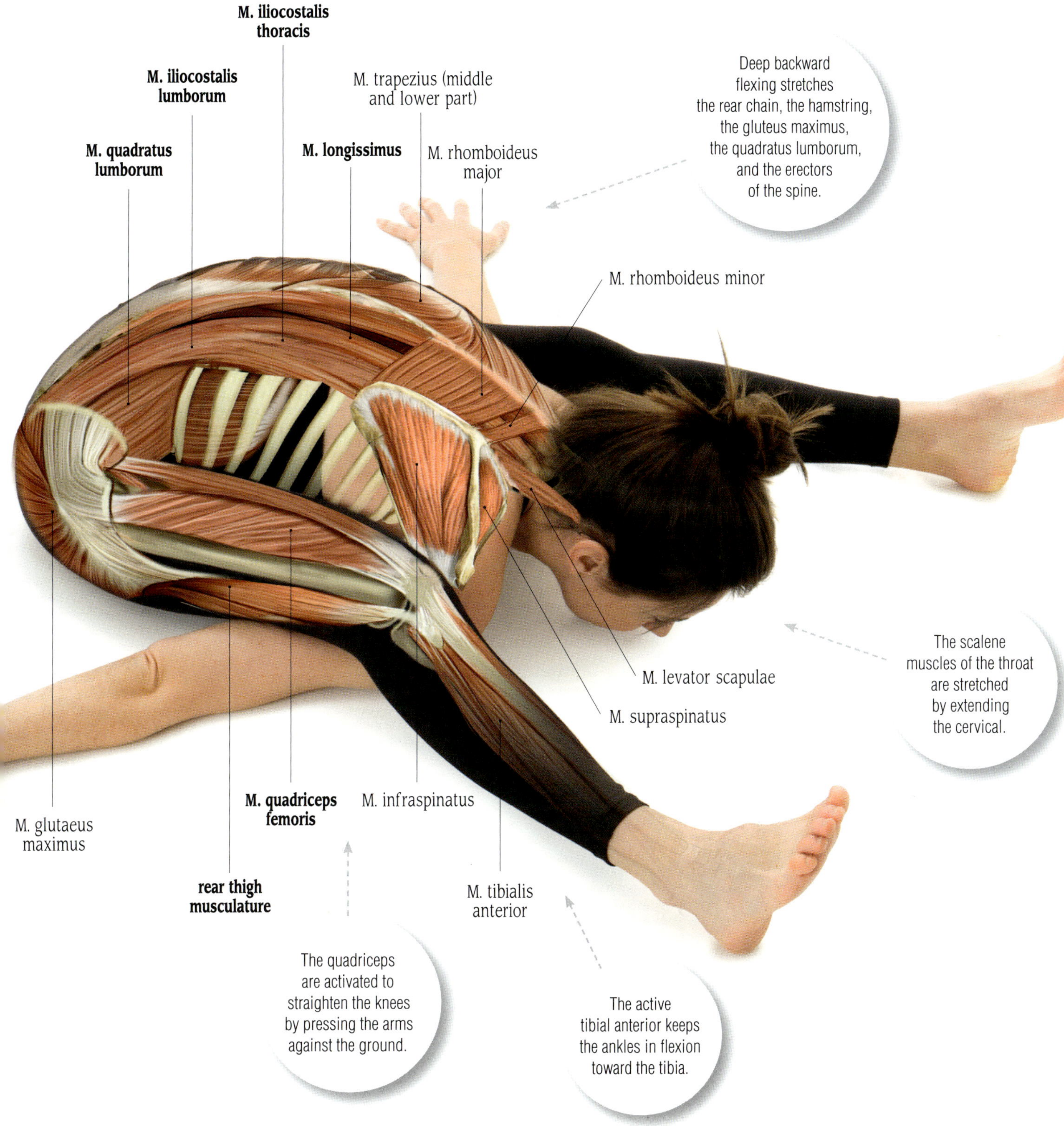

- **M. iliocostalis thoracis**
- **M. iliocostalis lumborum**
- M. trapezius (middle and lower part)
- **M. quadratus lumborum**
- **M. longissimus**
- M. rhomboideus major
- M. rhomboideus minor
- M. levator scapulae
- M. supraspinatus
- M. glutaeus maximus
- **M. quadriceps femoris**
- M. infraspinatus
- **rear thigh musculature**
- M. tibialis anterior

Deep backward flexing stretches the rear chain, the hamstring, the gluteus maximus, the quadratus lumborum, and the erectors of the spine.

The scalene muscles of the throat are stretched by extending the cervical.

The quadriceps are activated to straighten the knees by pressing the arms against the ground.

The active tibial anterior keeps the ankles in flexion toward the tibia.

Asanas

TWISTING ASANAS

# Ardha Matsyendrasana

This is a pose dedicated to Matsyendranath, the Lord of fish, the legendary founder of Hatha Yoga, who in the form of fish spied on Shiva while teaching yoga to his wife Parvati. It is a pose of medium spinal twisting.

**BENEFITS**
- Flexes the muscles of the back and hips. Strengthens the joints of the shoulders.
- Massages and tones the digestive organs and improves their function.
- Relieves back pain. Recommended for lumbago or scoliosis.
- Stimulates and strengthens the nervous system.

**WARNINGS**
- Herniated discs.
- Peptic ulcer, inguinal hernia.
- Knee problems: use adapted variations.

**CLASSIFICATION**
A twisting pose, asymmetric, seated.

**TECHNIQUE**
We start in the Dandasana pose. We bend the left knee and raise the heel to the right buttocks so that the leg, the thigh, and the foot are resting on the floor. We bend the right knee and place the sole of the foot on the ground with the external side of the ankle touching the left knee. We take the right knee with both hands and straighten the spine as vertically as possible. We rotate the trunk to the right and place the left elbow against the exterior face of the right thigh. We use the right arm like a lever on the right leg. We breathe in and twist from the bottom up. The head remains rotated to the right. The right hand goes behind the back, while the left fits into the space of the left leg. Intertwine the hands on the back. We make the Jñana mudra with the right hand. The back should be vertical and relaxed, the shoulders at the same height, and the two ischium bones should touch the ground. To release this pose, we make the inverse movement. We proceed to do the same on the other side.

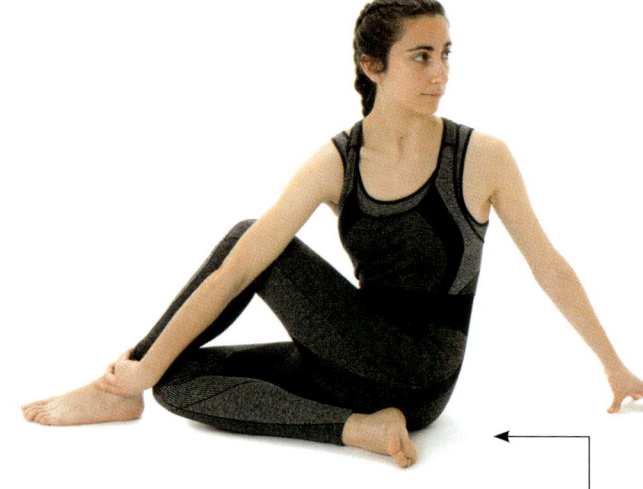

By moving the left arm we can use it like a lever with the same arm on the right leg. We reach for the right ankle with the hand.

We bend both legs and place them in the same direction. As we stretch the spine and rotate in the opposite direction of the legs, the hand reaches for the knee. This variation makes it easier to straighten the spine in a more natural way.

**VARIATIONS**
For a more simple variation, the right hand is supported on the ground, behind the back, while the left forearm is supported on the left thigh.

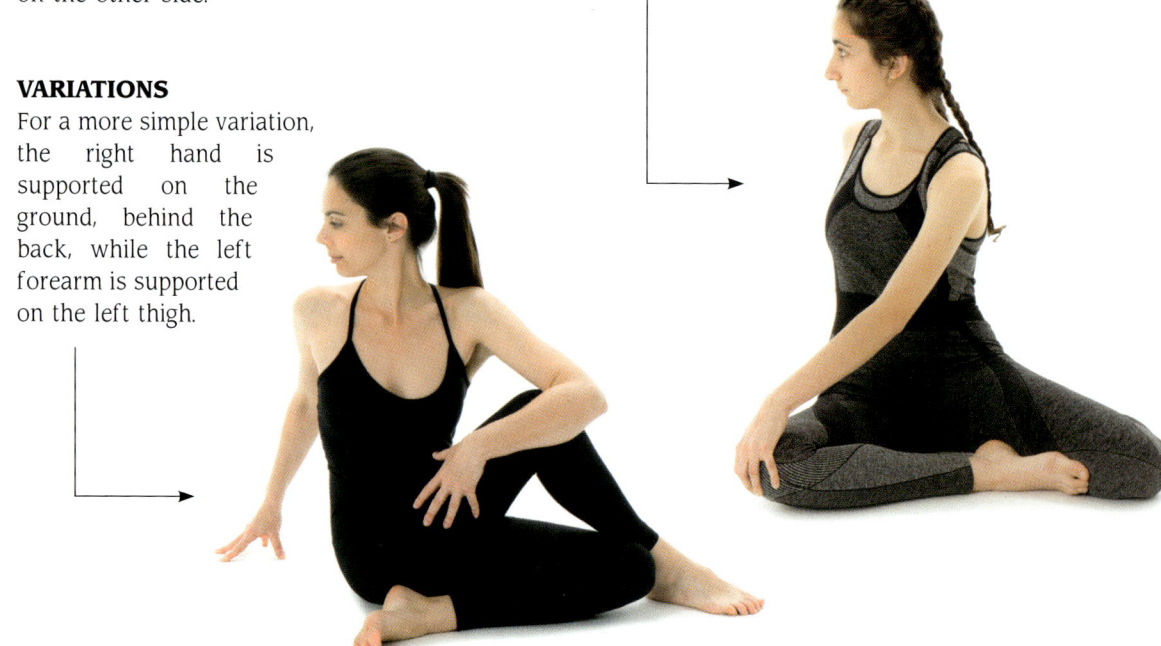

# TWISTING ASANAS: Ardha Matsyendrasana

Ardha Matsyendrasana allows energy to flow through both sides of the spine, thus balancing the Ida and Píngala nadis. In addition, it balances the polarized forces of the elements water/fire, symbolized by *matsya* (fish/water) and *indra* (fire). It stimulates the Manipura, Vishuddha, and Ajna Chakras.

The abdominal oblique on the side of the twisting is lengthened while the other contracts.

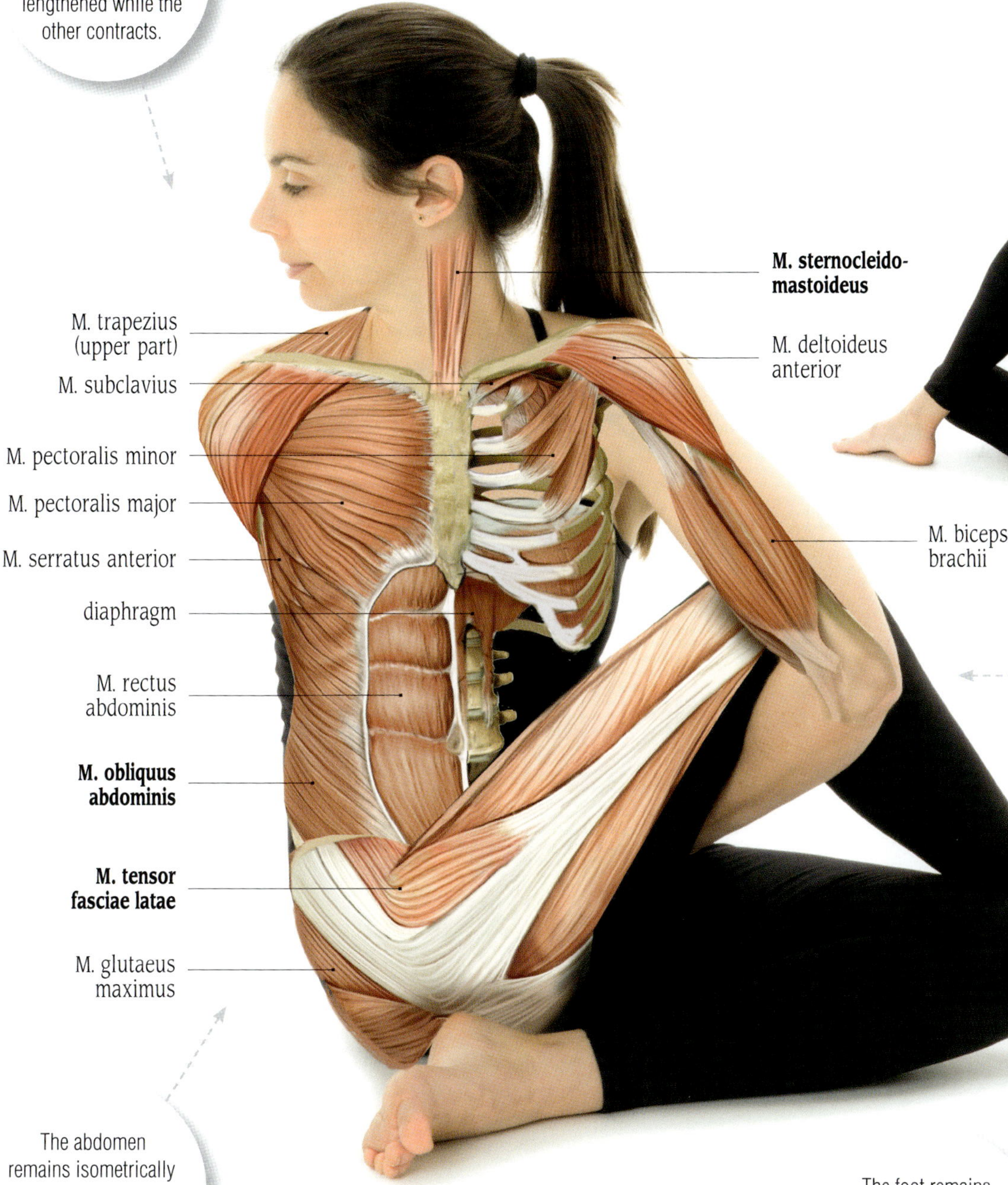

- M. trapezius (upper part)
- M. subclavius
- M. pectoralis minor
- M. pectoralis major
- M. serratus anterior
- diaphragm
- M. rectus abdominis
- **M. obliquus abdominis**
- **M. tensor fasciae latae**
- M. glutaeus maximus

- **M. sternocleido-mastoideus**
- M. deltoideus anterior
- M. biceps brachii

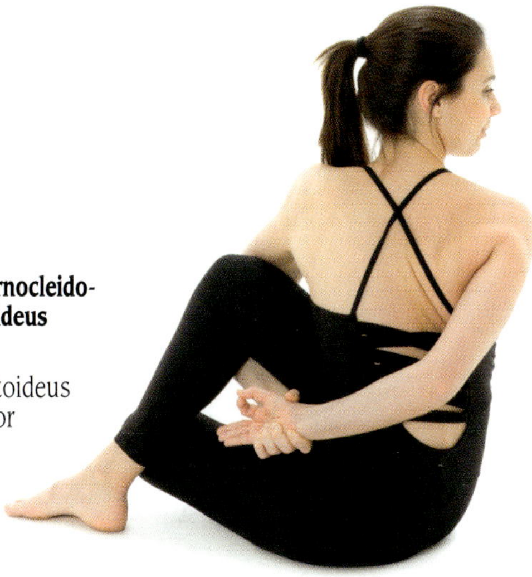

The tensor facia latae (upper thigh) is activated isometrically, with the knee pressing against the elbow.

The abdomen remains isometrically activated to straighten the torso.

The foot remains activated, pressed into the floor by the gastrocnemius and the soleus.

Asanas

TWISTING ASANAS

# Jatara Parivartanasana

*Jatara* means "stomach" or "belly", and *parivartana* means "rotate" or "roll." The spine twists in a spiral in this pose.

**BENEFITS**
- Compensates for deviations in the spinal column.
- Offers mobility to the thorax, affecting respiratory capacity.
- Stimulates the digestive processes.
- Relaxes the nervous system.

**WARNINGS**
- Severe back pain, severe sciatica, or herniated discs.

### CLASSIFICATION
A twisting pose, asymmetric, a face-up position.

### TECHNIQUE
We start in Savasana, placing the hands in a cross, in line with the shoulders and with the palms facing up (some schools have the palms facing down). With flexed legs and the feet on the ground, we lift the pelvis a little and advance it laterally to the left. We lift up both legs together while vertically extended and let them lower slowly, diagonally, toward the right side of the body, the feet reach for the hand. The abdomen and chest move to the other side, and the scapulae and shoulders stay in contact with the floor. Hold this pose for a while, utilizing abdominal breathing. To release it, bend the legs a little and lift the up vertically. Complete on the opposite side.

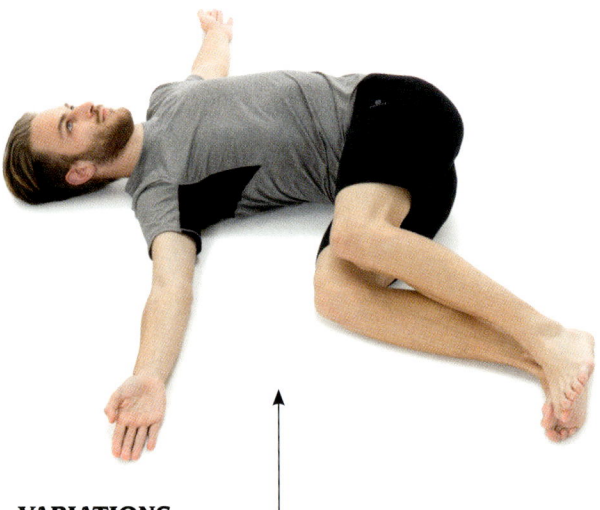

### VARIATIONS
Twisting with bent legs. We can practice this pose with the knees close to or far away from the chest, which will affect the joints of the hips, lumbar, and thoracic regions in different ways. Bringing the knees closer to the chest will cause more twisting in the thorax, eliminating tension in the hips and lumbar.

We cross one knee over the other and rotate the lower part of the body slowly so that both knees come close to the ground. We can relax in this pose.

### ADAPTATION
We proceed with a stretched leg. We can use a mat or cushion to adapt the poses and allow the body to advance further in them.

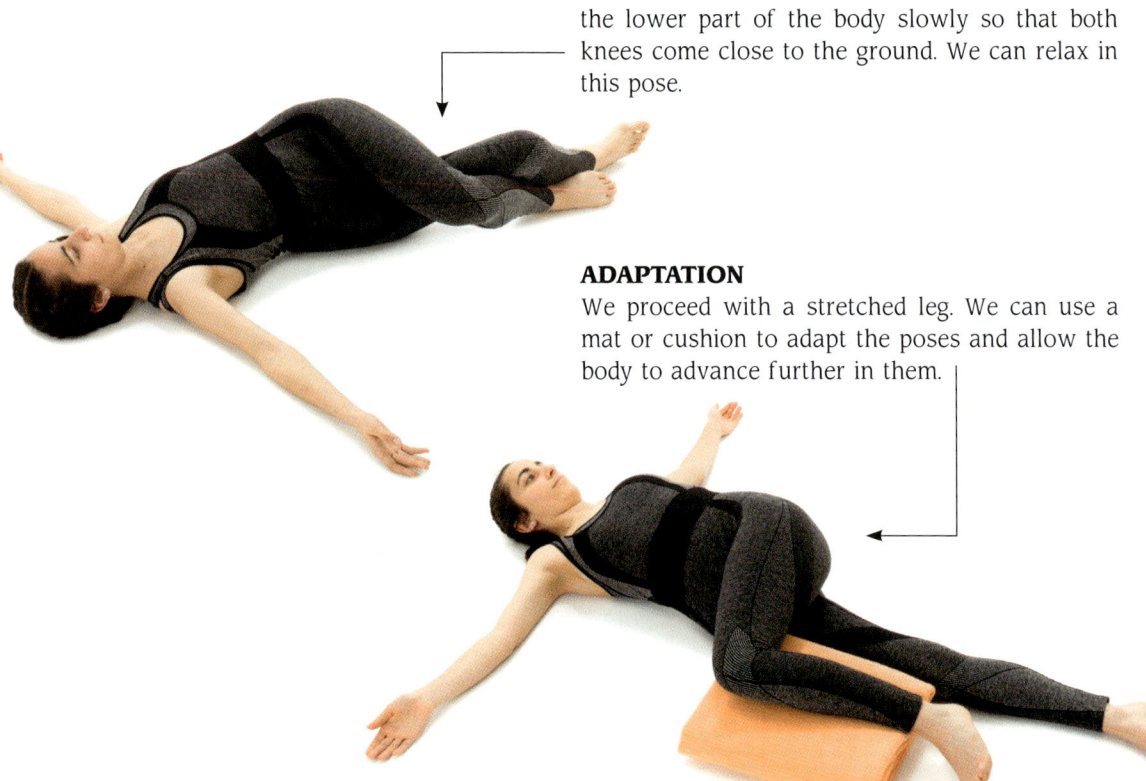

TWISTING ASANAS: Jatara Parivartanasana    103

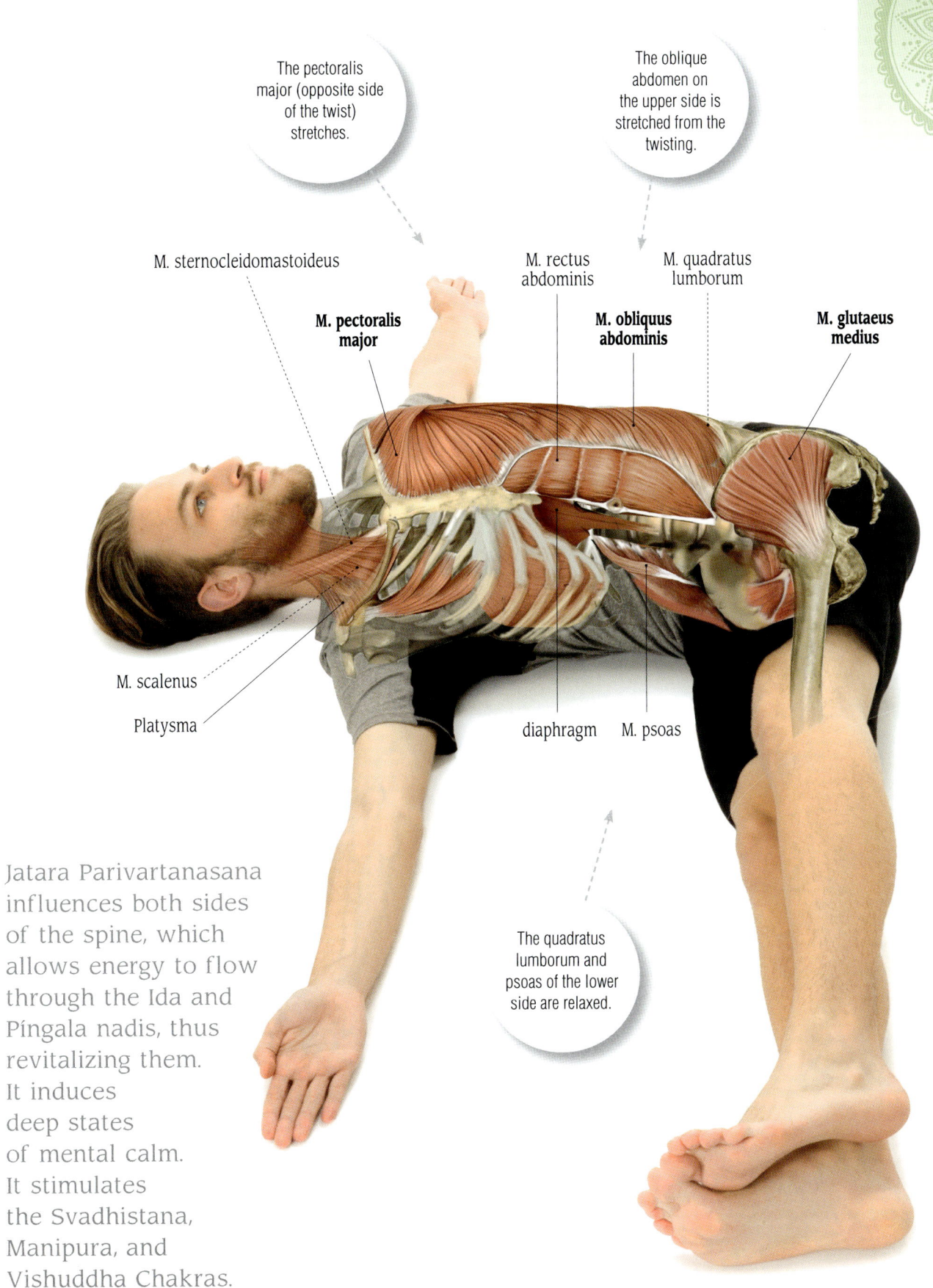

The pectoralis major (opposite side of the twist) stretches.

The oblique abdomen on the upper side is stretched from the twisting.

M. sternocleidomastoideus — M. rectus abdominis — M. quadratus lumborum

**M. pectoralis major** — **M. obliquus abdominis** — **M. glutaeus medius**

M. scalenus
Platysma

diaphragm — M. psoas

The quadratus lumborum and psoas of the lower side are relaxed.

Jatara Parivartanasana influences both sides of the spine, which allows energy to flow through the Ida and Píngala nadis, thus revitalizing them. It induces deep states of mental calm. It stimulates the Svadhistana, Manipura, and Vishuddha Chakras.

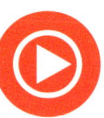

SEMI-INVERTED AND INVERTED ASANAS

# Prasarita Padottanasana

*Prasarita* means to "expand" or "extend" and *pada* means "foot" or "leg." In this pose, you will stretch and strengthen your legs and bring your feet, hands, and head in contact with the floor.

## BENEFITS

- Intense stretching of the entire back of the body.
- Indicated in case of shortening of the posterior muscles, hyperlordosis, and hyperkyphosis.
- Increases blood flow to the head and promotes concentration and intense mental work. Combats stress and depression.
- Invigorates venous return and normalizes blood flow through the muscles and internal organs.

## WARNINGS

- Herniated discs, sciatica. If there are disc problems in the lumbar area, practice with the legs slightly flexed.
- Hypertension.
- Cataracts or intraocular pressure.

### CLASSIFICATION
Semi-inverted pose, symmetric, flexed from the waist to the feet.

### TECHNIQUE
We start in the Tadasana pose, with the legs separated and flexed.. On an exhale, we place our hands on our hips and lean forward until the back is flat. Bending our waist opens the joints of the hips. Next, we put the palms of our hands on the ground, between our feet and separated as wide as our shoulders. Our hands stay open and our fingers point forward. If we have enough flexibility, we bend our elbows and try to put the crown of our head on the ground. Feet, hands, and head should be in line. Keep this pose for a few breaths and release from the pose.

### VARIATION
We flex the body forward and hold the big toes with the middle and index fingers on both hands.

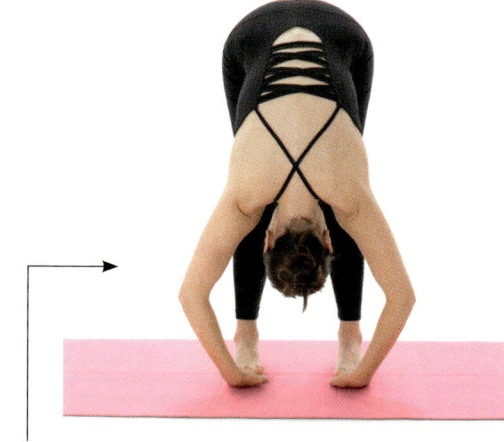

### RELATED ASANA PADA HASTASANA.
This is another flexing exercise for the feet. We start with Tadasana and, while raising our arms upward, extend our body. With an exhale, flex downward. We place our hands under the soles of our feet. This asana helps to relax the back of the neck and vertebra.

### ADAPTATIONS
If there is tension in the hamstrings or tightness of the back, we can try using cork blocks. This way we can progress with the pose.

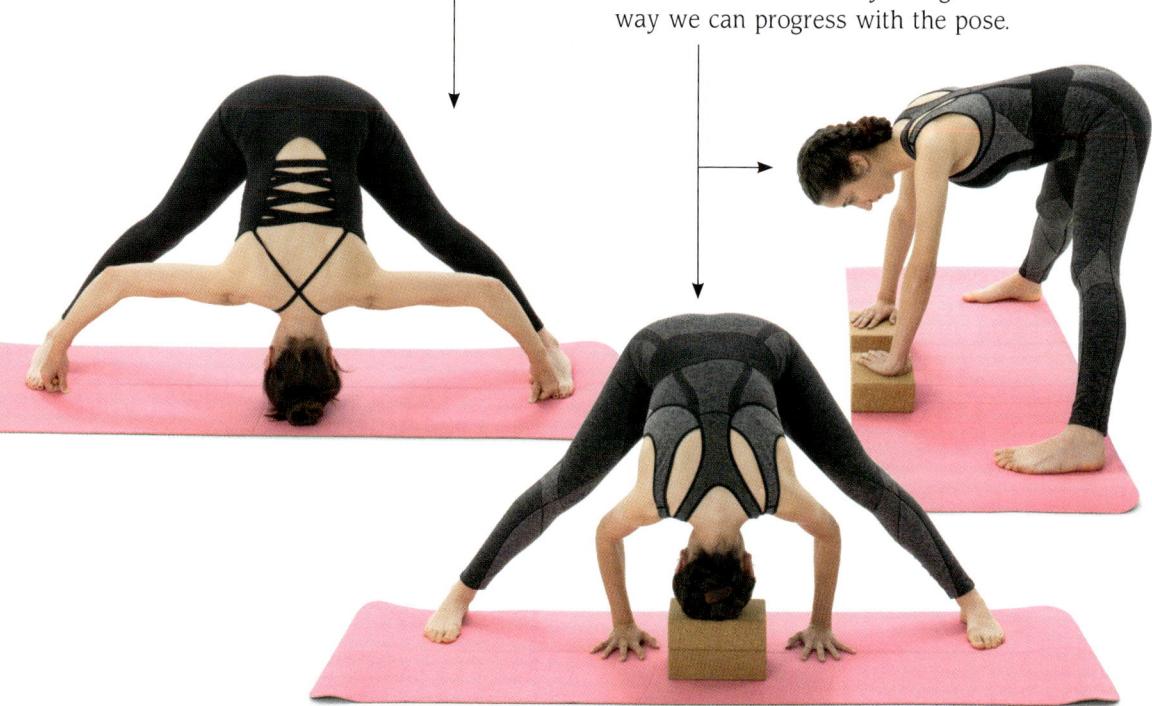

SEMI-INVERTED AND INVERTED ASANAS: Prasarita Padottanasana 105

Prasarita Padottanasana helps us perceive how close we are to the Earth with the upper part of our body. It offers us mental clarity and emotional balance. This asana stimulates the Sahasrara Chakra.

The erectors of the spine, the hamstrings, the gluteus maximus, the soleus, and gastrocnemius are stretched thoroughly.

The quadriceps are active and straighten the knees.

**M. glutaeus maximus**

M. sartorius

M. psoas

M. glutaeus medius und minimus

**rear thigh musculature**

**M. quadriceps femoris**

M. quadratus lumborum

M. teres minor

M. iliocostalis lumborum

M. tibialis anterior

diaphragm

M. fibularis longus

M. iliocostalis thoracis

M. longissimus

**M. gastrocnemius**

**M. soleus**

**M. trapezius (lower part)**

M. deltoideus (upper part)

M. infraspinatus

M. supraspinatus

M. trapezius (middle part)

M. levator scapulae

M. spinalis

The anterior and posterior tibialis maintain the elevation of the plantar arch. In turn, the peroneus longus is stretched eccentrically, anchoring the outer edge of the foot to the floor.

The trapezoids are stretched with concentration to open the scapulae of the shoulders, thus opening up the space of the neck.

Asanas

SEMI-INVERTED AND INVERTED ASANAS

# Sasangasana

*Sasaka*, in Sanskrit, means "bunny." This is a posture reminiscent of the rounded spine of a rabbit or a hare.

**BENEFITS**
- Stretches the spine and cervical area.
- Increases blood flow to the head, thereby oxygenating the brain, face, and neck.
- Relieves mental fatigue.
- Stimulates the immune and endocrine systems.

**WARNINGS**
- Hypertension.
- Intraocular pressure.
- Inflammations in the head.

**CLASSIFICATION**
Semi-inverted pose, symmetric, flexed from the trunk to the knees.

**TECHNIQUE**
We start in the Vajrasana pose, seated on the heels. We flex the trunk forward until the belly is resting on the thighs, and we place the forehead on the ground. We place the arms on both sides of the body; each hand reaches for the heel of the corresponding foot. While inhaling, we raise the pelvis and, at the same time, slide the head toward the body, tucking the chin in until the crown of the head rests on the ground. The weight of the body should fall on the hands and heels. It is important to hold the heels firmly. We hold this asana for a few breaths. To release the pose, we bring the pelvis back to the heels and slide the head out to rest in the Balasana pose for a moment.

**COUNTER POSE**
Relaxed in Balasana.

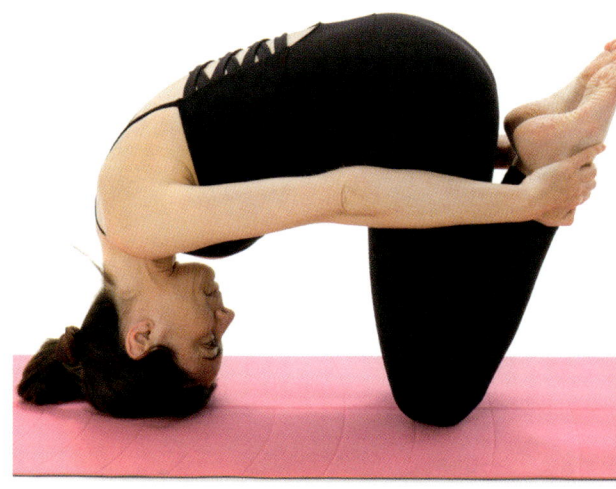

**VARIATION**
It is an intense variation. We hold the ankles with both hands. The weight is distributed between the knees and the crown of the head.

**ADAPTATION**
The hands are supported on the ground. We push the hands forward and to both sides of the body. With a breath, we raise the pelvis while we lower the head to support it on the floor. The hands and arms push down slightly so that all the weight of the body doesn't fall on the head.

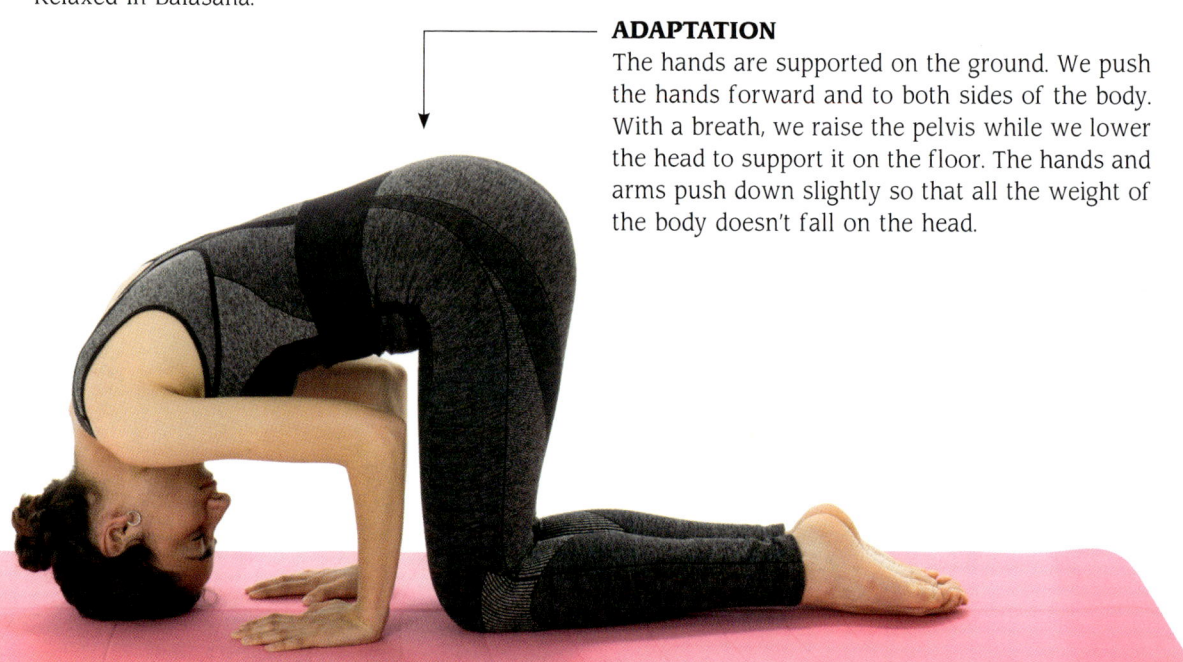

## SEMI-INVERTED AND INVERTED ASANAS: Sasangasana

Sasangasana is a pose that stimulates the Sahasrara Chakra. It allows us to enter into a state of mental calm and relaxation. It is appropriate for correcting mental disorders.

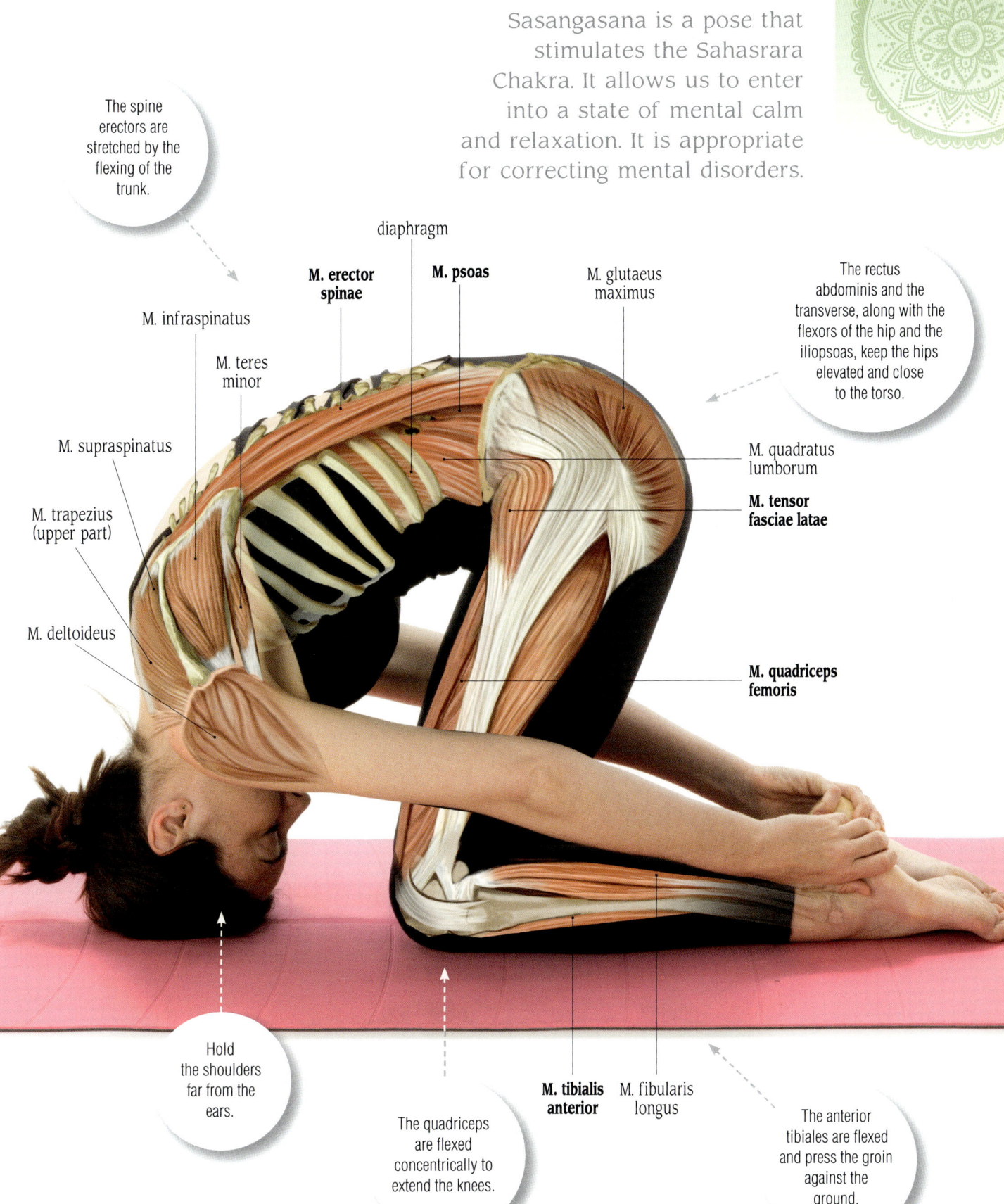

- The spine erectors are stretched by the flexing of the trunk.
- The rectus abdominis and the transverse, along with the flexors of the hip and the iliopsoas, keep the hips elevated and close to the torso.
- Hold the shoulders far from the ears.
- The quadriceps are flexed concentrically to extend the knees.
- The anterior tibiales are flexed and press the groin against the ground.

Labels: M. infraspinatus, M. teres minor, M. supraspinatus, M. trapezius (upper part), M. deltoideus, diaphragm, **M. erector spinae**, **M. psoas**, M. glutaeus maximus, M. quadratus lumborum, **M. tensor fasciae latae**, **M. quadriceps femoris**, **M. tibialis anterior**, M. fibularis longus

Asanas

SEMI-INVERTED AND INVERTED ASANAS

# Salamba Sarvangasana

*Salamba* means "supported," *sarva* means "entire" or "complete," and *anga* means "member" or "extremities." It is a pose on the shoulders with the support of the arms, popularly known as the candle pose.

**BENEFITS**
- Improves blood circulation and venous return in the legs and pelvis, thus improving varicose veins and hemorrhoids.
- Stimulates the digestive system.
- Improves the symptoms of bronchitis and asthma.
- Calms and rests the mind.

**WARNINGS**
- Displaced vertebral discs.
- Thyroid inflammation.
- Liver, spleen, or heart problems.
- Inflammations or ailments in the head (e.g., otitis, angina, glaucoma).
- Vertigo.

### CLASSIFICATION
Inverted pose, symmetrical.

### TECHNIQUE
We start in the Savasana pose, with the hand facing the ground. We bend the knees and raise the thighs to the belly. With a breath, we raise the pelvis and, while bending the shoulders, we support the hands on the hips. We raise the trunk until the sternum touches the chin. With another breath, we raise the legs up with the toes pointing up. We place the arms on the center of the back, the hands press firmly. The legs and trunk make a straight line that is perpendicular to the ground. Only the occipital area, the nape, the shoulders, and the arms should be in contact with the ground. We establish abdominal breathing. We can remain in this pose for a maximum of ten minutes. To release it, we bend the legs again and place the back slowly on the ground.

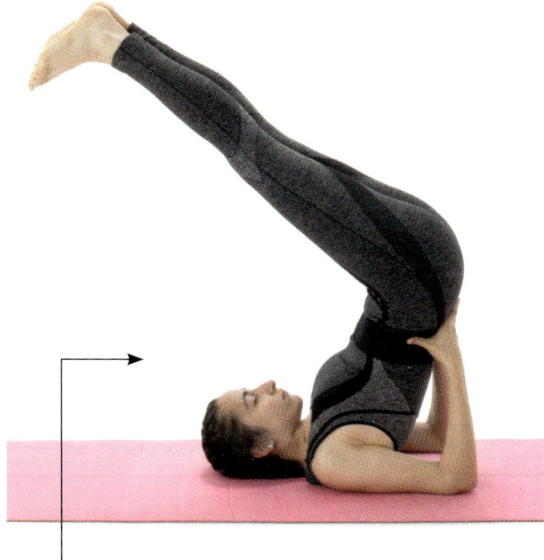

### RELATED ASANA
Viparita Karani Mudra. In this pose, the body is supported by the scapulas, the arms support the weight of the hips, and the chin is not blocked. It is a purifying and calming mudra.

### COUNTER POSE
Matsyasana.

### VARIATIONS
Variation with the soles of the feet together.
Variation of the lotus pose.

### ADAPTATION
With the feet supported on a wall, we progress up to the pose.

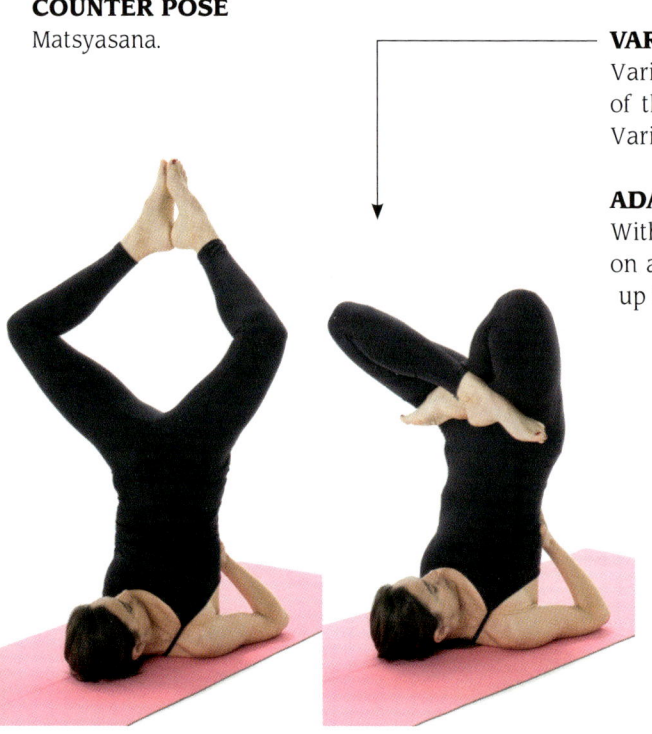
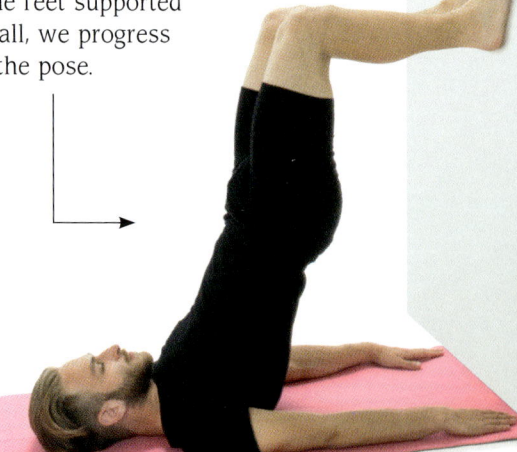

# SEMI-INVERTED AND INVERTED ASANAS: Salamba Sarvangasana

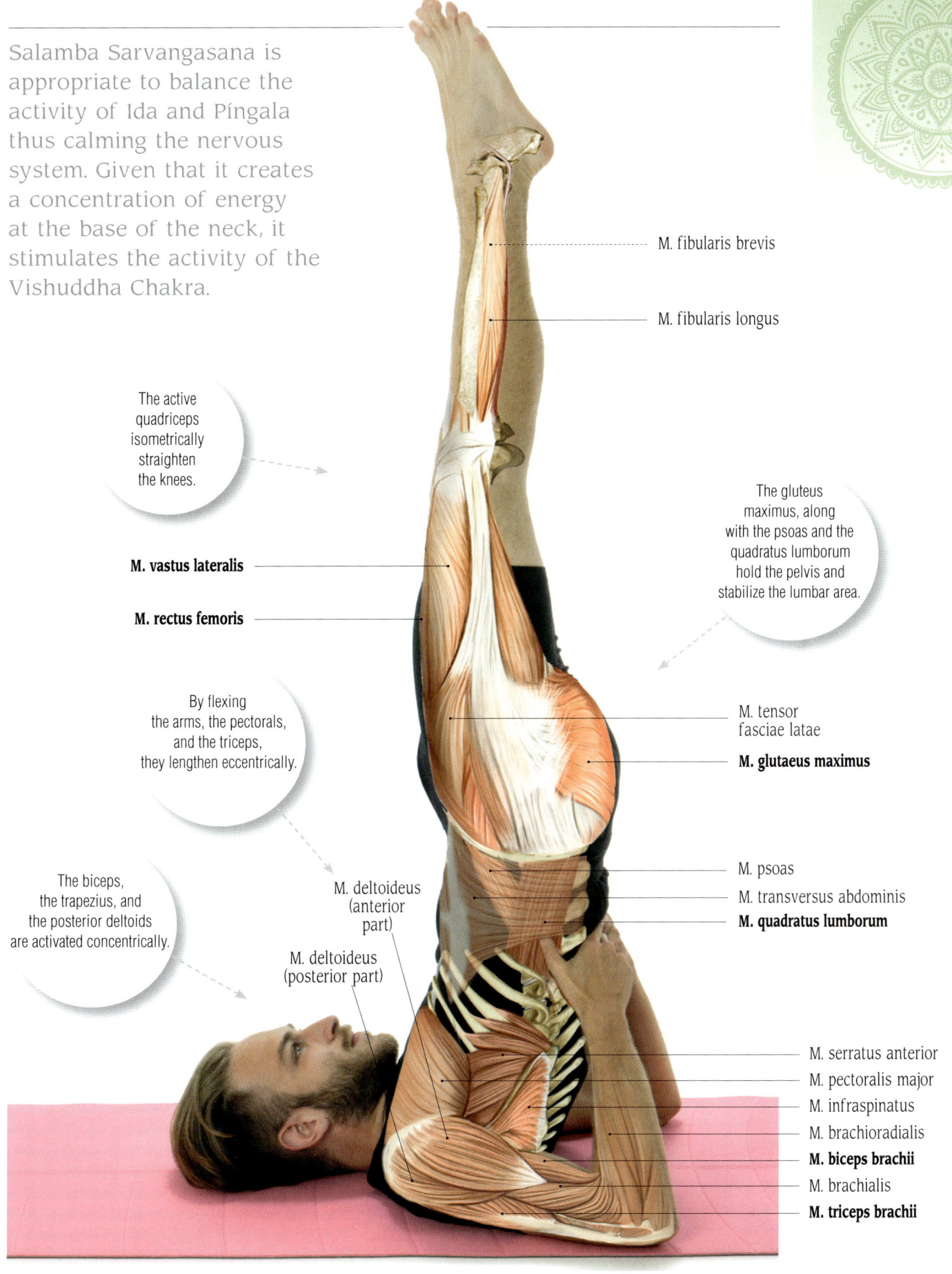

Salamba Sarvangasana is appropriate to balance the activity of Ida and Píngala thus calming the nervous system. Given that it creates a concentration of energy at the base of the neck, it stimulates the activity of the Vishuddha Chakra.

The active quadriceps isometrically straighten the knees.

**M. vastus lateralis**

**M. rectus femoris**

By flexing the arms, the pectorals, and the triceps, they lengthen eccentrically.

The biceps, the trapezius, and the posterior deltoids are activated concentrically.

M. deltoideus (anterior part)

M. deltoideus (posterior part)

M. fibularis brevis

M. fibularis longus

The gluteus maximus, along with the psoas and the quadratus lumborum hold the pelvis and stabilize the lumbar area.

M. tensor fasciae latae

**M. glutaeus maximus**

M. psoas

M. transversus abdominis

**M. quadratus lumborum**

M. serratus anterior

M. pectoralis major

M. infraspinatus

M. brachioradialis

**M. biceps brachii**

M. brachialis

**M. triceps brachii**

Asanas

SEMI-INVERTED AND INVERTED ASANAS

# Halasana

*Hala* means "plow." This is the plow pose. It is often done after, or in combination with, Sarvangasana. Since the heart and legs are above the head, it is considered an inverted pose.

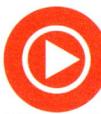

**BENEFITS**
- Stimulates the thyroid gland.
- Increases flexibility of the spine.
- Massages the abdominal muscles, thus favoring digestion.
- Stimulates brain activity and reduces stress.

**WARNINGS**
This asana can cause a lot of tension in the cervical spine, it is recommended to practice with the direction of a yoga teacher or to perform the adapted variation.
- Back and neck pain.
- Hypertension.
- Cervical problems, herniated disc, sciatica.
- Hiatal hernia.
- Advanced pregnancy.

### CLASSIFICATION
Inverted pose, symmetric, flexed waist.

### TECHNIQUE
We start the pose in Savasana, with the arms stretched along the length of the body and the palms facing down. The cervical column should be lengthened and the chin tucked. We breathe and lift the legs until they make a right angle with the spine. With a breath, we press the hands into the floor and raise the pelvis, moving the legs in the direction of the trunk and leaving the soles of the feet anchored to the floor behind the head. The trunk remains perpendicular to the floor and the feet at a right angle with the legs. We fold the hands together. We hold this pose for 10 to 20 breaths. To release it, we stretch the arms again and let the spine drop vertebra by vertebra, moving the legs close to the face.

If we start the pose from Sarvangasana, we should lower the legs together and slowly stretch them until the toes touch the ground behind the head.

### COUNTER POSE
Matsyasana. Balasana.

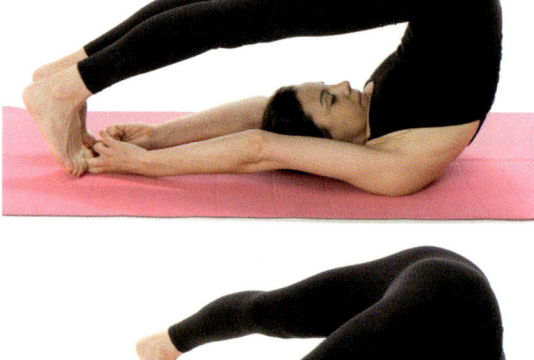

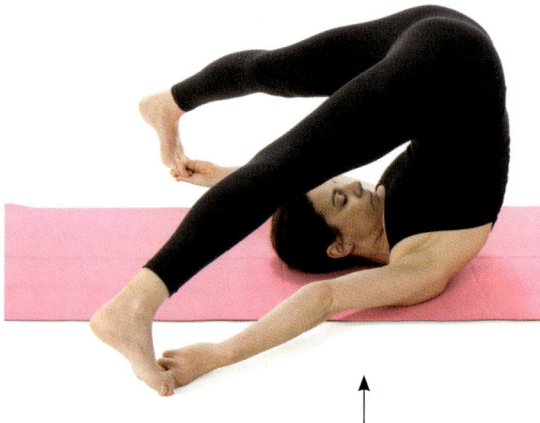

### VARIATIONS
With the legs together, the hands reach for each corresponding foot. The index and middle fingers grab the big toe of the respective foot. The legs are open and the index and middle fingers grab the big toes.

### ADAPTATION
If there is cervical tension, and to advance in the pose, we can support the legs on a stool.

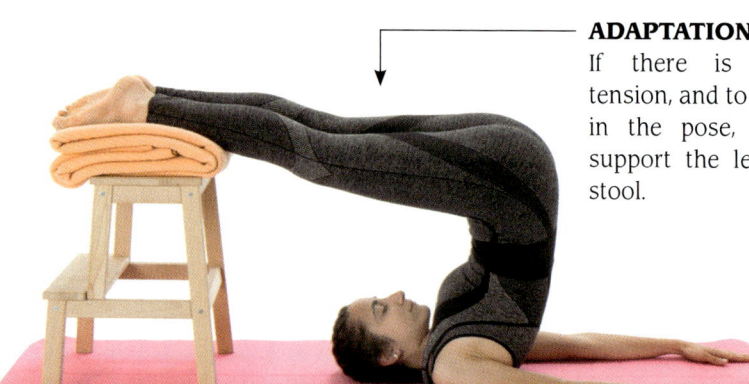

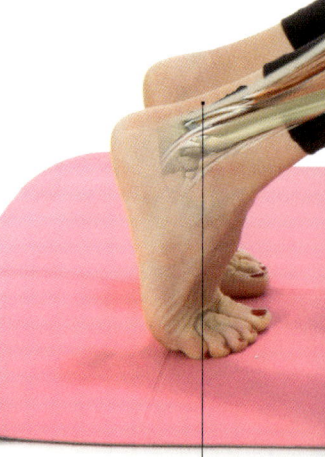

Achilles tendon

# SEMI-INVERTED AND INVERTED ASANAS: Halasana

Halasana stimulates the Vishuddha Chakra. This asana calms the mind, induces internalized states, and prepares for meditation.

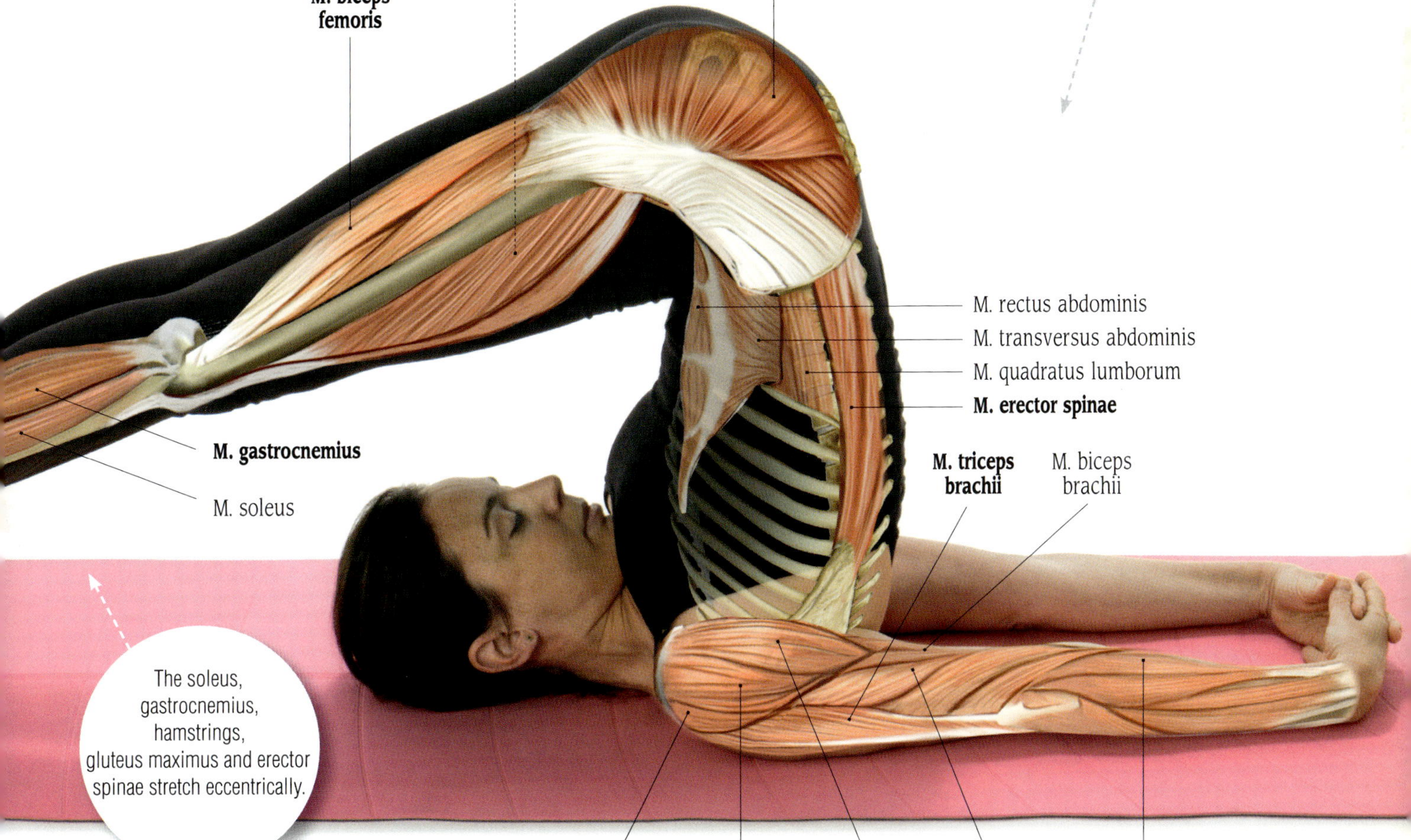

The concentric action of the quadriceps extends the knees.

The action of a straight abdomen directs the pelvis toward the torso.

The triceps contract concentrically, pressing the arms toward the ground; this causes a stretch of the anterior deltoid.

**M. quadriceps femoris**

M. glutaeus maximus

**M. biceps femoris**

M. rectus abdominis
M. transversus abdominis
M. quadratus lumborum
**M. erector spinae**

**M. gastrocnemius**

M. soleus

**M. triceps brachii**

M. biceps brachii

The soleus, gastrocnemius, hamstrings, gluteus maximus and erector spinae stretch eccentrically.

M. deltoideus (posterior part)   M. deltoideus (middle part)   M. deltoideus (anterior part)   M. brachialis   M. brachioradialis

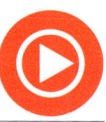

Asanas

SEMI-INVERTED AND INVERTED ASANAS

# Salamba Sirsasana

*Salamba* means "with support," and *sirsa* is translated as "head." It is a vertical pose over the head with support. This is one of the most important asanas of Hatha Yoga.

### CLASSIFICATION
Inverted pose, symmetric, with support from the arms. Balanced pose.

### TECHNIQUE
We start in a kneeling pose, with the forearms supported on the ground and separated the same distance as the knees, making a triangle. We intertwine the fingers in a way that makes a basin; the fingers should be closed and firm. We support the crown of the head on the ground so that the posterior part of the head is in contact with the palms of the hands. We bend the toes and raise the hips. We stretch the legs and raise the weight of the body with the forearms and the head. We walk the feet toward the head and, with a soft impulse, we raise the legs and the feet off of the floor, moving the bent legs toward the chest. All the weight of the body falls on the arms with a little falling on the head. We slowly raise the legs toward a vertical position. We remain in this pose for 20 to 30 breaths and release, inversely and slowly. In order to advance the pose, we can practice next to two angled walls.

### COUNTERPOSE
Balasana. Tadasana.

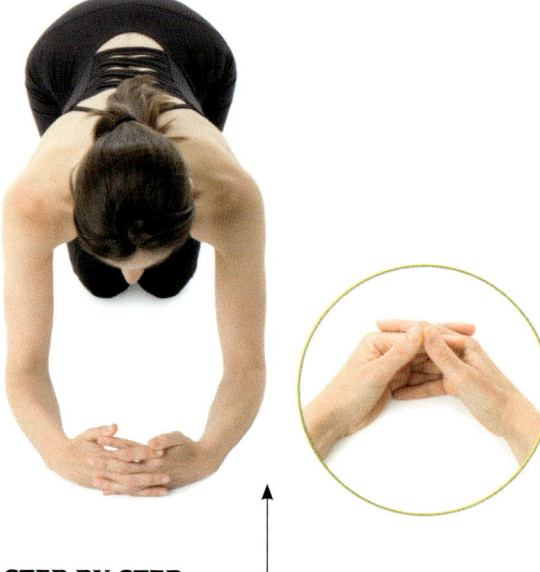

### STEP BY STEP
Starting position on forearms and hands.

We place the head and adjust the hands so that they are well positioned. We move the weight toward the arms and the head. The forearms push on the floor, raising first one leg and then the other.

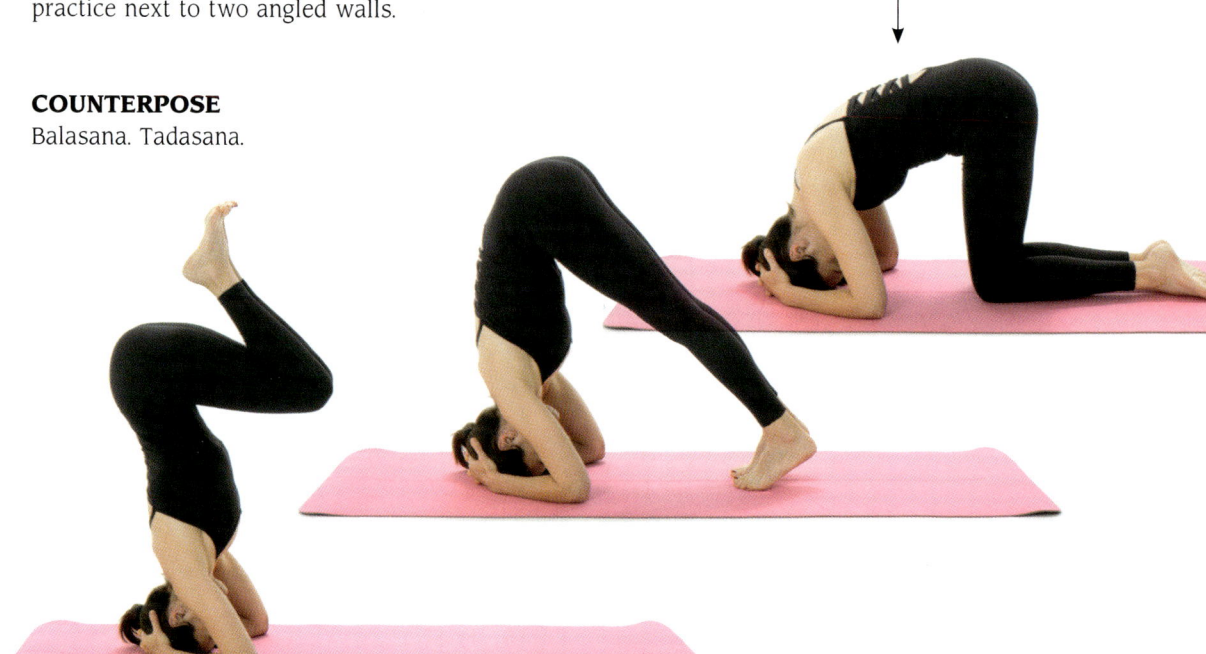

**BENEFITS**
- Improves venous return in the legs, as well as lymphatic drainage.
- Regulates the activity of the circulatory system.
- Rejuvenates the entire organism.

**WARNINGS**
- High or low blood pressure, heart problems.
- Arteriosclerosis.
- Headache, migraines, intraocular pressure, cataracts, or retinal detachment.
- Deviations in the spine or injury in the cervical area.
- Advanced pregnancy.

SEMI-INVERTED AND INVERTED ASANAS: Salamba Sirsasana

The name Sirsasana offers a calm mind, and strengthens self-esteem and self-confidence. It regulates the Ida and Pingala nadis, balancing them. It stimulates the Sahasrara Chakra.

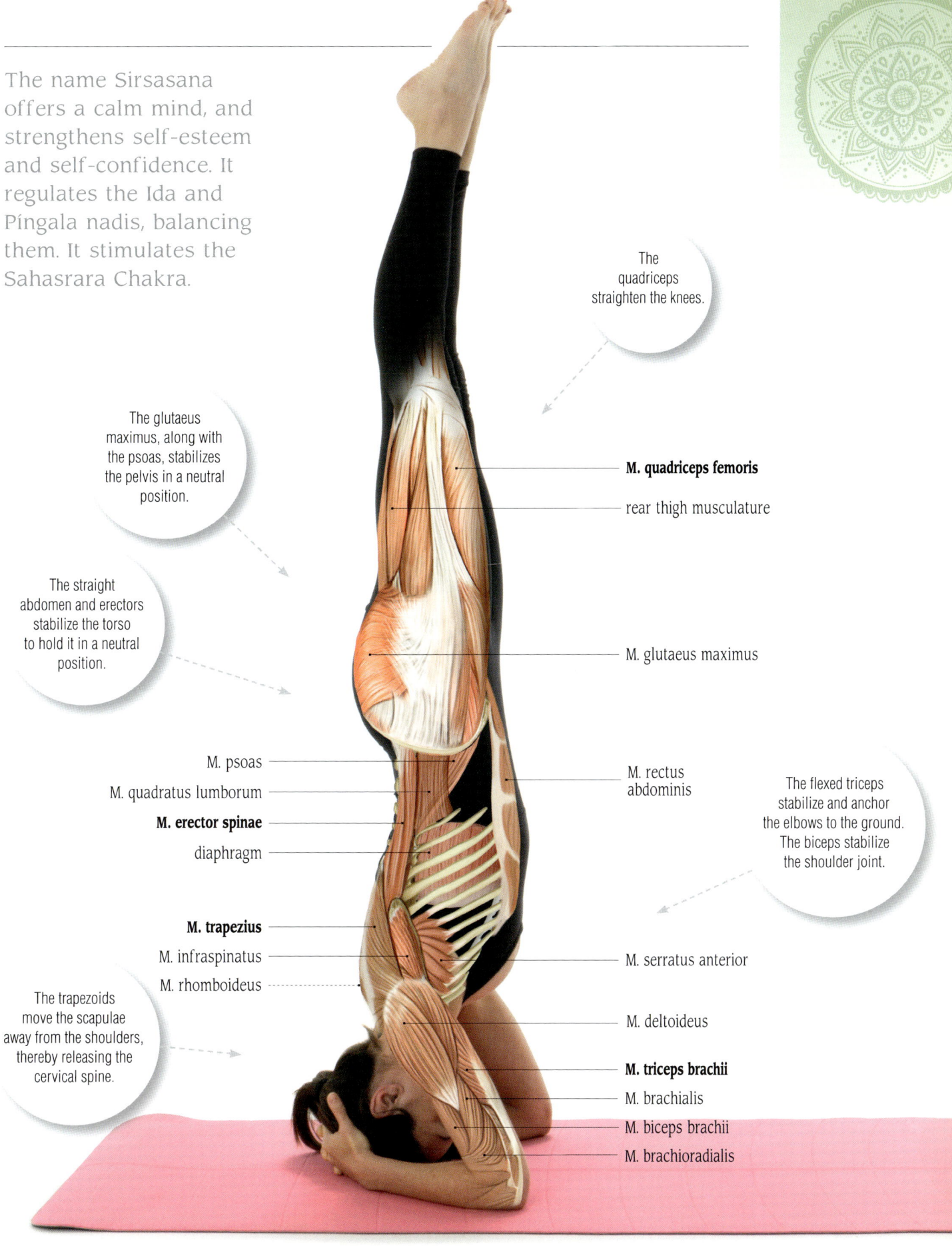

The quadriceps straighten the knees.

**M. quadriceps femoris**
rear thigh musculature

The glutaeus maximus, along with the psoas, stabilizes the pelvis in a neutral position.

M. glutaeus maximus

The straight abdomen and erectors stabilize the torso to hold it in a neutral position.

M. psoas
M. quadratus lumborum
**M. erector spinae**
diaphragm

M. rectus abdominis

The flexed triceps stabilize and anchor the elbows to the ground. The biceps stabilize the shoulder joint.

**M. trapezius**
M. infraspinatus
M. rhomboideus

M. serratus anterior
M. deltoideus
**M. triceps brachii**
M. brachialis
M. biceps brachii
M. brachioradialis

The trapezoids move the scapulae away from the shoulders, thereby releasing the cervical spine.

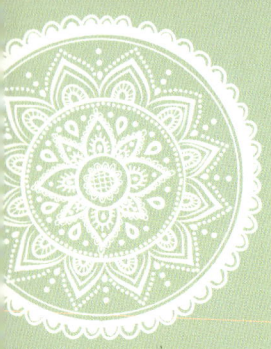

# Suryanamaskar, the Sun Salutation

Sun Salutation is a dynamic succession of 12 poses that are repeated with each movement synchronized with a breath. This series of exercises can be practiced independently or before a session of yoga.

## BENEFITS

- Acts on the whole organism, invigorating and strengthening all muscles.
- Mobilizes the joints, which makes the back flexible.
- Tones the digestive system, providing a massage to all internal organs responsible for digestion. Avoids constipation and dyspepsia.
- Stimulates and tones the nervous system, regulating the functions of the sympathetic and the parasympathetic nervous systems.
- Continued practice returns serenity.
- Increases cardiac activity and allows a good blood supply throughout the body.
- Oxygenates and detoxifies the whole body by synchronizing movement with breathing.

As tradition dictates, Suryanamaskar is done at dawn, when the sun is rising. The exercise is repeated, and can be completed 12 times in a row, maintaining an internal attitude of prayer and gratitude in the light of the sun. It is also done at the beginning of a session of asanas, since it is the best way to warm up and prepare the muscles and the joints.

There are many different variations, depending on the succession and speed. We have chosen one of the most traditional as it is easy to execute and learn.

### TECHNIQUE

To learn the Sun Salutation, you only have to memorize the first movements, since they are repeated inversely.

### 1. Pranamasana.
### Prayer pose

We start in Tadasana. The feet together or lightly separated, we spread out the weight of the body equally between the heels and the anterior part of the feet. With the legs firm, we place the pelvis in a neutral position, bent neither backward nor forward, and we lengthen the straight spine and the cervical column. With a breath, we put the hands into a position of greeting *(namasté)*, with the thumbs touching the sternum. We breathe deeply.

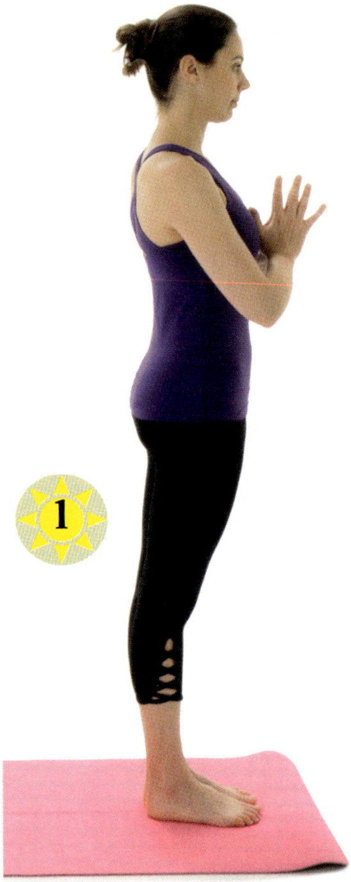

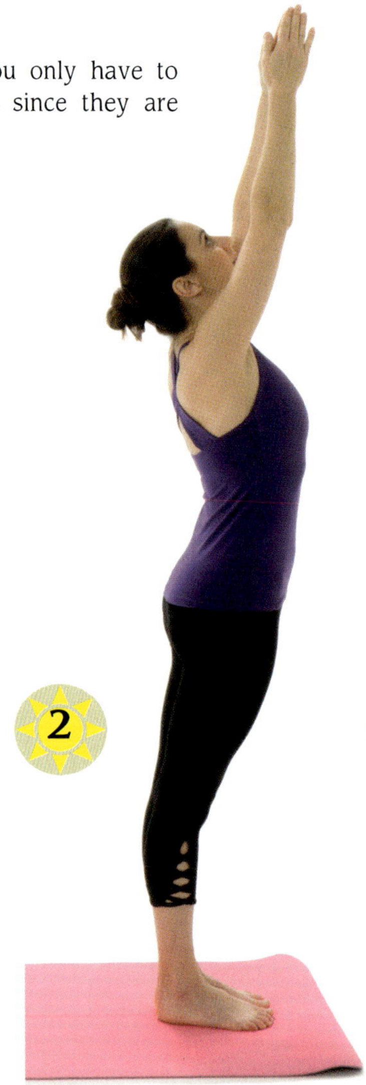

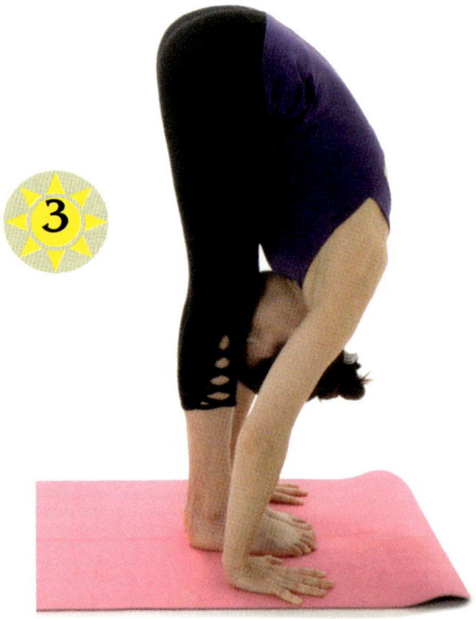

Suryanamaskar, the Sun Salutation

## 2. Hasta Uttanasana.
### A pose with the arms raised
Breathing in, we raise the arms forward and up. The head follows the movement. The sternum also makes a movement upward at the same time that we lean the spine slowly backward. The buttocks and thighs remain flexed.

## 3. Padahastasana.
### A forward flexing pose
With a breath we lower the arms and bend the trunk forward The back is straight and lowers and the palms reach for the ground, we place them on both sides of the feet, making a line between them with the toes pointing forward. If we have limited flexibility, we can bend the knees. The trunk and head move close to the thighs. The head remains relaxed.

## 4. Ashwa Sanchalanasana.
### Horse pose
We breathe in while bending the left knee, without passing the ankle, and lengthening the right leg backwards. The right knee and the toes of the right foot are based on the floor. The hands and left foot are held on the ground. The head is facing forward, although some schools leave the head slightly back.

## 5. Chaturanga Dandasana.
### Table pose
While exhaling, we bring the left leg back, next to the other, so that both legs are parallel. The pelvis should not fall down. The body makes an inclined plane, from the head to the feet.

## 6. Ashtanganamaskara.
### Salutation with the eight members
With the lungs empty, we hold our breath, while first resting our knees on the ground, then the chest and, lastly, the chin. In the final position, the spine is slightly arched and the pelvis is raised.

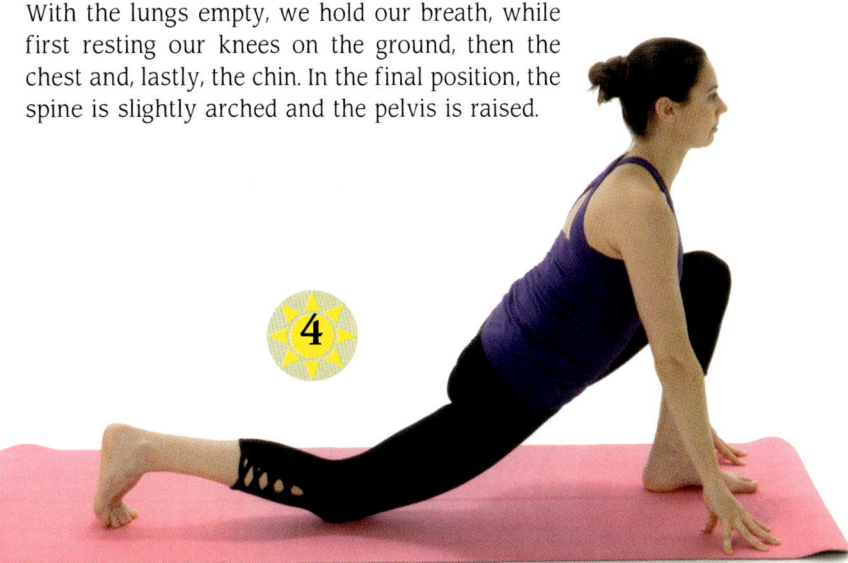

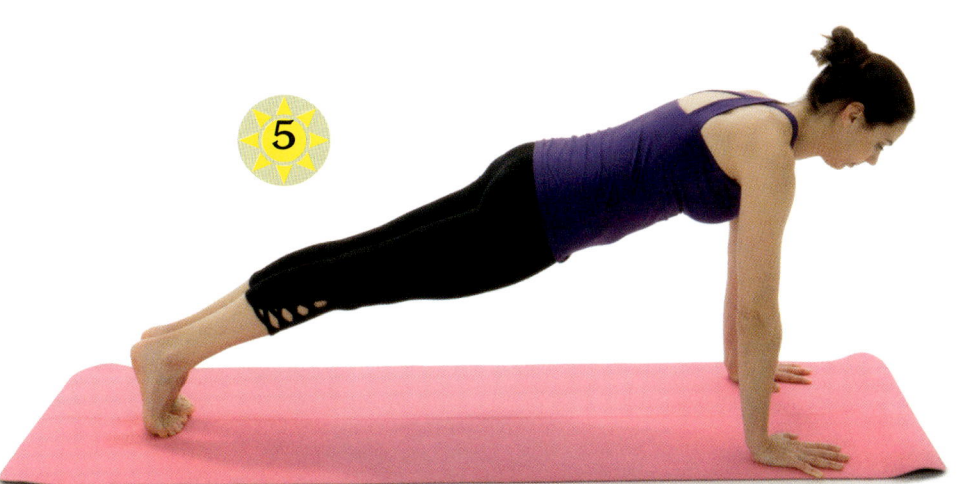

The Sun Salutation allows us to fully integrate the body, mind, and breathing.

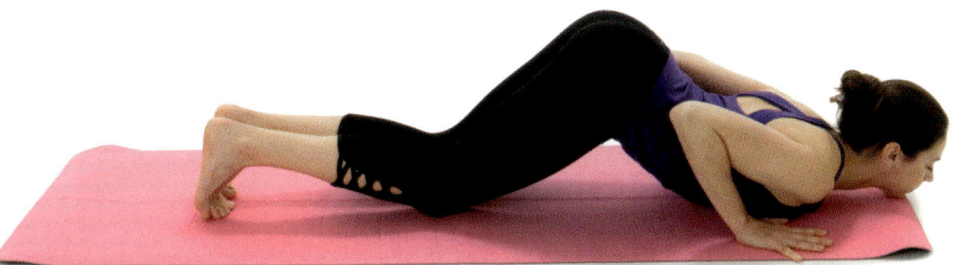

## WARNINGS

- Severe problems or chronic back pain.
- Hernias.
- Inflammation in the abdomen.
- Hypertension and eye problems.
- Pregnancy in advanced stage.

### 7. Bhujangasana.
**Serpent pose**

With an inhale, we move the body forward, sliding the chin and the chest on the ground. The palms of the hands are pressed against the ground and while using the strength of the arms and the back, we first lift the head and then the thorax, focusing on raising one vertebra at a time. The buttocks and thighs are contracted. The shoulders should remain back and down, in a way that creates broadness in the thorax. The pubis keeps contact with the ground and the spine extension should be spread equally, making sure not to create any pronounced lumbar lordosis.

### 8. Adho Muka Svanasana.
**Dog pose** (also called Parvatanasana or mountain posture)

With an exhalation, we press our hands hard against the ground, and raise the knees and the pelvis, which we project backwards and upwards. We move the weight to the soles of the feet and stretch the legs, pushing the heels toward the floor.

### 9. Ashwa Sanchalanasana.
**Horse posture**

As we inhale, we bend the right knee (or the left one, but remembering to always bend the same knee in one series, and the other knee in the next series), without exceeding the ankle, and stretch the left leg towards behind. The right knee and the toes of the right foot are based on the floor. The head is facing forward.

### 10. Padahastasana.
**Forward flexing pose**

With one breath, we bring back the leg that is stretched forward, placing it next to the other, and stretch both legs. The arms are low with the trunk flexed forward. The trunk and head move close to the thighs. The head is relaxed.

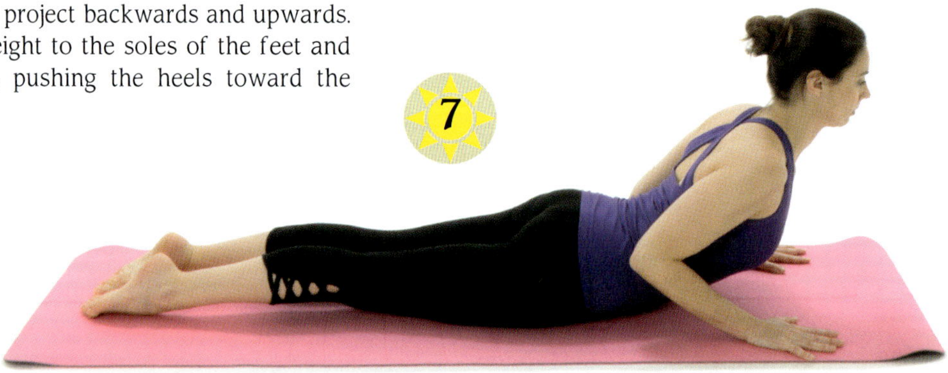

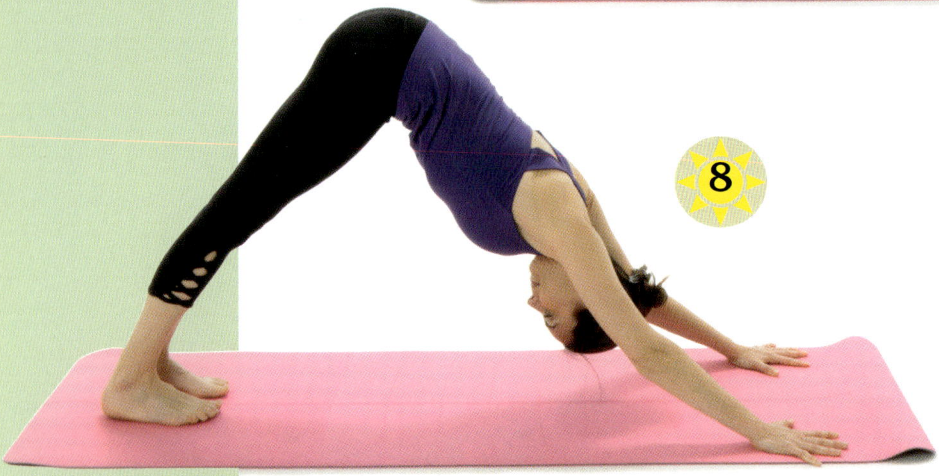

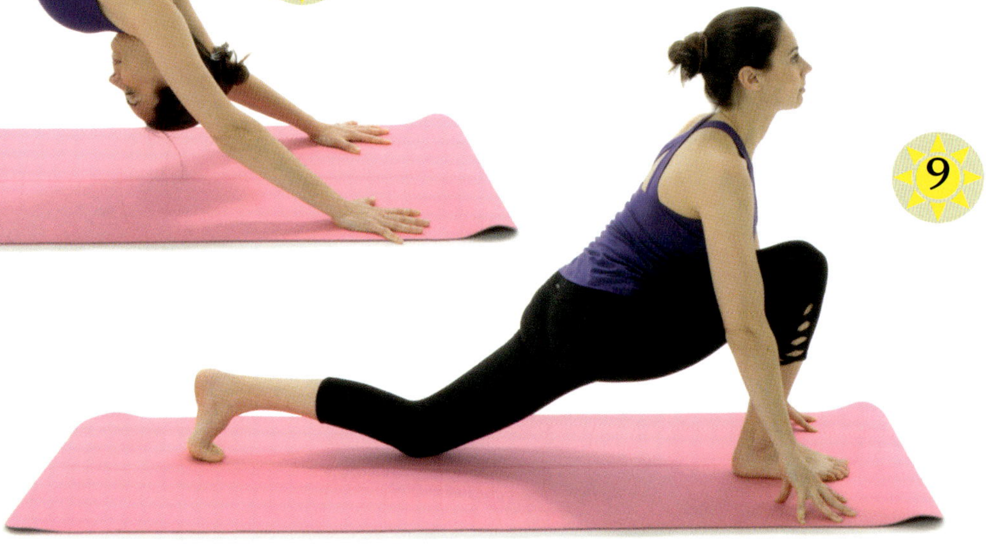

Suryanamaskar, Sun Salutation

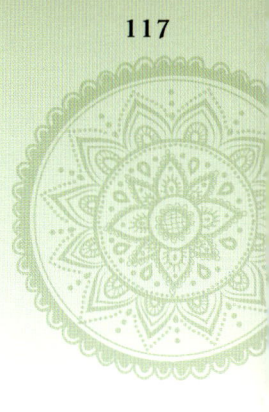

## 11. Hasta Uttanasana.
### Arms raised pose

While breathing in, we bend our legs slightly and carry our arms and trunk forward and up. While we raise the trunk, it remains straight and the leg muscles are active. The head follows the movement. The sternum also makes a movement upward, the spine leans slowly backward. In the final position, the buttocks and thighs remain flexed.

## 12. Pranamasana.
### Prayer pose

We breathe in and return to the starting position. The arms drop with the hands together in *namasté*; they pass by the face and the thumbs make contact with the sternum.

We can do two to twelve series, while considering that the leg that we move forward in the 4th position should alternate with the other leg in the next series. When finishing the series, we remain in Tadasana for a moment and then relax by sitting or stretching out on the floor. We become aware of the benefits that the Sun Salutation provides us.

### ADAPTATION

We can completed a half Sun Salutation by combining the poses in a short series, for example:
**a)** poses 1, 2, 3, 11, 12
**b)** poses 1, 2, 3, 4, 10, 11, 12
**c)** poses 1, 2, 3, 4, 8, 9, 10, 11, 12

These combinations are an alternative for people who, for various reasons, cannot complete the full Sun Salutation.

### KEY ASPECTS

- Use a non-slip mat to perform the asanas and practice with bare feet.
- Perform the exercises giving full attention, to the movements linking them in a smooth and harmonious way and avoiding sudden changes in speed.
- Start slowly if the body is a little stiff or sore, and increase speed little by little.
- The speed will depend on the circumstance of each person.
- To get maximum benefits, exercise must be synchronized with breathing.
- After practice, we relax for a few minutes in Savasana, and we become aware of what the exercise has brought us.

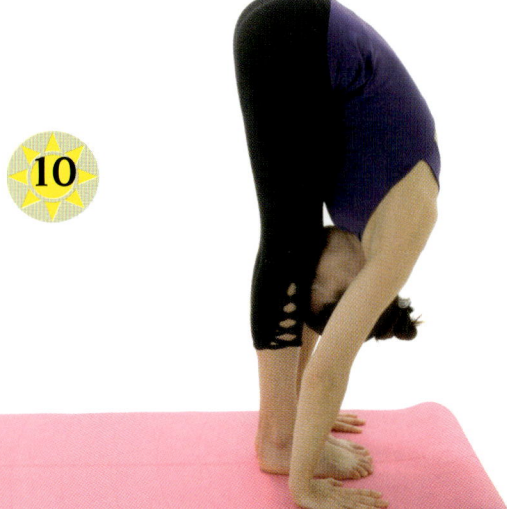
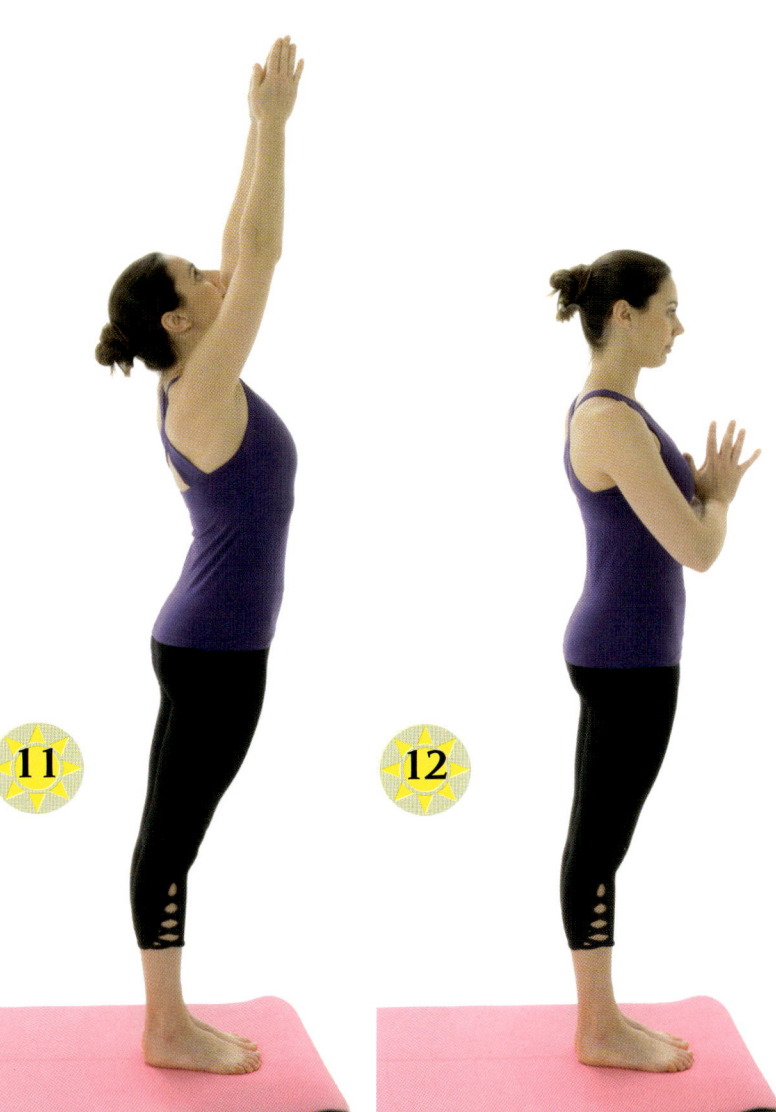

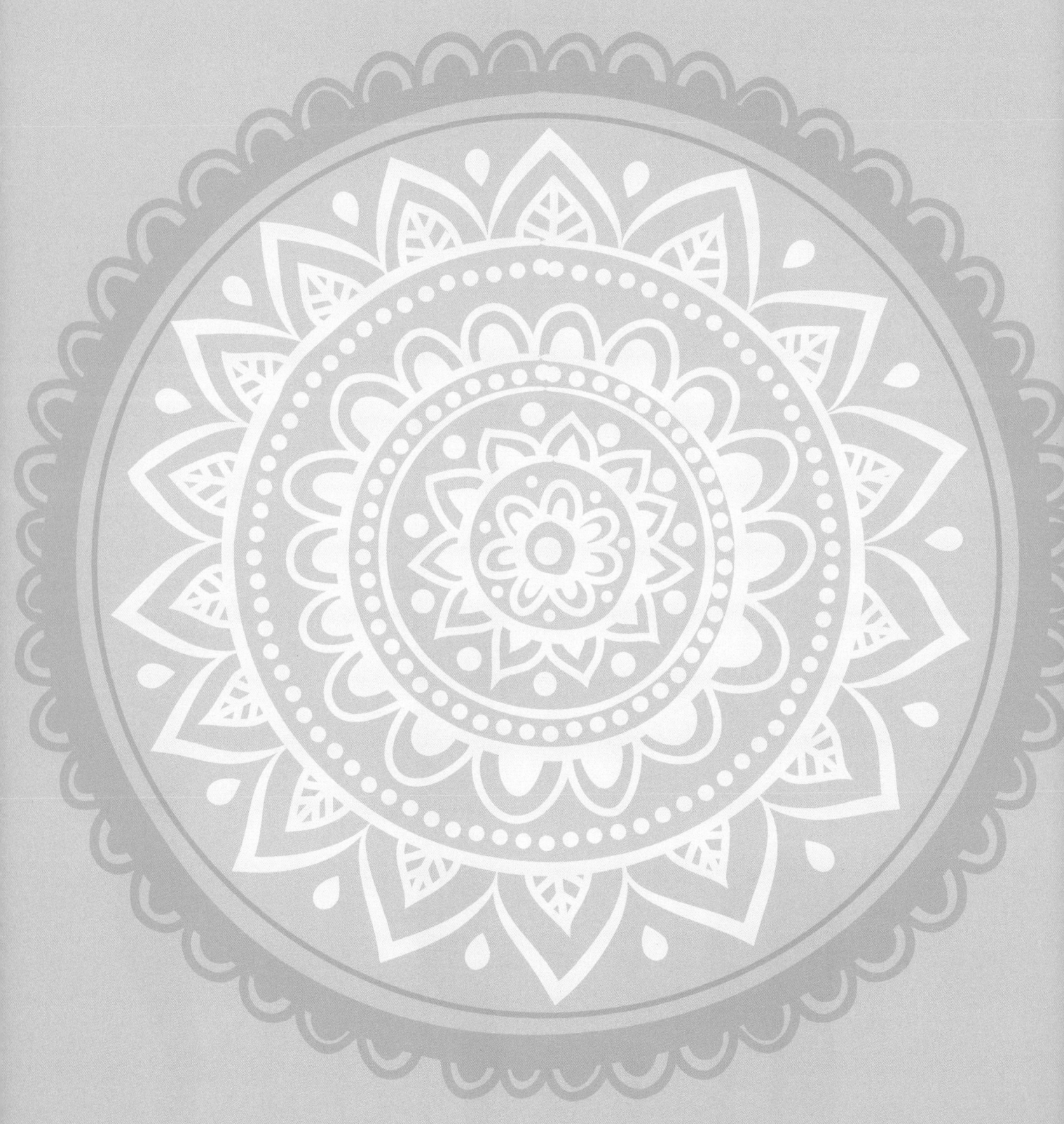

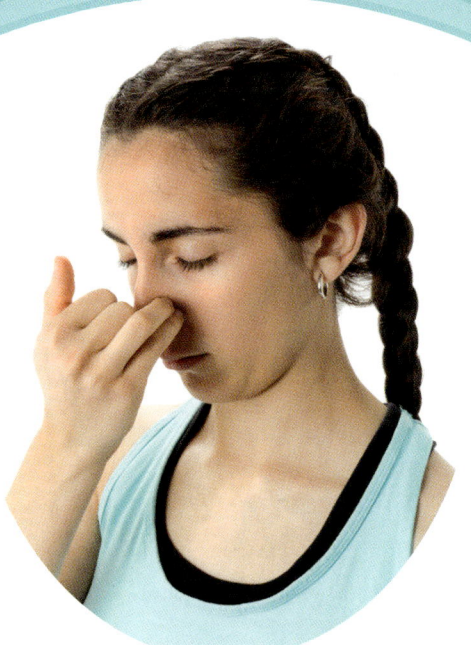

# PRANAYAMA AND BANDHAS

Pranayama is a set of techniques that make it possible to voluntarily control the respiratory process. The primary goal is to dominate the mental states and balance the flow of energy in the body. As for the bandhas, their voluntary muscular contractions allow us to control and channel energy. In the first part of this chapter, the anatomy and biomechanics of the respiratory system are described, which are necessary to introduce the proposed exercises. The following will explain some basic techniques that are commonly used when practicing pranayama. Lastly, the three most important bandhas are described.

PRANAYAMA

# The respiratory system

The respiratory system works in cooperation with the cardiovascular system to provide oxygen to our body and eliminate carbon dioxide. The exchange, which occurs at the cellular level, is called cellular respiration. Oxygen is obtained from the atmosphere and goes to the lungs, and from there into the blood, which, thanks to the pumping of the heart, transports it through the organism until it reaches all the cells where the exchange takes place. Conversely, carbon dioxide is removed from the body.

**THE ORGANS OF THE RESPIRATORY SYSTEM**

The respiratory system is made up of various organs: nasal cavities, pharynx, larynx, trachea, bronchii and lungs, the latter of which contains the alveoli. The primary function of all of them is to transport, humidify, heat, and purify the air that enters the lungs. The exchange of gases occurs in the alveoli.

**The nasal cavities.** They are covered with a mucus whose function is to filter, heat, and humidify the air that we breathe. The olfactory receptors are found in this mucosa. The air that enters is pushed toward the rear of the nose, where it rotates 90º to enter the pharynx.

**The pharynx.** Commonly called the throat, it is made up of three regions: the nasopharynx, the oropharynx, and the laryngopharynx. Only the first area is exclusive of breathing, the other two are shared with the digestive tract. In the pharynx we find the tonsils, which perform a defensive function in the body.

**The larynx.** It directs air to the trachea and stops food from entering while swallowing, thanks to the glottis. In addition, it is the phonation organ; its folds, or vocal cords, have the ability to vibrate and generate the sound for the voice.

**The trachea.** It is a tube that is reinforced by some cartilaginous rings and smooth muscles. It is responsible for transporting air from the larynx to the primary bronchus.

**The primary bronchus.** The trachea is subdivided into the right and left bronchial tubes. From these, air passes into the lungs.

**The lungs.** Each lung is primarily comprised of elastic tissue and respiratory tracks. Each one contains 10 bronchial-lung segments that are subdivided into secondary and tertiary bronchus and bronchiole. All of this makes up the bronchial tree.

The alveoli is where gas exchange occurs.

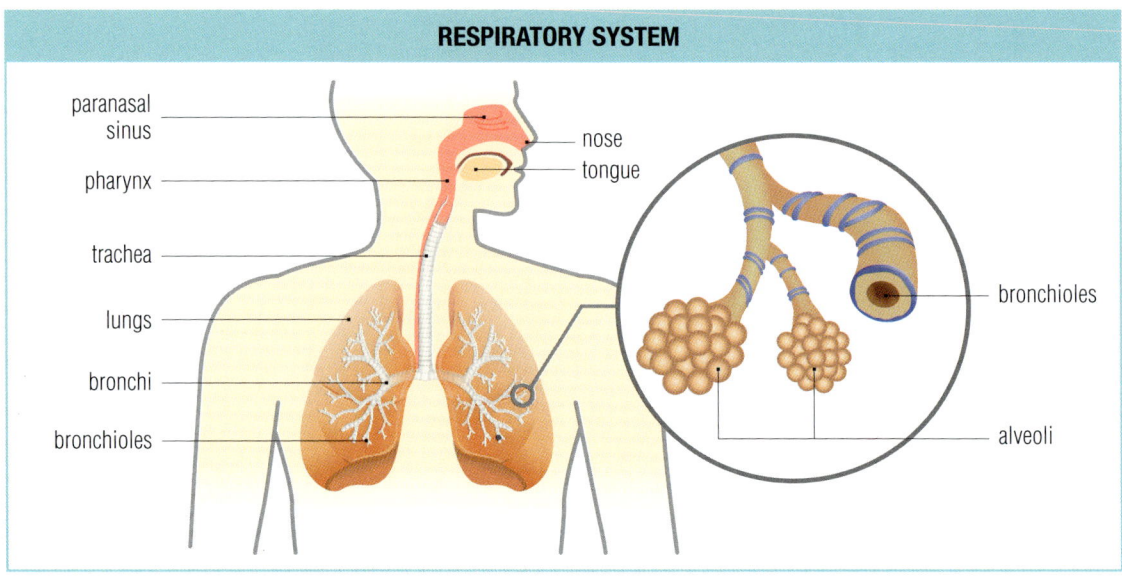

RESPIRATORY SYSTEM

PRANAYAMA: The respiratory system

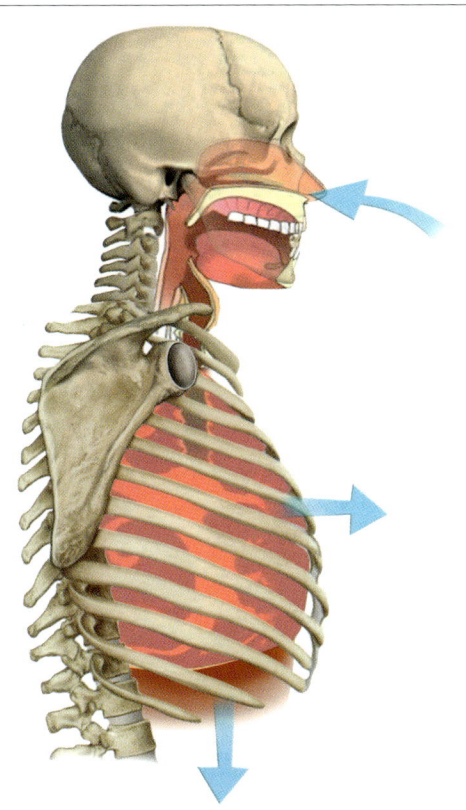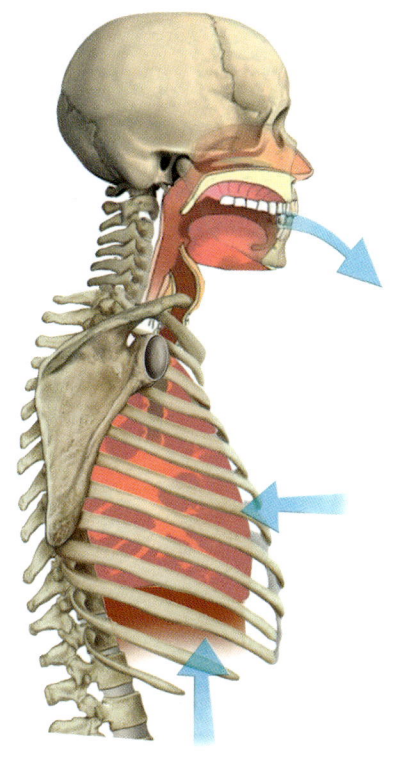

The lungs are formed by an elastic tissue that adapts to the dimensions of the rib cage. On the inhale, the ribs are raised by the contraction of the external intercostal muscles, the diaphragm descends, and the air enters the lungs. On the exhale, the intercostal muscles relax, the diaphragm rises, and the air leaves the lungs.

**The alveoli.** The minor bronchioles end up in the alveoli or air sacs. This is where gaseous exchange occurs, that is, the oxygen obtained from the atmosphere passes from the alveolus to a tiny blood capillary and the carbon dioxide from the capillaries passes into the alveoli.

## THE MUSCLES OF BREATHING

Inhalations are produced by a combined muscular action, while in the exhalation the lung, which is elastic, recovers its natural state by contracting next to the rib cage. There are three main muscle groups involved in respiration:

**The intercostal muscles** are involved in the expansion and contraction of the chest. In inhalation, the external intercostal muscles widen the rib cage. In a forced exhalation, it is the internal intercostal muscles that contract the thorax.

**The abdominal muscles** are involved in deep and consciously forced exhalations. In yoga, they are very important and we use them in pranayama.

**The diaphragm** is a large umbrella-shaped muscle located between the thoracic and abdominal cavities. It forms a central tendon attached to muscle fibers, forming muscle bands around it.

## BIOMECHANICS OF BREATHING

Changes in the volume of the rib cage cause a continuous change of pressure between the inside and outside of the lungs. These pressure changes are compensated through the incoming or outgoing air flow.

**Inspiration** occurs when air enters the lungs, thereby increasing the thoracic cage due to contraction of the diaphragm and the external intercostal muscles. The diaphragm, when contracting, moves down and flattens, while the intercostal muscles elevate the ribs. This operation generates more intrapulmonary volume, as well as a slight vacuum, which makes the air flow into the rib cage.

**Expiration** is usually a passive process. The natural pulmonary elasticity, together with the relaxation of the inspiratory muscles, decreases the intrapulmonary and thoracic volume. The diaphragm ascends. The intrapulmonary pressure is higher than the atmospheric pressure and the air exits to the outside in order to equalize the pressure inside and outside the rib cage.

When expiration becomes an active process, it is called forced expiration. The intercostal muscles are activated and the abdominals are contracted, and the combination of both helps to expel the air outwards.

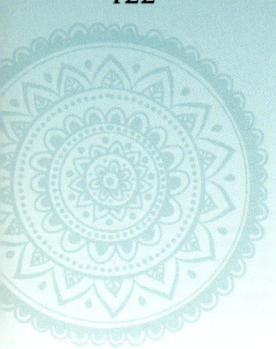

## PRANAYAMA

# Basic types of breathing

Before introducing pranayama we present the four basic types of breathing that we can consciously perform: diaphragmatic breathing, chest breathing, clavicular breathing, and paradoxical breathing.

It is necessary to become aware of our natural breathing before starting any exercise. The observation of the breath allows us to obtain a lot of information about our physical and psychological state.

These first breathing exercises that we propose will facilitate the later practice of pranayama.

### OBSERVING NATURAL BREATHING

Before any conscious modification of our breathing can take place, we must listen to our interior and observe how we are breathing before and after exercise. In this way, we can focus on the present, the here and now of our respiratory process.

### Technique

To become aware of how we breathe, we sit in Sukasana or we lie down in Savasana. We close our eyes and, without modifying our respiratory process, we perceive how the air enters and exits our nostrils. The observation must be passive: we notice where it arises, what part of our body expands, which is contracted, as well as the touch and temperature of the air that enters and exits through the nose.

Let us accept our breath as it is, without trying to modify it. We stay like this for a few minutes. If a blockage appears or we tire, we stop and yawn by stretching the body.

### DIAPHRAGMATIC BREATHING

This is the simplest and most natural breath, the one we observe in a baby when he sleeps peacefully. However, diaphragmatic breathing is not only a relaxed abdominal breathing, it must be performed taking into account the abdominal waist.

### Technique

Stretched in Savasana or posture of the corpse, we place the hands on both sides of the abdomen. At first, we establish an abdominal breathing so that on an inhalation, the abdomen rises and on an exhalation, it lowers toward the floor.

Once this relaxed abdominal breathing is achieved, we focus the attention on the abdominal waist. For this, it is necessary that we maintain a slight muscle tone below the navel. When inhaling, only the upper part of the abdomen widens. The volume of inhaled air is the same as in relaxed breathing, but now the back pressure of the abdominals widens the upper abdomen, creating an adequate intra-abdominal pressure. This is important in order to avoid permanent deformation of the lower abdomen.

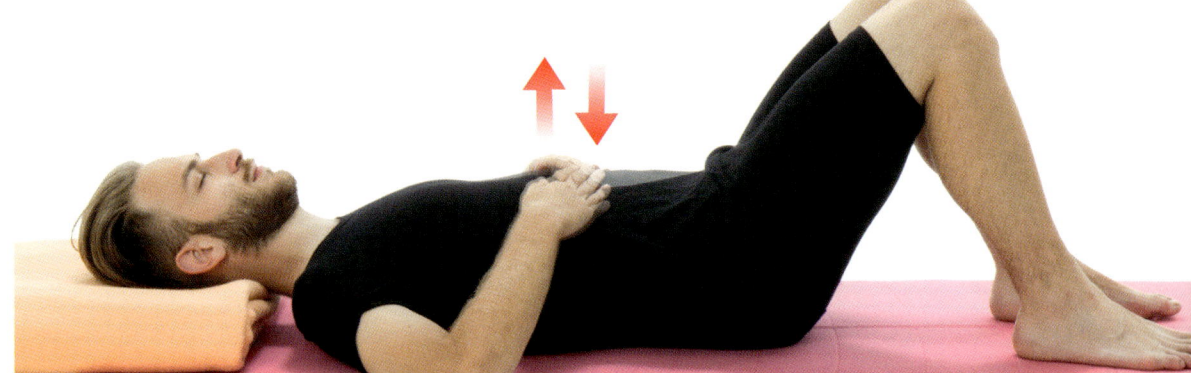

Observation of abdominal breathing.

PRANAYAMA: Basic types of breathing

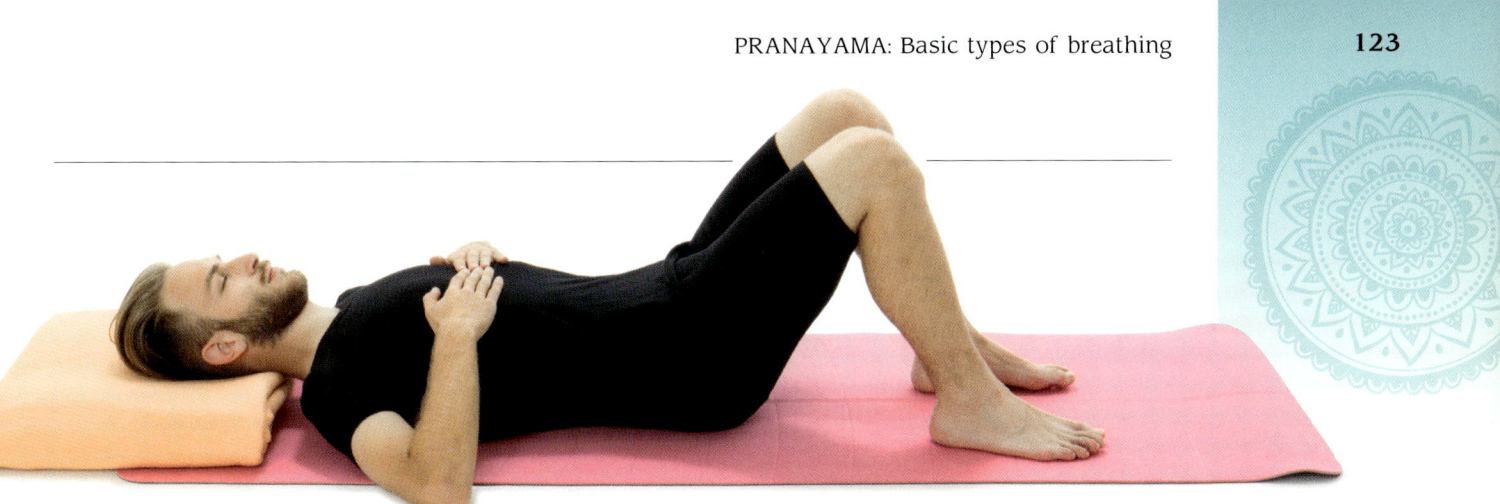

## THORACIC BREATHING
It is a deep breath. The air enters the thorax, and it expands upwards and to the sides. The breast is lifted by the intercostal muscles.

### Technique
The Savasana position is ideal for experiencing thoracic breathing. We place both hands at the level of the ribs and inhale, trying to feel the thorax expand toward the sides and upwards. The abdominal wall remains relaxed, but at the same time retains a smooth muscle tone. When inhaling, the thoracic cage widens to the maximum and the diaphragm only intervenes so that its vault is not pressed upwards (as would happen in an exhalation or in reverse or paradoxical breathing).

## CLAVICULAR BREATHING
It is a very shallow breathing in which only the upper part of the chest rises. The muscles responsible for this breathing are the scalenes, which originate in the cervical spine, and are inserted into the first and second ribs. We observe our clavicular breathing during the course of a full breath (see Maha Yoga Pranayama).

## PARADOXICAL BREATHING
Paradoxical breathing appears after having a scare or suffering an unexpected situation. In stressful situations of great intensity, we also adopt this breath.

It is called paradoxical because the abdominal wall moves inward during inhalation, and outward in exhalation. This is the opposite of what happens in diaphragmatic breathing. The external intercostal muscles create a vacuum in the rib cage that pushes the diaphragm up.

This breathing stimulates the sympathetic nervous system and prepares us for a stressful fight-or-flight situation in an emergency.

Observing thoracic respiration.

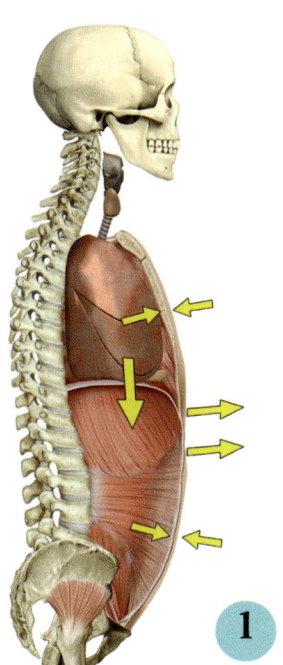
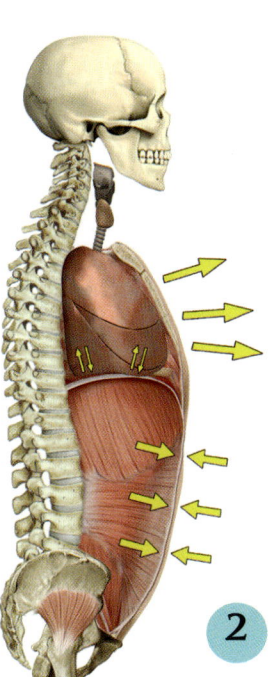
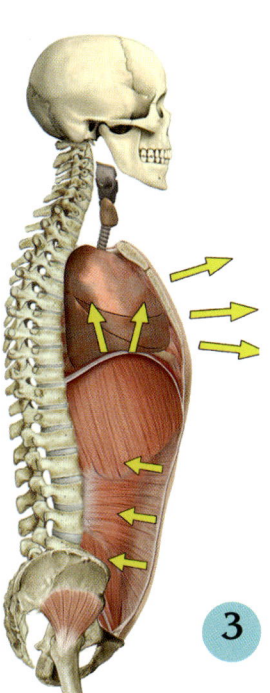

1. Diaphragmatic breathing

2. Thoracic breathing.

3. Paradoxical breathing.

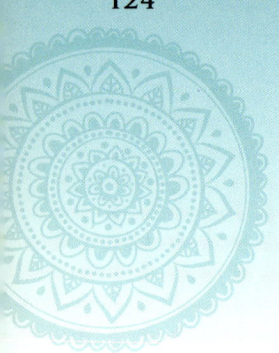

PRANAYAMA

# The practice of pranayama

The ancient yogis of India devised pranayama, which is a set of techniques that allow self-control of the respiratory process. With its continued practice, mental states can be mastered and the energy fluxes of the body balanced.

**THE PRANA**

The term *prana* has been translated in many different ways: breath, air, life, life force, and energy. Other interpretations describe prana as the essence of the energy principle of the universe. From this definition, prana would be found everywhere, manifesting itself in constant movement and transformation. Breathing, in addition to providing oxygen to all the cells of the body and eliminating carbon dioxide, is the main source of obtaining prana. We also absorb prana through the skin.

Prana is the vital, pure, and subtle energy that permeates the entire universe.

**THE PRANAYAMA**

The term *pranayama* comes from the word *prana*, which is translated as "vital energy," and from *ayama*, which means "to contain" or "to control." The pranayama is, then, a set of techniques that, through the regulation of the respiratory process, allow us to control the prana. This control of breathing occurs consciously, through the prolongation of inhalation, retention, and exhalation.

Its main objective is the collection, accumulation, and distribution of prana throughout our body. With continued practice, it increases and balance the vital energy flows. In addition, by controlling the breath, we can, at the same time, control the mental states.

The prana that we absorb is a specialization of *cosmic prana*. In the human body, prana performs 10 functions known as *pranavayus* (vital airs). The five *pranavayus* that work within the body are called *vayus* or *pancha pranas*. These are: *prana, apana, samana, udana,* and *vyana*.

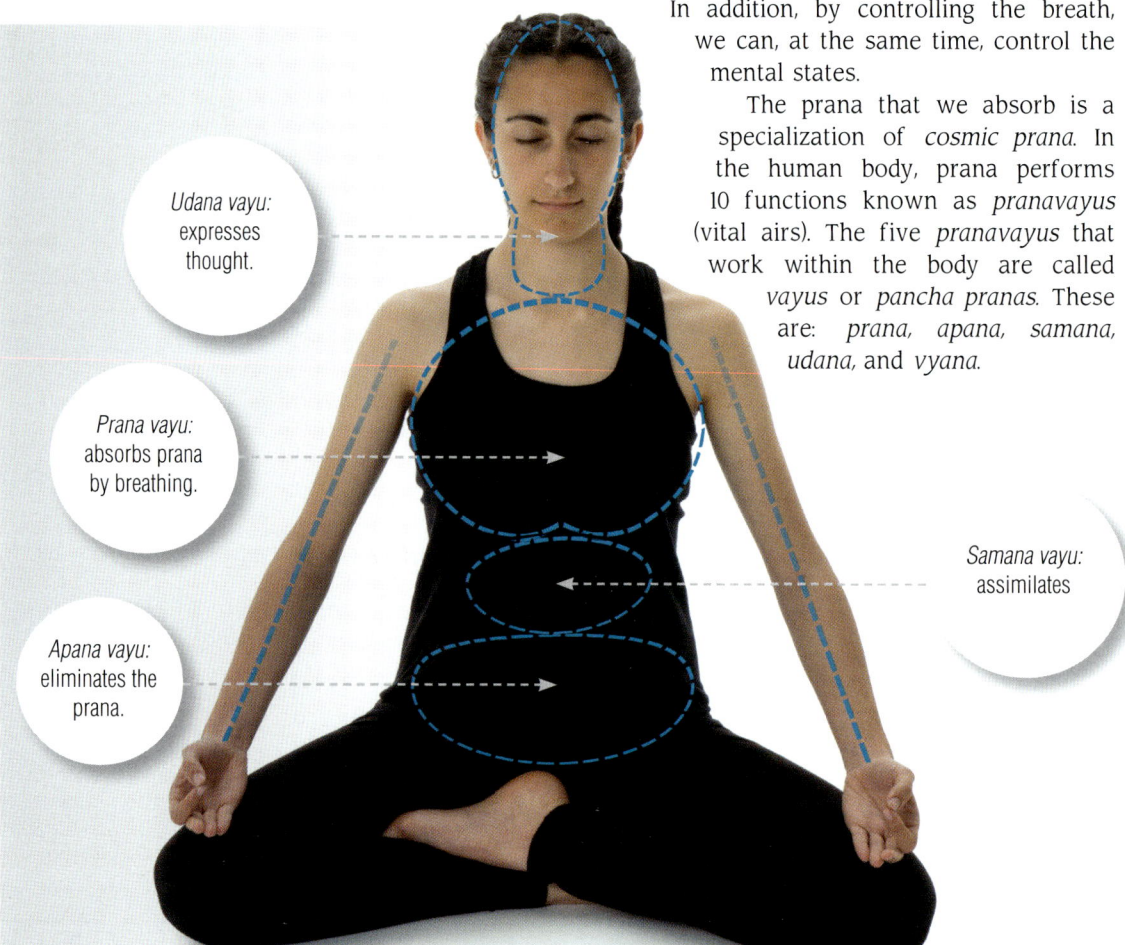

*Udana vayu:* expresses thought.

*Vyana vayu:* distributes the prana in the body, and coordinates the other vayus.

*Prana vayu:* absorbs prana by breathing.

*Samana vayu:* assimilates

*Apana vayu:* eliminates the prana.

# PRANAYAMA: The practice of pranayama

## BENEFITS OF PRANAYAMA

- Positively influences the physical, mental, and energetic body of the human being.
- Favors better oxygenation of the blood and elimination of carbon dioxide.
- Develops a stable and balanced mind.
- Benefits the nervous, respiratory, and circulatory systems.
- Tones the heart.
- Provides vitality, increases the level of energy, and activates the chakras.
- Balances the activity of the nadis, purifying them and eliminating their possible blockages.

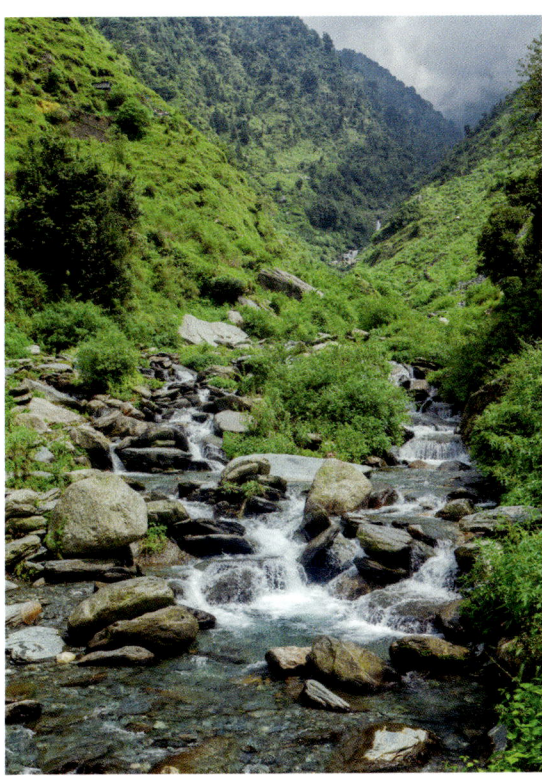

## PHASES OF BREATHING

Yogic breathing comprises four phases: the inhalation *(puraka)*, the retention of the breath with the lungs completely filled *(antara kumbhaka* or *puraka kumbhaka)*, exhalation *(rechaka)*, and breath retention with empty lungs *(bahya kumbhaka* or *rechaka kumbhaka)*.

In *puraka* we participate in the environment that surrounds us; the attitude must be open to reception. In *antara kumbhaka*, the universal energy merges with the individual energy, and the experiences are assimilated and retained. In *rechaka* we let go all that we no longer want; it is a process of detachment. In *bahya kumbhaka*, we abandon our own being to merge with the universal Prana; it is a moment of calm and recollection with oneself.

## JALA NETI

Respiration is usually done through the nose, so it is necessary to have clean and clear nostrils. For this, it is advisable to perform *Jala Neti*, using a neti pot and salt water.

The process is simple. Fill the saltwater pond to a warm temperature. It is best to use distilled water or saline in the water of the neti. It is important to make sure the water is pure. Alternately, we first pass water through one nostril to the other and vice versa. The mouth remains open throughout the process. When finished, it is important to dry the nostrils well.

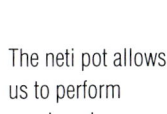

The neti pot allows us to perform nasal washes.

## CONSIDERATIONS BEFORE STARTING PRACTICE

- The best time to practice pranayama is in the morning, after performing an asana session or the Sun Salutation.
- We will practice in a ventilated place or in the open air.
- We will choose a firm and comfortable posture, and keep our eyes closed.
- We will avoid practicing after eating or and when we feel hungry.
- Before beginning a practice of pranayama, we will observe our natural breathing.
- Our breathing must be (except in some practices) silent, soft, slow, and deep.
- After performing pranayama, it is necessary for us to relax in Savasana for a few minutes.

Bhagsu Waterfall, northern India. Air in nature is loaded with *prana*.

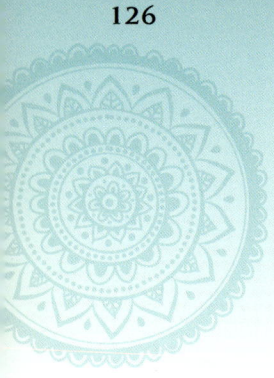

## PRANAYAMA

# Initiation to pranayama

There is a deep connection between breathing and our emotional, mental, and energetic states. Through pranayama, we can modify and balance our internal state, so that we can activate, calm, and balance it. The continued practice will develop new capabilities and allow us to strengthen those we need.

**FREQUENCY AND RESPIRATORY RATE**

**The frequency** is the number of breaths we perform at a specific time. In a healthy adult, the normal frequency is between 12 and 20 breaths per minute. The frequency varies with age and mood. Rapid breathing can be a symptom of emotional agitation or anxiety, while slow breathing indicates psychic and mental tranquility.

**The rate** is the regularity of the time we invest in the phases of inhalation and exhalation. The continued practice of pranayama will allow us to modify our own rhythm at will to obtain different breaths: balancing, stimulating, and tranquilizing. When the duration of exhalation is similar or equal to inhalation (1:1), we say that breathing is balancing. If exhalation is slower and longer than inhalation, we obtain a calming breath (1:2); and if, on the other hand, the inhalation is passive and slow and the exhalation short and powerful, it is a stimulating breath (2:1).

the jaw, and the tongue remain relaxed. Unlike meditation, pranayama can be practiced with the tip of the nose toward the sternum, that is, with the head slightly tilted downward.

During the practice, the eyes remain closed, but if necessary, they can be opened from time to time to observe the posture and readjust it. The ears are attentive to the sound of our breathing. The gaze is directed toward our interior.

The graph shows normal breathing in a relaxed state, at which time the expiration is slightly longer than the inspiration. The rhythm would be (breathe in 5 : breathe in 6).

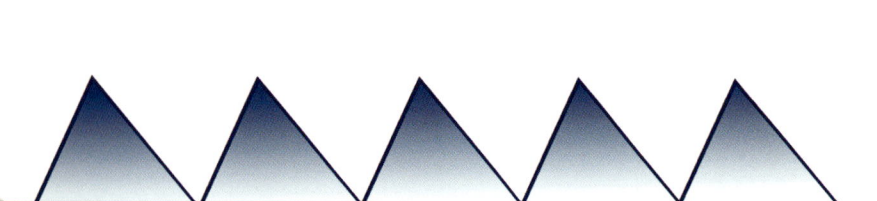

**THE RIGHT POSITION FOR PRACTICE**
To practice pranayama, it is essential to sit in a correct posture, that is, in a posture of meditation (see next chapter). Depending on our flexibility, we choose one position or the other.

We sit with the back straight and the trunk active, while the arms rest on the legs. Shoulders fall down, away from the neck. The lips, the face,

Practicing pranayama. We maintain the body stable and firm, while the mind remains alert, though calm.

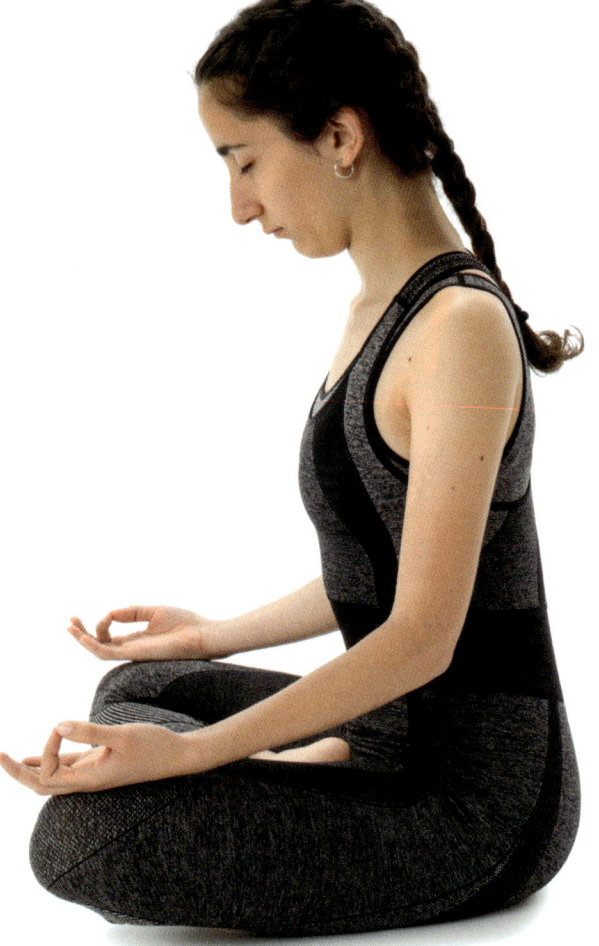

## MAHA YOGA PRANAYAMA

*Mahat* means "great," "powerful," or "abundant." It can also mean the first principle of consciousness from which all other phenomena arise. It is the complete breathing, the great breathing of yoga.

### Technique

Sitting in meditation posture or in Savasana, we observe our natural breathing. With a slow and uniform movement, we establish a new breath that will affect the three respiratory zones. We begin the inhalation in the abdominal area, which spreads smoothly to the thoracic area and ends in the clavicular. When we exhale, we proceed in the same way: we remove the air first from the abdominal area, then from the thoracic, and finally from the clavicular.

## SUKHA PRANAYAMA

This is an easy breath, that allows us to match the breathing rhythms.

### Technique

Seated in pranayama posture, with the chin slightly tucked in, we observe our natural breath without modifying it. A few minutes later, we match the duration of Puraka (inhalation) and Rechaka (exhalation). At first, we concentrate on counting the time we spend on exhalation (one, two, three...) and we match it with the inhalation time (one, two, three...).

We perform Suka Pranayama for a few minutes and then let the breath flow naturally again.

We see the effects of this practice.

### BENEFITS

- Oxygenates the body.
- Eliminates toxins.
- Relaxes the nervous system, calms the mind.
- Eliminates tiredness, tension, and stress.
- Massages the internal organs.
- Increases lung capacity, and allows the heart to rest.
- Rejuvenates the entire body.

### BENEFITS

- Balances the whole organism.
- Accompanied by complete breathing, the same benefits are added.
- Prepares us for meditation.

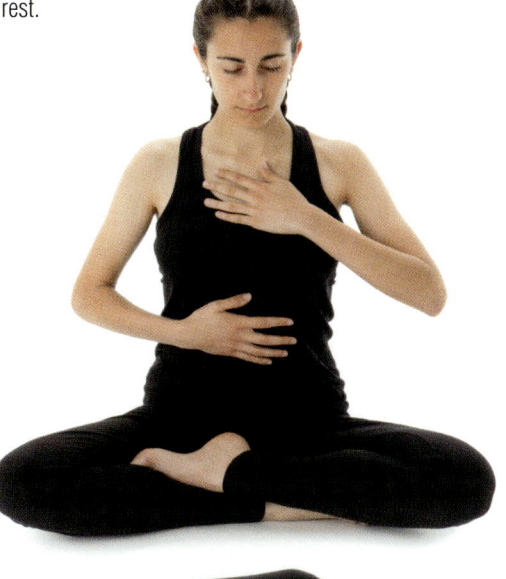

Sitting in meditation posture, with one hand on the abdomen and another on the thoracic area, we become aware of the flow of the breath through the three breathing spaces.

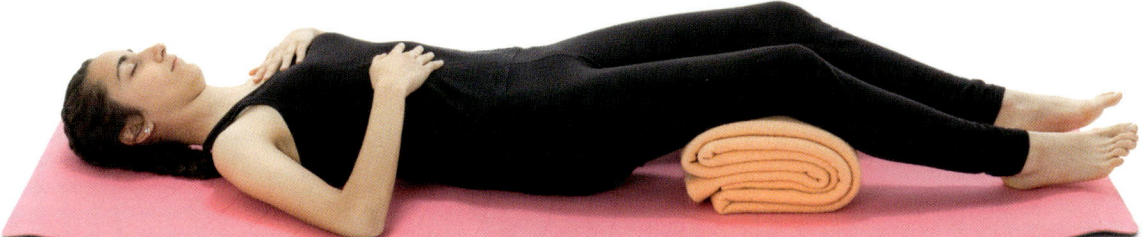

In Savasana, the practice of Maha Yoga Pranayama allows us to better observe the three breathing spaces.

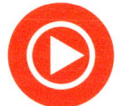

PRANAYAMA

# Basic techniques of pranayama

The various techniques of pranayama that exist exert numerous beneficial effects on our organism. Some are reassuring and act as a sedative on the nervous system; others are revitalizing. The continued practice will bring us a state of physical-mental balance preparatory to meditation.

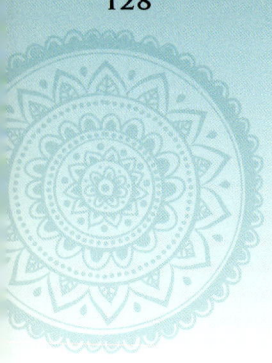

Detail of the position of the fingers in the nose. To find the exact position, we slide our fingers up and down on both sides of the nasal septum. When we reach the soft zone, the nostrils, we find the exact place to press to cover the air way.

We present three basic and simple techniques that will bring us balance and mental calm: Nadi Sodhana, Ujjayi, and Bhramari pranayama.

### NADI SODHANA PRANAYAMA

*Nadi* means "conduit" or "channel," and *sodhana* is synonymous with "purify." Nadi Sodhana Pranayama is, therefore, the breath that purifies the *nadis*. It is a breath without retentions where air passes, alternately, through each nostril.

### Technique

Sitting in meditation posture, we observe our natural breathing. We place the right hand with the index and middle fingers folded inwards, leaving free the thumb, the ring finger and the little finger. With the thumb we cover the right nostril, and with the ring finger and the little finger we cover the left nostril. The left hand is in Jñana mudra.

With the thumb we cover the right nostril so that we breathe out and breathe in from the left. Next, with the ring finger and the little finger we cover the left nostril, and then we breathe out and breathe in from the right. We go back to covering the right nostril and in this way we alternate the breathing for each nostril.

We breathe relaxed and without interruptions. Maintain the exercise until it's comfortable. When we acquire practice in the technique, we will be matching the rhythm between exhalation and inhalation.

### BENEFITS

- Balances the flow of prana that passes through both nostrils.
- Purifies the nadis.
- Regulates the digestive function.
- Calms the mind, calms the nerves.

### WARNINGS

- Deviated septum.

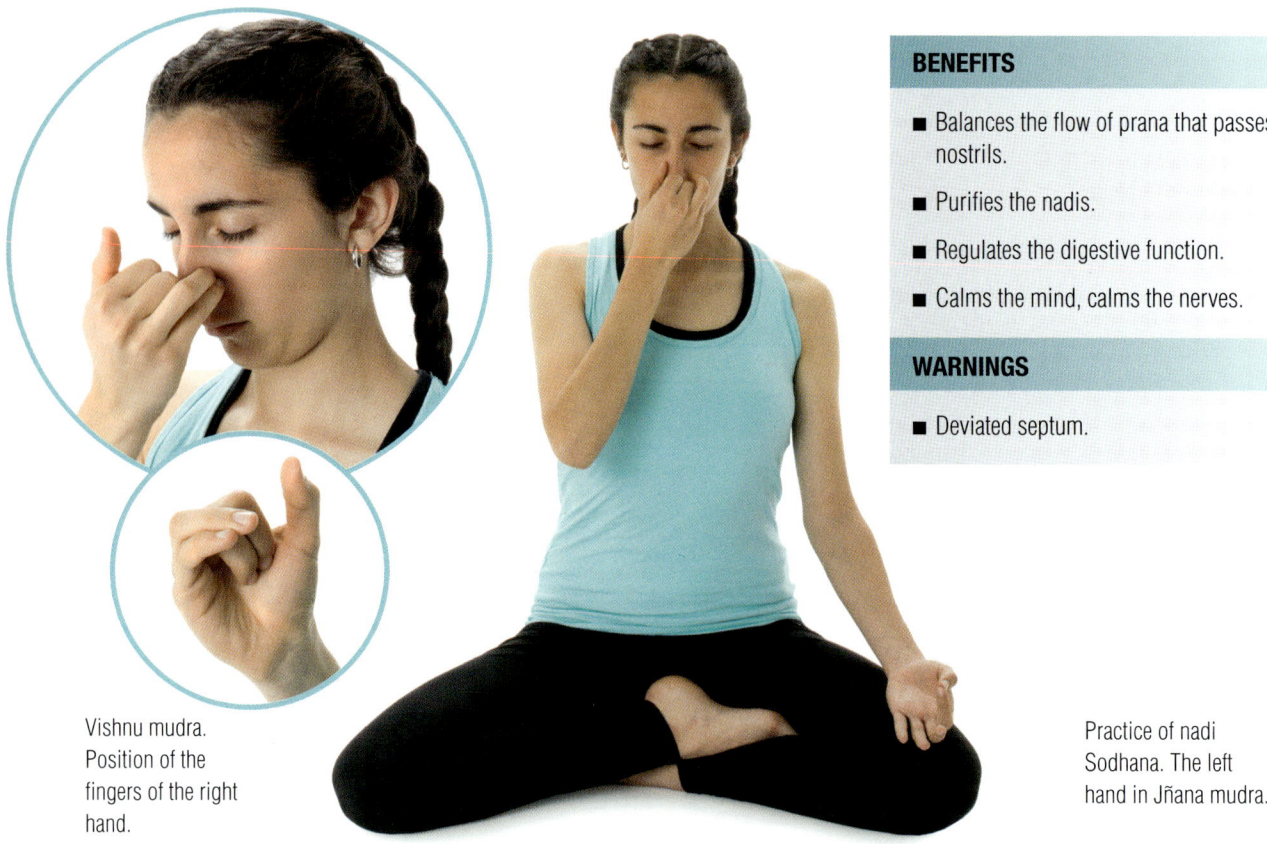

Vishnu mudra. Position of the fingers of the right hand.

Practice of nadi Sodhana. The left hand in Jñana mudra.

PRANAYAMA: Basic techniques of pranayama 129

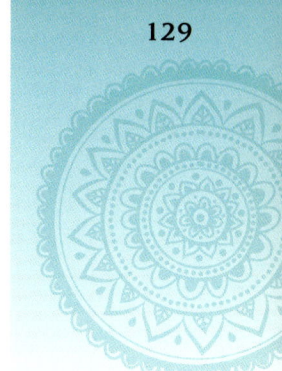

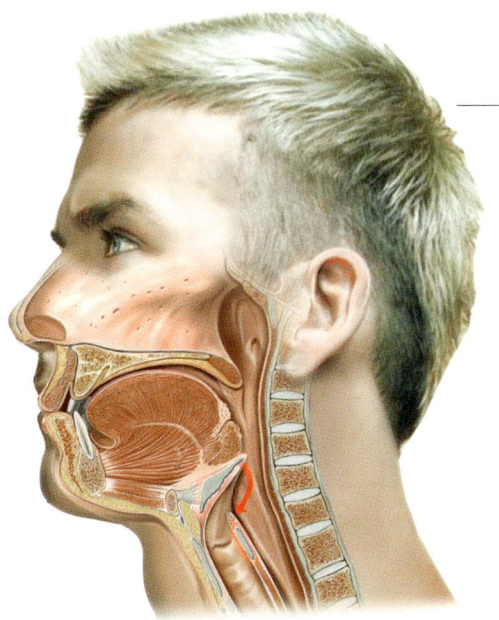

Anatomy of the larynx, with the location of the glottis.

## BHRAMARI PRANAYAMA

It is the breathing of bees.

### Technique

Seated in meditation posture, we become aware of our breathing for a few minutes. We exhale and make a great inhalation. With the lungs full, we retain the air for a few seconds. We can perform Jalandhara and Mula bandha (see the next page) for a few seconds and then undo them. We place the arms at the height of the shoulders, and plug the ears with the index fingers of each corresponding hand. We expel the air little by little, emitting a sound similar to the buzzing of a bumblebee. We undo the position of the hands and recover the initial position of meditation.

We can repeat the exercise several times.

## UJJAYI PRANAYAMA

*You* means "up." *Jaya* is translated as "victory" or "success." It is the breath that leads to success. It is a breath in which the glottis partially closes on inhalation and exhalation.

### Technique

Sitting in meditation posture or in Savasana, we observe our natural breathing. We partially close the glottis, so that the air that enters and exits stops gently. We make an inhalation that is mainly thoracic, wide, slow, and deep. With the lungs full of air, we close the glottis for a second to retain it. Upon exhalation, the glottis becomes ajar again, we contract the muscles of the abdominal wall, and the air comes out more slowly than in the inhalation. The rhythm must be 1:2, that is, the exhalation must last twice as long as the inhalation.

We observe the noise that occurs throughout the inhalation-exhalation process. We can extend this process from a few minutes to a much longer time, and practice Ujjayi when performing the Sun Salutation or while doing some asanas.

### BENEFITS

- Lowers blood pressure.
- Provides physical and mental calm.
- Induces meditative states.

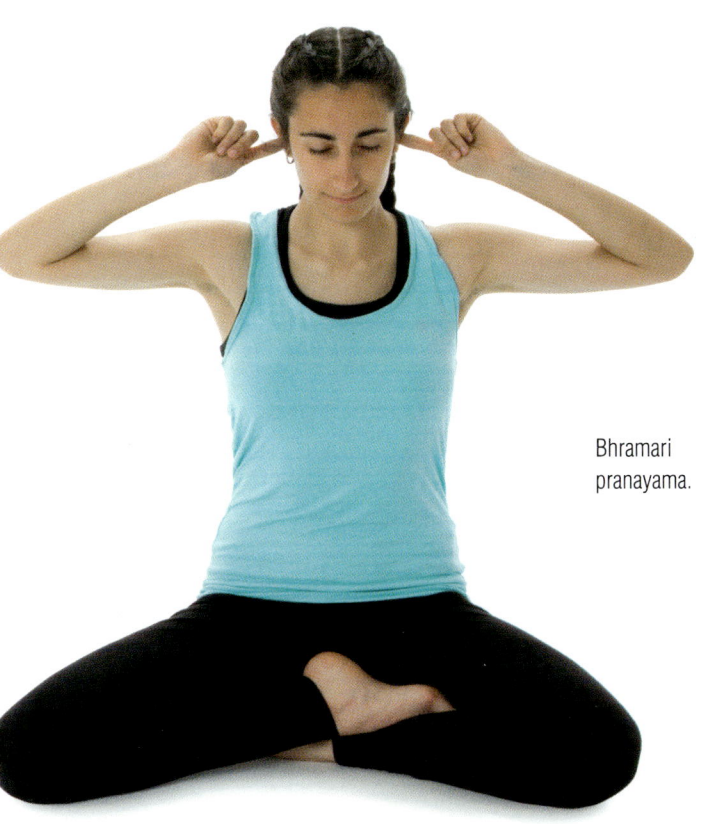

Bhramari pranayama.

### BENEFITS

- Increases strength and respiratory volume.
- Slows heart rate, lowers blood pressure.
- Provides great mental calm and a deep sense of relaxation.
- Increases the capacity for concentration and internalization.

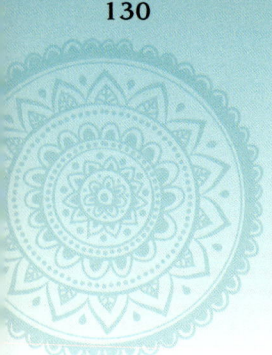

## BANDHAS

# Bandhas. Energetic keys

The word bandha means "closing" or "key." Bandhas are muscle contractions, performed voluntarily, that affect a specific part of the body. From an energetic point of view, they are in charge of controlling and channeling the prana that circulates through the nadis, directing them toward Sushumna nadi. They also relieve knots (granthis) that block the prana and prevent it from flowing freely into the central channel.

The three most important bandhas are the Jalandhara bandha, the Uddiyana bandha, and the Mula bandha. Normally, they are combined by practicing mudras and pranayama. An experienced yoga teacher should help guide anyone who wants to correctly practice this yoga.

### JALANDHARA BANDHA

*Jala* means "net," "screen," or "mesh," and *dhara* means "upward traction." Jalandhara seals the breath in the throat.

### Technique

Seated it in a meditative pose, with the hands resting on the knees. We breathe and complete a full breath. With the lungs full *(antara kumbhaka)*, we make the gesture of swallowing saliva and we bow the head forward, placing the chin between the hollow of the two clavicles and the start of the sternum. The clavicles stretch. The hands press against the knees. The shoulders lean slightly forward and up, to help seal off the throat.

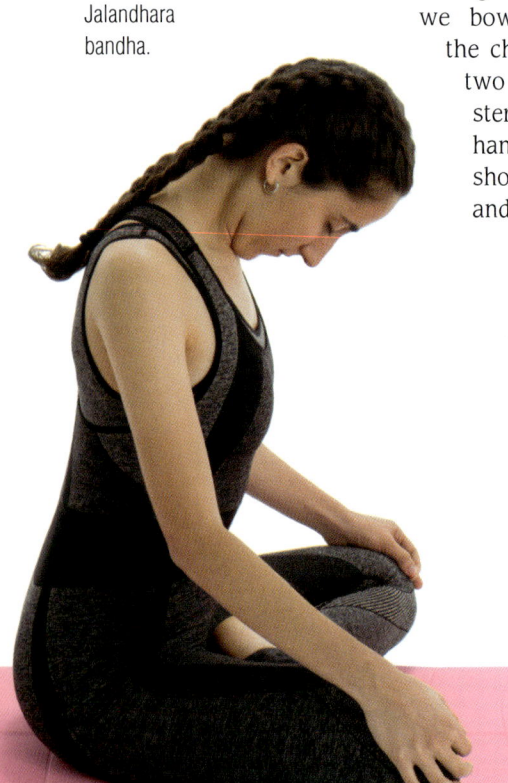

Jalandhara bandha.

We keep the closure as long as it is comfortable for us. To finish, relax the shoulders and neck. We let the glottis free to circulate the air.

| BENEFITS |
|---|
| ■ Stimulates the thyroid gland. |
| ■ Regulates the flow of blood to the heart. |
| ■ Decreases the heart rate. |
| ■ Calms the whole organism in general. |

| WARNINGS |
|---|
| ■ Hyperthyroidism, high blood pressure, heart problems. |

### UDDIYANA BANDHA

*Uddiyana* means "flying upward." In this bandha, the contraction of the abdominal muscles raises the diaphragm towards the thorax. It should always be done on an empty stomach.

### Technique

This bandha is practiced in the sitting postures of Sukhasana, Siddhasana, or Padmasana. To start in the bandha, we can also do it standing up. We should only perform this exercise with completely empty lungs *(bahya kumbhaka)*.

We stand with our legs slightly apart and our knees slightly bent. We support the hands on the thighs, with the fingers toward the inside. We breathe in and out to empty all the air from the lungs. The exhalation can be done forcefully through the mouth. We retain the breath with the empty lung and we contract the abdominal muscles inwards and upwards, making a cup with the stomach. We hold the pose until it isn't comfortable. We release this position by releasing the abdominal muscles and returning to the starting position. We breathe slowly.

We can also start in a meditation pose, with the hands resting on the knees. We breathe in and out deeply. We close our eyes, completing the Jalandhara bandha and, following this, we contract the abdominal muscles and complete a false breath in order to raise the diaphragm. The hands press on each knee and the shoulders lift slightly. We hold the pose until it isn't comfortable. We first release Uddiyana bandha, then the Jalandhara, and we breathe slowly.

### BENEFITS

- Tones and massages the abdominal organs.
- Revitalizes.
- Channels the energy upwards and toward the central channel.
- Stimulates the Manipura Chakra.

### WARNINGS

- Ulcers in the digestive track, cardiac conditions, pregnancy, menstruation.

## MULA BANDHA

*Mula* means "root," "source," "origin," or "base." In Mula bandha, the perineum (the area between the anus and the genitals) is contracted. In women, it can be located in the cervix. The most appropriate posture is Siddhasana.

### Technique

Sitting in meditation posture, we observe our natural breathing. We close our eyes and relax. We pay attention to the muscle of the perineum, and we contract it (the cervix for women), trying not to contract the anal sphincters *(aswini mudra)* or the urogenital muscles *(vajroli mudra)*. We relax the area and repeat several more times.

We can also practice it with full lungs, along with Jalandhara bandha, or with empty lungs.

### BENEFITS

- Increases blood circulation in the perineal area.
- Directs the prana upward, propelling apana vayu towards prana vayu.
- Stimulates the Muladhara Chakra and induces the awakening of Kundalini energy.

### WARNINGS

- Hypertension, pregnancy, menstruation.

## MAHA BANDHA

*Maha* means "large," "strong," or "powerful." This bandha, also called *Bandha Traya*, is done with the three previous bandhas simultaneously. Before performing it, it is necessary to practice the technique of the three bandhas separately.

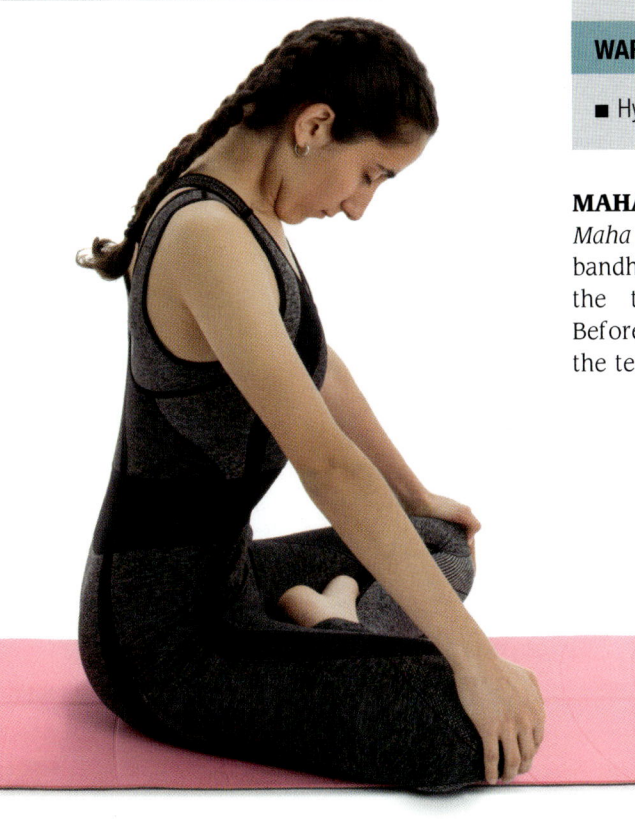

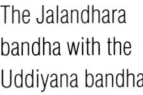

The Jalandhara bandha with the Uddiyana bandha.

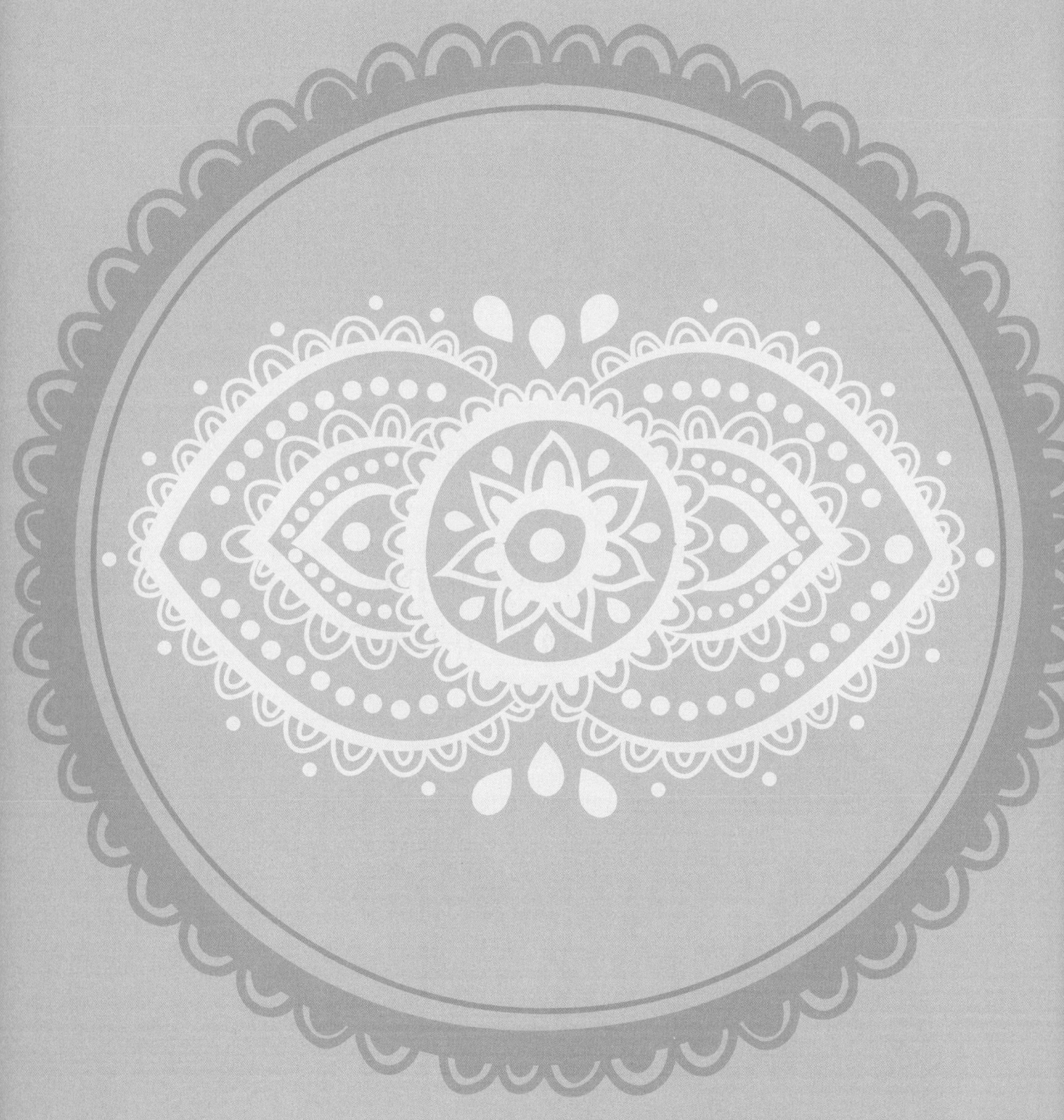

# RELAXATION, MUDRAS, MEDITATION

Relaxation is a moment in which we allow the body and mind to rest after a session of asanas. Meditation is a state in which the mind is silenced and we observe, in depth, our own inner being. *Mudras* are symbolic gestures made with the hands that allow us to channel energies and enter into meditative states. This chapter is, then, an introduction to relaxation techniques, the practice of some mudras, the appropriate postures for meditation, and, finally, the last stage of yoga: inner silence.

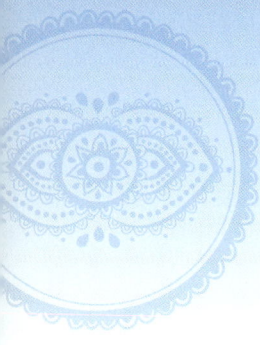

Relaxation, mudras, meditation

# Relaxation

At the end of the practice of the asanas, we are liberated from deep tensions through relaxation. This space of time, to which we dedicate about ten minutes, has the purpose of loosening the body, creating a state of physical and mental calm. This moment of tranquility allows us to assimilate the benefits of the practice of asanas.

By remaining in complete bodily quietude, relaxation gives us the opportunity to perceive our inner state clearly. All our internal mental movement surfaces, therefore, it is a good opportunity to become aware of whether there is any physical or mental tension. Relaxation will allow us to release tensions so that, little by little, the problems lose their strength.

There are many specific relaxation techniques (see the works of Dr. Coué, Dr. Jacobson, or Dr. Schultz). It is also practiced in various positions, although the best known, and the one that is normally used, is Savasana, the posture of the corpse. Others are performed in a prone position: Advasana, Makarasana, or adapted variants.

**PHYSICAL AND MENTAL TECHNIQUE**
Stretched on the floor, we spread our legs slightly and let our feet fall out. The arms are slightly separated from the body, with the palms of the hands facing upwards. We close our eyes and observe our body, our breathing, and our thoughts, without judging or modifying anything; we only intensify consciousness.

**To enter into relaxation**, we install the breath in the abdominal area; we breathe spontaneously and freely. We begin by becoming aware of our feet, their shape, their sensations, their contact with the ground, their weight. When we exhale, we lose them, we relax them. We become aware of our ankles, their shape, their sensations, their weight, and we also lose them. We continue with the calves, the knees, the thighs, the buttocks; from bottom to top, we are becoming aware, in parts, of the form, the interior and exterior sensations, and we are loosening them. Once the legs are relaxed, we continue with the pelvis, hip, and lower abdomen, and we are loosening the muscles, relaxing the internal organs. Then we focus our attention on the thorax, the back, the spine, always from the bottom up, relaxing and loosening the whole trunk. We continue with the arms; we start with the fingers, the hands, noticing their shape and their sensations, perceiving the contact with the ground, and letting them loosen. Then we move on to the forearm, arm and shoulder, in this order; we feel the contact with the ground, and we let them fall relaxed. Finally, we focus on the neck, head, and face; we relax the jaw, the lips, the tongue, the cheeks, the eyelids, the eyes. The face is completely relaxed, and then an inner smile appears.

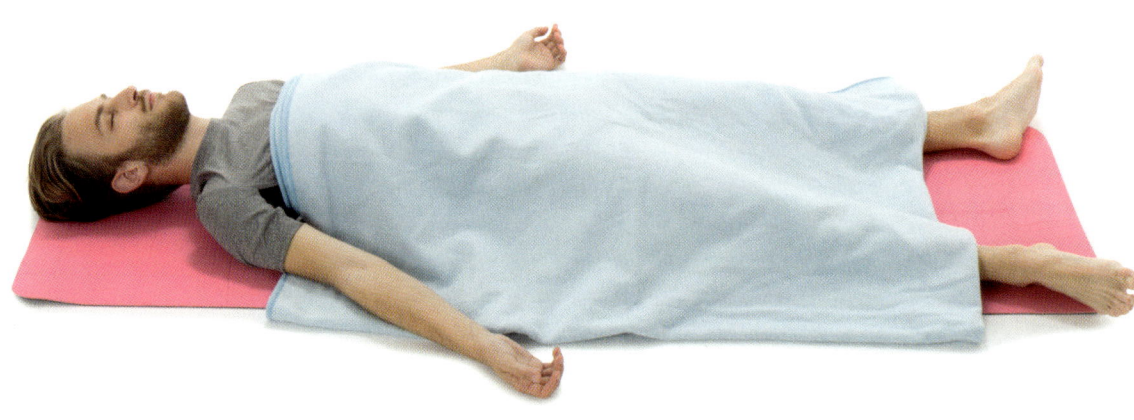

Relaxing in Savasana. During relaxation, body temperature usually drops a little, so it is advisable to cover the body with a blanket.

With the body deeply relaxed, we direct our attention to the breath. With each exhalation we release the mind of thoughts and with each inhalation we fill our body with light coming from the cosmos, a light that fills us with peace, calm, serenity, serenity, placidity, and inner joy.

**To get out of relaxation**, we lengthen our breathing a little. Very slowly, we move the fingers and toes. We transmit the movement very slowly to the arms and legs. We stretch the body, we open our eyes, we rub the palms of our hands and the soles of our feet. We remain seated a few minutes before we stand up.

## BENEFITS

- Helps to assimilate the work done with the asanas.
- Allows the body and mind to rest.
- Reduces physical and mental stress.
- Develops awareness of the body and breathing.
- Prepares the body and mind for meditation.

## WARNINGS

- Serious psychic disorders.

## PREMISES BEFORE AND DURING RELAXATION

Before starting each relaxation, we must prepare the place and foresee the material that we will need depending on the position.

The space where we make the relaxation must be a quiet place and have a pleasant temperature. It should be in the dark, as this will help our mind to relax. We need few accessories. For example, to support the head, we can use a cushion. It will also be very helpful to place a folded blanket under your legs.

The pose must be comfortable, and we will try to stay awake, with an attentive mind and a positive attitude. If we get sleepy, we can put our legs together and bring our arms to the body. If we normally fall asleep, we can try to change our position in the next session.

During pregnancy, it is advisable to lie on your side, with one leg bent.

Like a wave that breaks on the shore, which comes and goes, thus, in relaxation, we can inspire by bringing the attention from the feet to the head and exhale returning the attention from head to toe. We can also imagine that the waves are calming more and more at the same time that our mind is quieting.

Adapted relaxation pose, ideal if pregnant

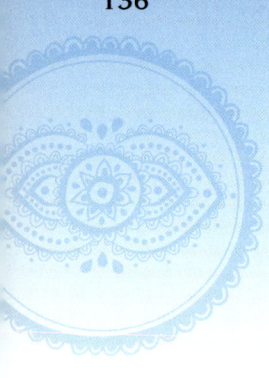

# Hasta mudras

The word *mudra* means "sign" or "symbolic seal." The mudras are symbolic poses that can be practiced with the body, the hands, the eyes, the legs, or the feet. In addition to being metaphoric representations of body language, it also is part of the control and regulation of energy in the body.

There is a wide variety of mudras, some are simple and other require a combination of asanas, pranayama, and bandhas. They are classified into three main groups: Hatha mudras (those done with the body), Prana mudras (those that relate to breathing), and Hasta mudras (those that are done with the hands). We will only deal with this last type.

## MUDRAS WITH THE HANDS

The origin of Hasta mudras goes back to early antiquity, probably the ancestors of Vedic ceremonies. They were used in tantric rituals and later had a direct influence on Indian dance.

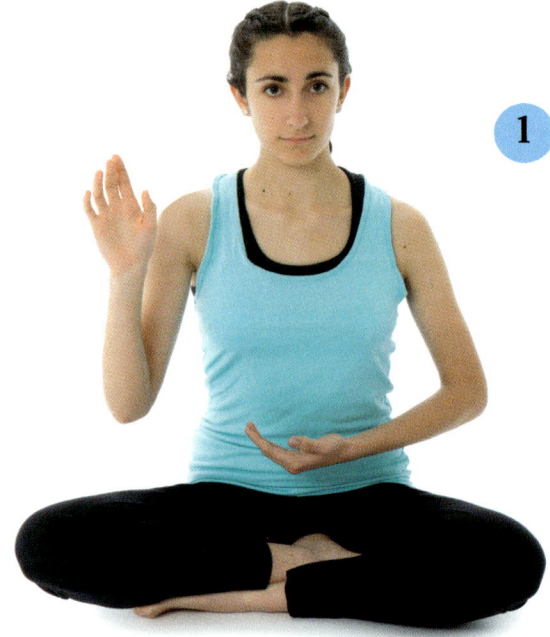

**Ring.** Its element is water. Related to abdominal or lower breathing. Energy channel of the lung.

**Index.** Symbolizes the human being, finite, limited. Its element is the air, and it is related to thoracic or middle breathing.

**Middle.** Its element is fire. Related to thoracic or middle breathing. Central energy channels: pelvis, abdomen, throat, solar plexus.

**Pinky.** Its element is Earth. When it connects with the thumb, it means a union of the earth and sky (material/spiritual). Related to abdominal or lower breathing. Energy channel for the heart or small intestine.

**Thumb.** It symbolizes the superior consciousness, unlimited and infinite. Related to clavicular or upper breathing. Its element is the ether.

While practicing yoga, Hasta mudras are often used to regulate the channels of energy and induce the practitioner to meditative states. They also have therapeutic properties.

We present some simple examples of Hasta mudras that will help us reach the optimal state of interiorizing and balancing internal energies.

**1. The Abhaya mudra, the symbol of promising protection.** The right hand is open with the palm forward. The left hand can rest on the thigh, or lap or at the height of the heart.

**2. The Namaskara mudra or Anjali mudra, the symbol of greeting or prayer.** We place the hands together in front of the heart. The right hand symbolizes heat, day, the light of the sun, the coming future; the left hand symbolizes night, cold, the moon, the past. The union of the two symbolizes the present moment and the balance between lunar and solar energy. This mudra provides calming, balance, harmony, and peace.

**3. The Jñana mudra and Chin mudra, the symbol of consciousness and wisdom.** The thumb and index finger touch to make a circle, while the other three are extended. The thumb symbolizes cosmic consciousness and the index finger, individual consciousness. The extended fingers represent the three gunas or qualities: Tamas (pinky), Rajas (ring), and Sattva (middle). If the fingers are facing up, it is the Jñana mudra; if we place the hand down, it is the Chin mudra. It is an excellent mudra to combat insomnia and nervous tension.

**4. The Bali mudra, a sign of an offering, generosity.** We bring the hands together on their sides forming a basin, with the palms facing up. We place them next to the chest.

**5. The Ksepana mudra, the symbol of spilling over.** We bring the index fingers together and intertwine the others, making a small cavity with the two hands. This mudra stimulates the evacuation of what is left over in the body as well as any negative energy.

**6. The Padma mudra I, the symbol of the closed lotus flower.** We touch the tips of the fingers and make a closed basin with the hands. Starting with this mudra, we open the fingers without separating the pinkies or the thumbs, thus appreciating the sign of the closed lotus.

**7. The Padma mudra II, the symbol of the lotus, the symbol of yoga.** It corresponds to the chakra of the heart, and it is the symbol of purity, love, and kindness. It provides many benefits, which include the opening up of abundance.

**8. The Shanka mudra, the symbol of the snail.** We encircle the thumb of the right hand with the four fingers of the left, which are extended. We support the right thumb in the middle of the left hand. We can place the hands next to the chest. It is a relaxing mudra for the nervous system and helps us remain in silence.

**9. The Tse mudra, the symbol of the three secrets.** We place the thumbs on the base of the pinky finger and close the hand slowly to form a fist. We can support them on the thighs. This mudra is helpful to reduce sadness, depression, and fear.

**10. The Dhyani mudra, the symbol of meditation and contemplation.** We place the right hand on the left, in the shape of a basin, with the thumbs touching. We place both hands in the lap. It induces meditative states, inner peace, and the well-being of others.

### BENEFITS OF THE HASTA MUDRAS

- They alternate the flow of mental, physical, or emotional energy, opening and connecting with the nadis.
- They balance and stimulate energy in the body.
- They induce the states of mental serenity and meditation.

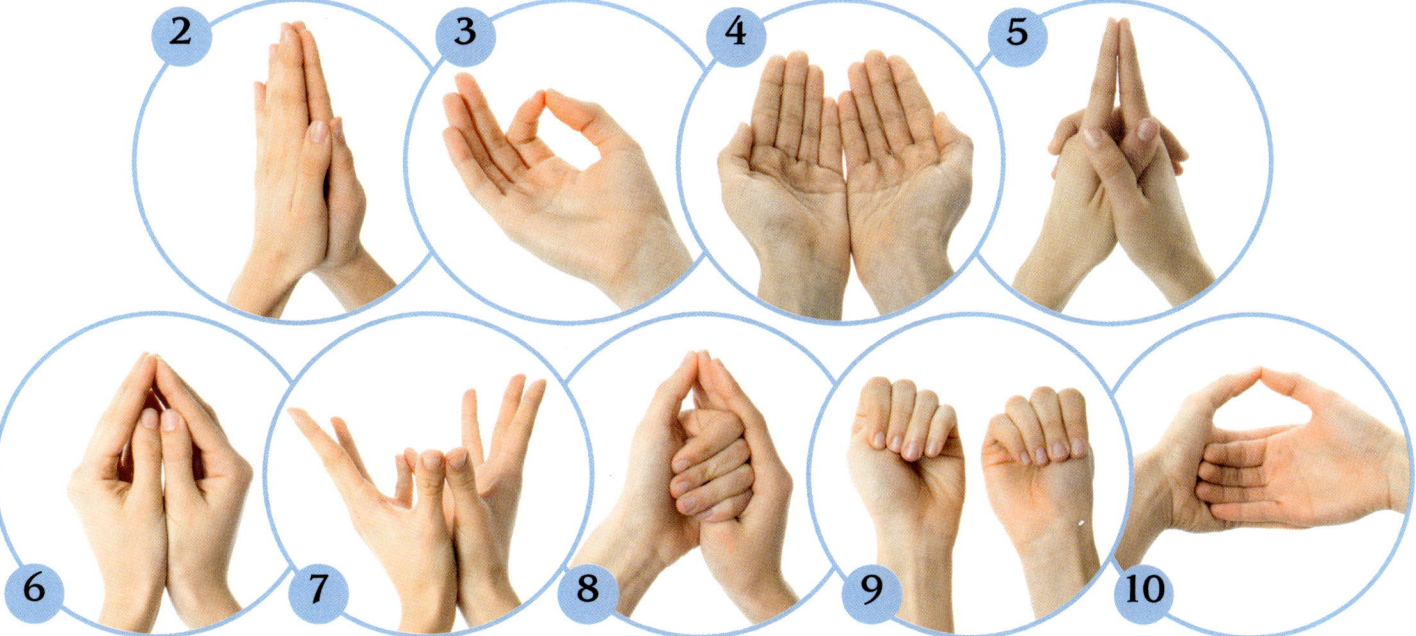

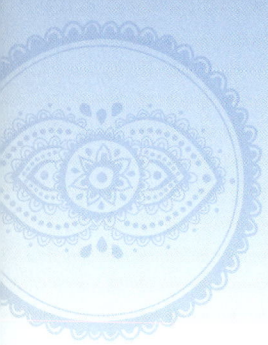

# Meditation

Meditation allows us to deeply observe our inner being. It is an intimate experience that prevails over any mental movement or rational thought. Through meditation we find absolute silence, inner peace, and inner happiness.

To reach the most elevated state of yoga, it is necessary to have worked through these middle stages. The asanas, pranayama, relaxation, and concentration make up part of the preparation of the body and the mind to reach this serene state of spiritual liberty.

**POSES**

To meditate, it is ideal to be seated on the ground with the legs crossed, but this is not always possible; since we are not accustomed to sitting this way so shortly after starting meditation, we will be uncomfortable. At the beginning, we can use some support, such as a doubled-up towel under the buttocks in order to sit with a more straight back and with the thighs leaning down.

We can adopt one of the six poses for meditation that we will show from the easiest to the most intense, with the last three being traditional poses.

**Maitryasana, the friendly pose.** This is done while sitting in a chair. It is appropriate for someone starting to practice yoga or for someone who cannot sit on the ground. In this pose, there is no tension at the base of the pelvis (created by the adductor muscles and the hamstrings), and it is easy to keep the lumbar area in a neutral position. The hands rest on the thighs and the feet rest on the floor. Its main drawback is that, as it does not offer a wide base for the floor poses, the body can tend to wobble forward and backward.

**Vajrasana, the pose of the diamond.** We kneel with the legs and the feet together and the groin against the floor. We sit on our heels with a straight back. In this position, we exert pressure on the common peroneal nerve, so that blood circulation is restricted. It is not advisable if you have varicose veins and weakness in the knee ligaments; if you do, it is recommended to sit on a low bench with the seat tilted forward.

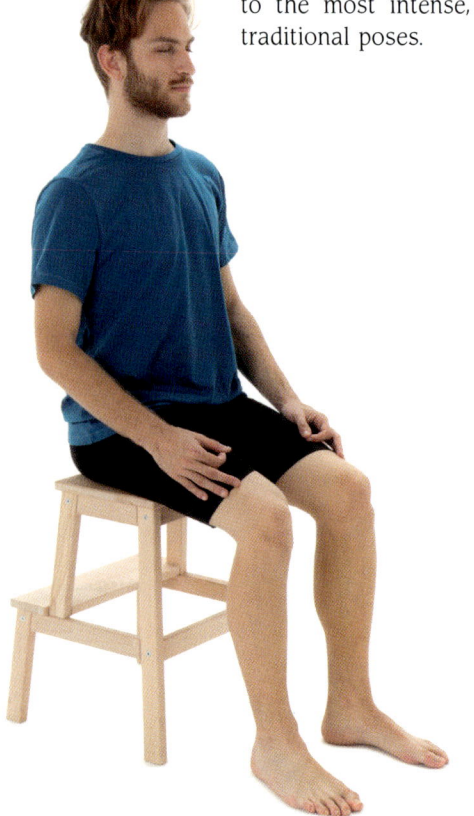

Maitryasana, the friendly pose.

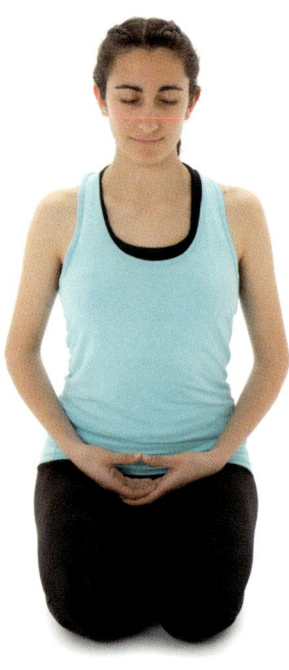

Vajrasana, the pose of the diamond.

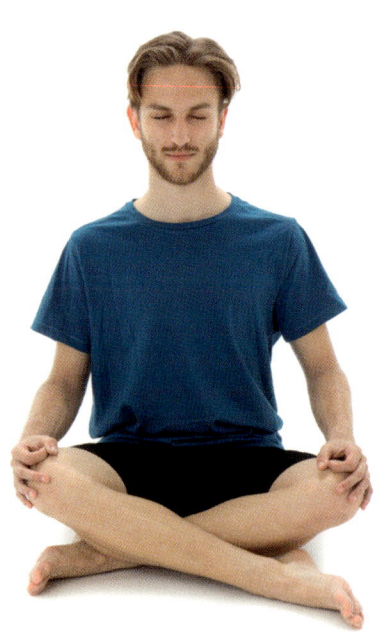

Sukasana, the easy pose.

# The meditation

**Sukasana, the easy pose.** We sit with legs crossed and each leg resting on the opposite foot. It is an appropriate pose to practice pranayama or to dedicate a few minutes to meditation. Without a base as broad as traditional positions, it ends up being unstable to maintain for a long time.

**Swatiskasana, the auspicious pose.** We place the left foot on the interior face of the right thigh, with the heel on the left side of the pubic bone. We place the right foot between the left leg and the thigh so that both ankles fall along the middle line of the body. If our hip is flexible enough, it is ideal to remain in this pose for a long while.

**Siddhasana, the perfect pose.** We keep the heel of the right foot next to the perineum, while the left foot is placed on the right foot, keeping the heel on the pubic bone. We place the sole of the left foot on the thigh of the other leg. To do this pose more comfortably, we can use a doubled-up blanket or small bench. It is helpful to alternate the two legs while doing this asana.

**Padmasana, the lotus pose.** We place the outer side of each ankle on the base of the opposite thigh, with the soles of the feet facing upwards. It is a difficult pose, but it is worth it to practice. You must alternate the position of the feet.

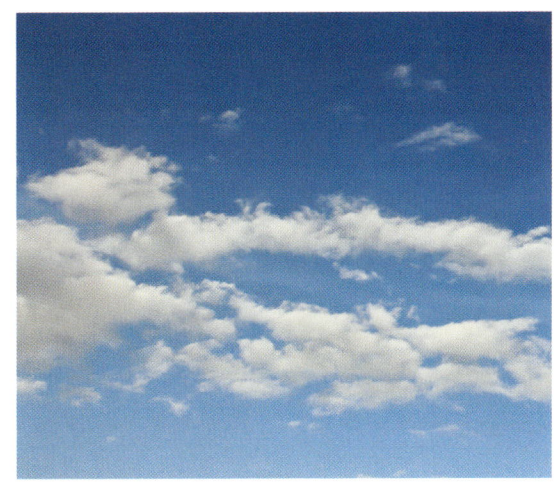

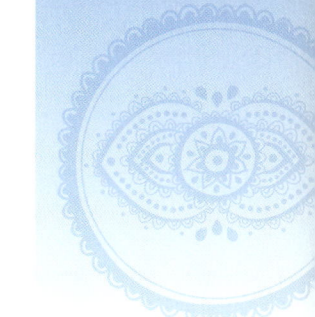

We create a mental image where thoughts become clouds: we observe them without judging and let them go...

### DHARANA: FIRST MEDITATIVE STATE

While seated on the floor, we adopt a meditative pose in which we feel comfortable and, at the same time, stable and calm. The back must remain straight, and the hands from a mudra (symbolic gesture). We observe what is around us: sounds, environment, and smells, and we integrate it into us. We relax the body without losing a stable pose and we concentrate on our breathing. Once we become aware of this, we observe our thoughts without judging; we imagine that they are clouds passing through the sky and leaving. With our senses and a calm mind, we focus on our consciousness, so that by emptying the mind, we keep it alert. Therefore, the first state of meditation is Dharana.

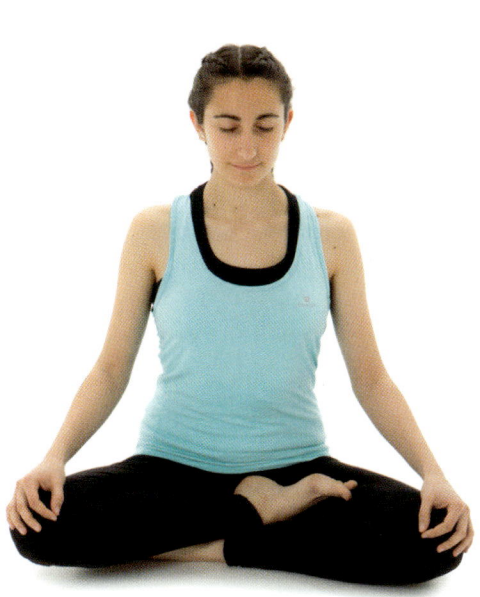

Swatiskasana, the auspicious pose.

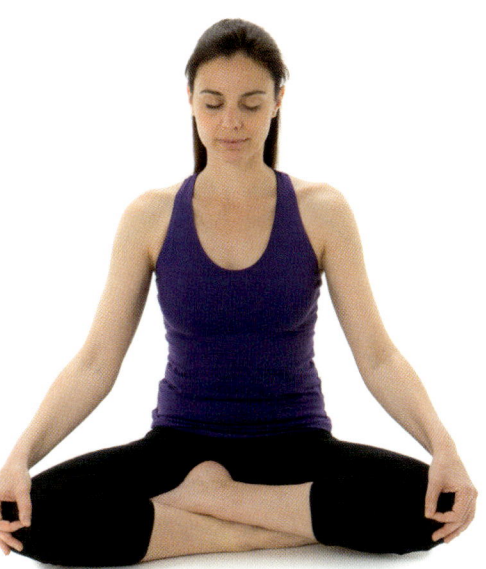

Siddhasana, the perfect pose.

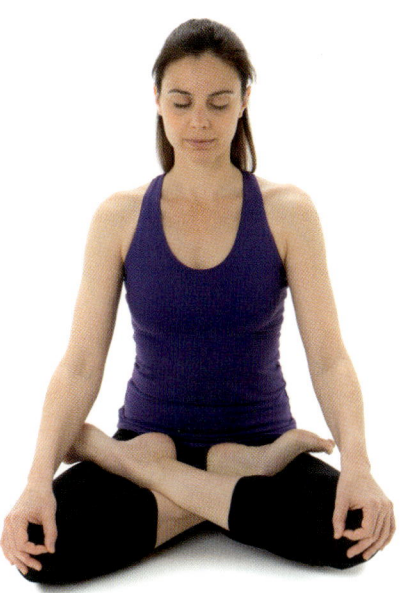

Padmasana, the lotus pose.

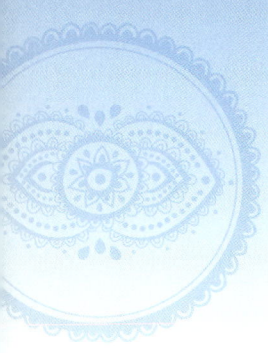

# Inner silence

Meditation is a state of being, an experience in which there is the dissolution of thoughts and any identification to them. First, it is a path of searching that leads us to the lucid perception of the present moment; little by little, we gain a deep understanding and, finally, the suspension of thoughts and images leads us to silence, to a discovery of one's own inner being.

**MEDITATION WITH SUPPORT: TRATAKA**

To advance in our meditative path, we can use various objects or elements to fix our attention on, for example: the sound of a mantra, the flame of a candle, an element from nature or the chakras. These objects work as anchors for us in order to develop constant attention and to keep it for more and more time with less effort.

The chosen object should always be the same. By fixing our eyes on this, everything else tends to fade away. First we can focus our attention with our eyes open, then, we can start to close them and create a mental image of the space between. Finally, after continued practice, we will visualize the chosen object permanently. A Trataka will develop our ability of prolonged concentration and will allow us to enter more deeply into these meditative states each time.

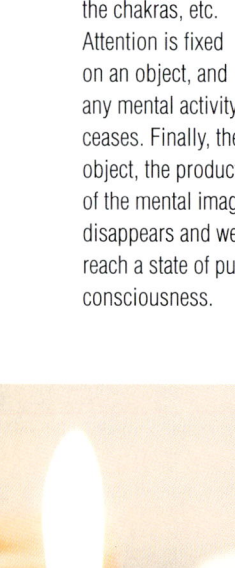

We can use any object to practice Trataka: a flower, a shell, the light of a candle, a mandala, the chakras, etc. Attention is fixed on an object, and any mental activity ceases. Finally, the object, the product of the mental image, disappears and we reach a state of pure consciousness.

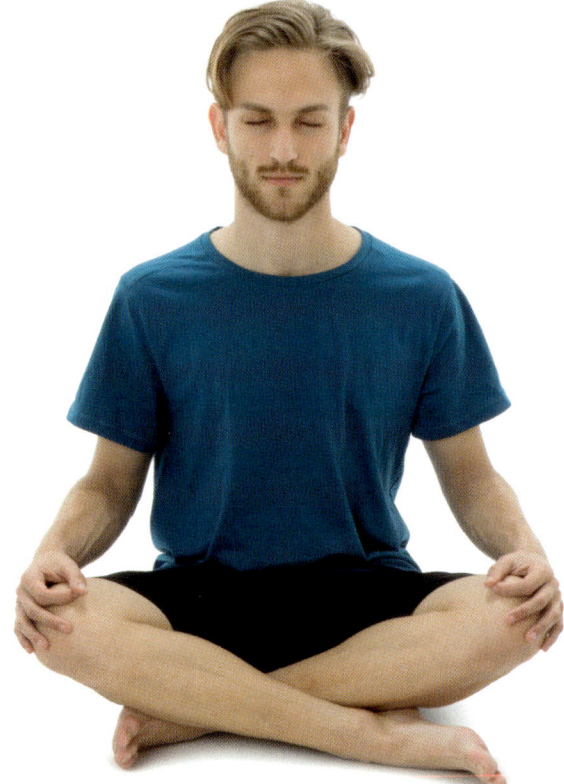

**DHYANA: SECOND MEDITATION STATE**

When we hold our concentration for a prolonged length of time, that is, when we observe our flow of thoughts, and we realize all our mental movement without distractions, we reach the second meditative stage: Dhyana.

Little by little, the thoughts and images that appear to us lose their strength, and dissolve by the very ability of the practitioner to hold their concentration without interruption. The mind is lucid and attentive; it becomes conscious of itself.

We can focus our mind on the question "Who am I?" And when thoughts attack us, ask "To whom is this thought coming?" "Who am I?"

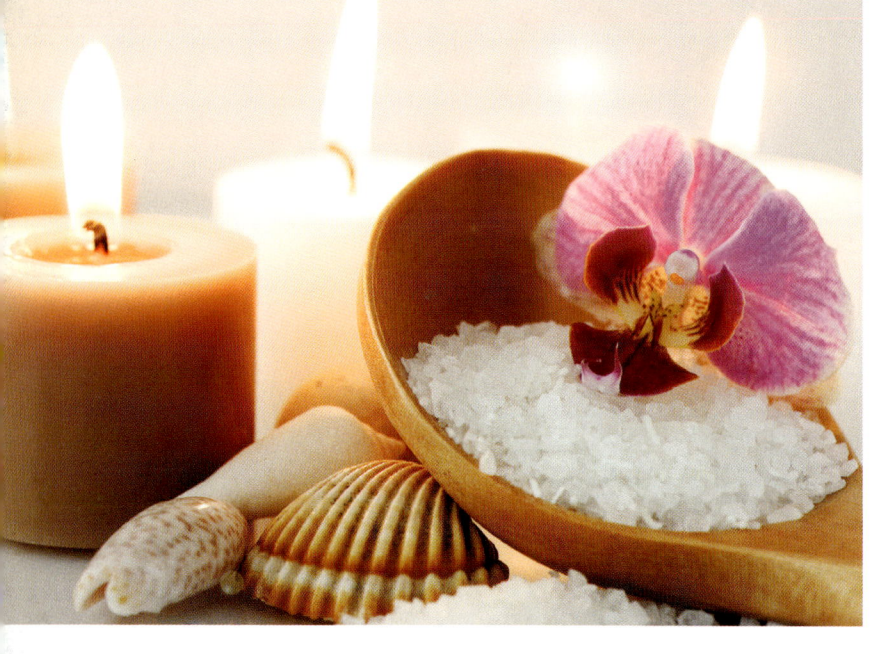

Inner silence 141

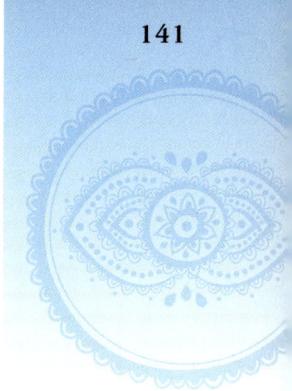

## SAMADHI:
## UNION WITH HIGHER CONSCIOUSNESS

Continued practice, usually over many years, opens up a deep understanding, the abandonment of all logical thought, the perception of internal movements, the disappearance of every image of the "I," of the ego, which will lead us little by little to the joyful experience of our inner silence.

In this total absence of images and thoughts, our true self will emerge, and we rediscover ourselves, obtaining all knowledge in a state of supra-consciousness, peace, and absolute happiness. All this will lead us to the end of our journey, to the last stage of Patanjali yoga: Samadhi, the union with Superior Consciousness.

### THE PHYSIOLOGICAL PROCESSES IN THE MEDITATIVE STATE

- Slows the entire metabolic process: the heart rate decreases, the breathing rhythm slows, oxygen consumption is reduced.

- Relaxes the sympathetic nervous system, which causes a decrease in the tone of the soft muscles that surround the arteries and arterioles, favoring blood flow to the skin and, consequently, increasing in temperature.

- Increases the temperature of the skin, which causes an irradiation of heat from the body to the outside, so that the body loses heat and cools down. (It becomes necessary to cover yourself in meditation.)

- Decreases arterial lactate (high levels of lactate indicate the existence of diseases in which lactic acid accumulates, for example stress).

- Penetrates the mind at a high state of consciousness, without falling asleep. Increases the potential for alpha waves (8-15 Hz) and theta waves (6-10 Hz) to appear. We can be awake and in states of deep sleep. When the mind is in deep sleep, in the state of delta waves (1.5-4 Hz) in the mind, a level of Samadhi consciousness appears.

A state of supra-consciousness from which an inner silence arises, leads to supreme happiness. Like a lake with perfect calm, a great mental clarity appears, in which the notion of the ego is lost.

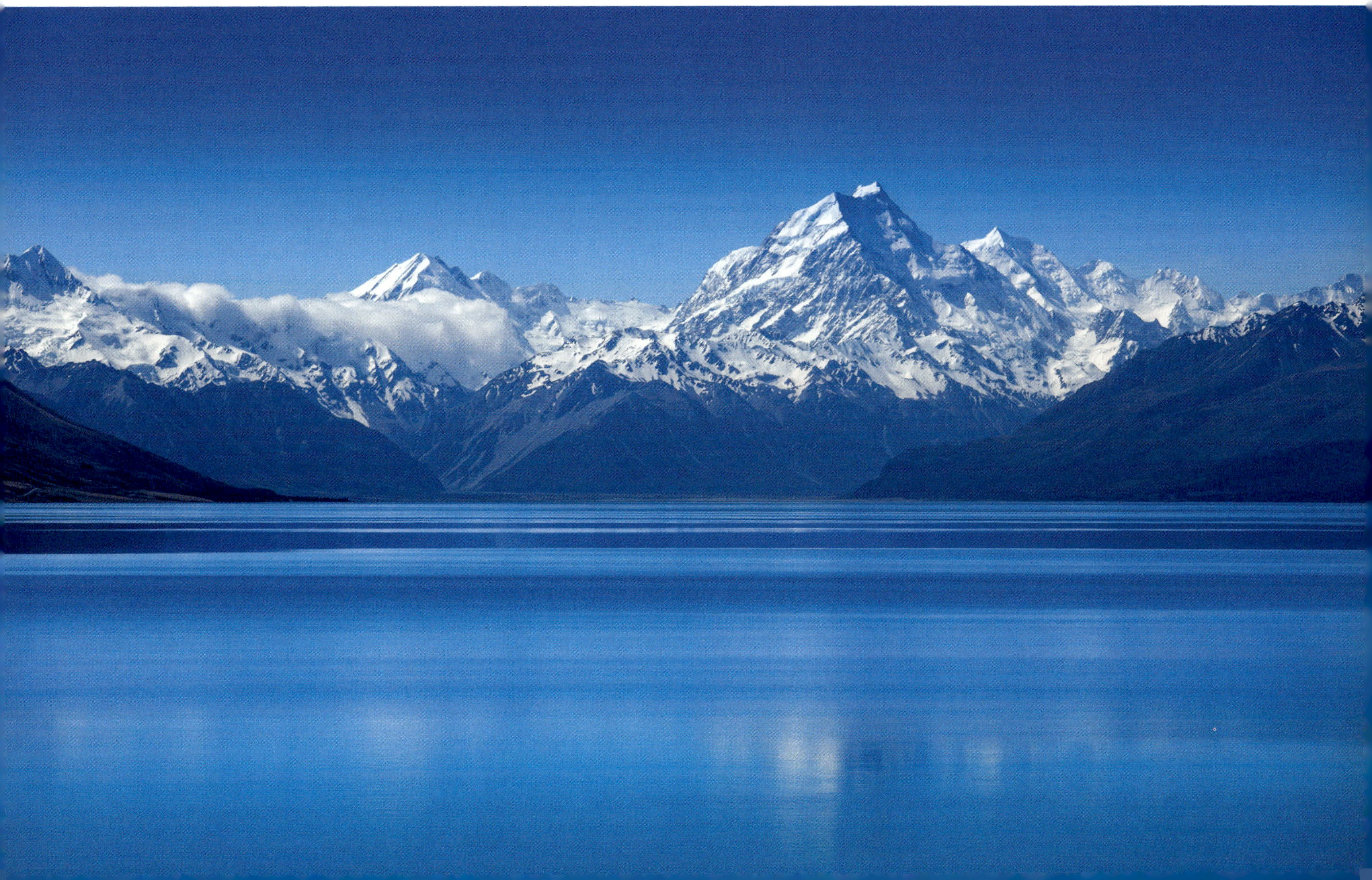

# Glossary

**Concentric muscular activity.** The muscle is activated by shortening; the muscle insertions come together and movement occurs.

**Eccentric muscular action.** The muscle is activated by lengthening; the muscle insertions move away from each other and the movement is stopped.

**Isometric muscular action.** The muscle is activated, yet no movement is produced; it fixes or holds the position.

**Ahimsa.** Non-violence. First of the yamas of Patanjali, the basis of yoga.

**Asana.** The pose of the physical body that is used while practicing yoga. It is the third state of Ahstanga Yoga in Patanjali.

**Ahstanga Yoga.** A system of Patanjali with eight branches.

**Asteya.** Do not steal. Third of the yamas of Patanjali.

**Bandha.** A key of yoga that is produced by means of muscular blocking by using any of the practices of pranayama.

**Bhakti.** Devotion, pure love, adoration.

**Bhagavad Gita**, or "The Lord's song." Philosophical poem that is the nucleus of the work *Mahâbhârata*. Written between the centuries V-II B.C.E., the work is a dialogue between Krisna (avatar of Vishnu) and Arjuna, a young prince who needs to fight a battle. The poem has great spiritual content.

**Chakras.** Centers of energy located in the primary energy axis of the body.

**Darsanas.** Means "points of view" or "vision of the world." These are the six classic systems, or orthodox philosophical schools, from the Hindu philosophy. It is based on the Vedas: Vaisheshika, Nyaya, Samkhya, Yoga, Mimansa, and Vedanta. Vedanta, or the "end of Veda," is the most important one; Samkhya is the oldest; and Yoga can be conceived as the praxis of the previous one.

**Dharana.** Concentration. Sixth state of Ahstanga Yoga of Patanjali.

**Dhyana.** Meditation. Seventh state of Ahstanga Yoga of Patanjali.

**Granthis.** Nests of subtle energy, which make it difficult for energy to flow.

**Gheranda Samhita.** Dated to the XVII century, this yoga manual is one of the three classic texts of Hatha Yoga, along with Hatha Yoga Pradipika and Shiva Samhita. Contemporary yoga is based on the techniques that it presents. It presents a sevenfold yoga: Shatkarmas, Asanas, Mudras, Pratyahara, Pranayama, Dhyana, and Samadhi.

**Gunas.** Basic qualities that impregnate all material and the universe. They designate the mode of existence. There are three: Sattva (intelligence, contemplation, purity, goodness, harmony), Rajas (dynamic, passion, energy), and Tamas (ignorance, darkness, inertia).

**Hatha Yoga.** Branch of yoga created between centuries XV-XVI. It is based on physical practices that purify the body and balance internal energy: the asanas, pranayama, the mudras, and the bandhas.

**Hatha Yoga Pradipika** (century XIV). Written by Swami Svatmarana, it includes the most important manual regarding Hatha Yoga. It combines Hatha Yoga with Raja Yoga, based on Ayurvedic medicine. The text is divided into four chapters: asanas and tridoshas, pranayama and kumbhaka, mudras and bandhas, and samadhi.

**Karma.** Action. Law of cause and effect.

**Kundalini.** Spiritual energy that is latent in the Muladhara Chakra.

**Kosha.** Layer or energy body.

**Mudra.** Gesture or pose, generally made with the hands, which creates a model of energy in the body and directs inner energy.

**Synergetic muscles.** They are activated to help move the agonistic muscles.

**Nadis.** Subtle channels through which energy flows.

**Neti.** Cleaning of the nostrils.

**Niyamas.** Depuration practices. Second state of Ahstanga Yoga of Patanjali.

**Prana.** Energy, vital strength that is found throughout the universe.

**Pranayama.** Technique for controlling breathing. It is the fourth state of Ahstanga Yoga in Patanjali.

**Samadhi.** Last state of yoga, where a union between individual consciousness and the Universal Consciousness or Supreme Spirit occurs.

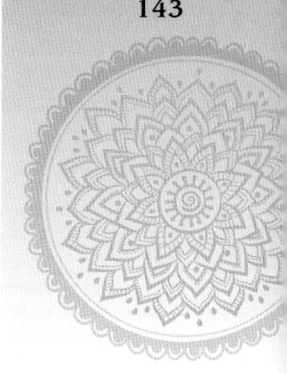

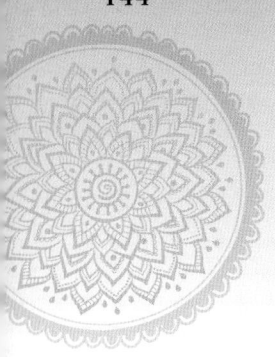

**Sutra.** Short phrases or aphorisms.

**Shiva-Samhita** (circa century XVIII). It is also called the "abstract of Shiva." Text written in Sanskrit that includes a synthesis of the tradition and praxis of yoga, and its asanas (it names 84), pranayama, tantric practices, mudras, and meditation.

**Surya.** Sun.

**Sushumna.** Central energy channel, located on the interior of the spine, which is included in the subtle part of the central nervous system. Tantra. Philosophical current whose goal is to expand consciousness.

**Upanishads.** Upa means "close," ni means "below," and sad is "to sit." It means to sit close to the master or guru to listen to their teachings. The Upanishads are ancient philosophical and esoteric texts composed between the sixth and fourth centuries B.C.E., although others were added later, as late as the fifteenth century A.D. Its main teaching is that the Atman, our immanent essence, and Brahman, the transcendent god, are the same.

**Yamas.** Universal ethical principles. It is the first state of Ahstanga Yoga in Patanjali.

**Yoga.** Means "union." It is the highest state of consciousness. It represents the union of the individual soul with the Supreme Spirit. Yoga is one of the six great philosophical systems from India.

**Yogui/Yoguini.** A person who follows the path of yoga or its practice.

# Bibliography

Anonymous *Bhagavad Gita*. Tola, Fernando (trad.). Biblioteca Nueva, Madrid, 2000.

Anonymous. *Los Yogasutras de Patañjali*. Vihari J., Rasik (trad.). Árbol editorial, México, 1992.

CALAIS-GERMAIN, Blandine. *Anatomía para el movimiento I*. Los libros de la liebre de Marzo, Barcelona, 2002.

CELLA, Gabriella. *I secreti dello Yoga*. Edizione Manuali Fabbri, Milán, 2001.

COULTER, David. *Anatomía del Hatha Yoga*. Obelisco, Barcelona, 2013.

ELAINE N, Marieb. *Anatomía y fisiología humana*. Pearson Educación, Madrid, 2008.

HALL, Jean and Doriel. *Enciclopedia práctica de Astanga Yoga y meditación*. Edimat books, Madrid, 2007.

HERNÁNDEZ, Danilo. *Claves del yoga*. Los libros de la liebre de Marzo, Barcelona, 1998.

HIRSCHI, Gertrud. *Mudras*. Urano, Barcelona, 1999.

IYENGAR, B. K. S. *Light above Pranayama*. Kairós, Barcelona, 2001.

IYENGAR, B. K. S. *The light of yoga*. Kairós, Barcelona, 2001.

JANAKIRAMAN-ROSSO, Yogacharya and Carolina. *Solar Yoga*. Ibis, Barcelona, 1992.

JENKINS-BRANDON, Nicky and Leigh. *Anatomía & Yoga para la salud y la postura*. Paidotribo, Barcelona, 2010.

JOHARI, Harish. *Los chakras*. Edaf, Madrid, 1989.

KAMINOF-MATTHEWS, Leslie, Amy. *Anatomía del yoga*. Tutor, Madrid, 2008.

LARSEN-WOLFF-HAGER FORSTENLECHNER. *Yoga terapéutico*. Paidotribo, Barcelona, 2014.

MARIEB, Elaine N. *Human Anatomy and physiology*. Pearson Educación, Madrid, 2008.
McCALL, Timothy. Yoga & Medicina. Paidotribo, Barcelona, 2010.

PANIKKAR, Raimon. *Hindu Spirituality*. Kairós, Barcelona, 2005.

ROMÁN, M. Teresa. *Enseñanzas espirituales de la India*. Oberon, Madrid, 2001.

WILLS, Pauline. *Chakras*. Gaia, Madrid, 2003.